Textbook of

Human Histology

Fourth Edition

Important note
for students reading this book

The matter given in this book is classified into two categories. Paragraphs dealing with main facts that every student must know are given in the typeface used for this paragraph.

Paragraphs containing more advanced matter are printed in a smaller type face (as used here). They are further distinguished by the presence of a broad pink stripe along the left side of the paragraph.

Such paragraphs should be omitted by beginners. They should be read only after the main facts have been clearly understood.

Paragraphs giving detail will interest good undergraduate students. They are essential for postgraduate students.

Textbook of

HUMAN
HISTOLOGY

Fourth Edition

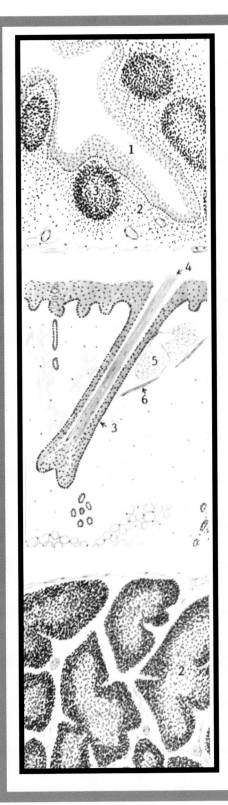

INDERBIR SINGH

52, Sector One, Rohtak 124001

JAYPEE BROTHERS

MEDICAL PUBLISHERS(P) LTD

New Delhi

Published by

Jitendar P Vij
Jaypee Brothers Medical Publishers (P) Ltd
EMCA House, 23/23B Ansari Road, Daryaganj
New Delhi 110 002, India
Phones: 23272143, 23272703, 2328202, 23245672, 23245683
Fax: 011-23276490 e-mail: jpmedpub@del2.vsnl.net.in
Visit our website: http://www.jpbros.20m.com

Branches

- 202 Batavia Chambers, 8 Kumara Kruppa Road, Kumara Park East,
  Bangalore 560 001, Phones: 2285971, 2382956 Tele Fax: 2281761
  e-mail: jaypeebc@bgl.vsnl.net.in
- 282 IIIrd Floor, Khaleel Shirazi Estate, Fountain Plaza
  Pantheon Road, **Chennai** 600 008, Phone: 28262665 Fax: 28262331
  e-mail: jpmedpub@md3.vsnl.net.in
- 4-2-1067/1-3, Ist Floor, Balaji Building, Ramkote, Cross Road
  Hyderabad 500095, Phone: 55610020, 24758498 Fax: 24758499
  e-mail: jpmedpub@rediffmail.com
- 1A Indian Mirror Street, Wellington Square
  Kolkata 700 013, Phone: 22451926 Fax: 22456075
  e-mail: jpbcal@cal.vsnl.net.in
- 106 Amit Industrial Estate, 61 Dr SS Rao Road, Near MGM Hospital
  Parel, **Mumbai** 400 012 , Phones: 24124863, 24104532 Fax: 24160828
  e-mail: jpmedpub@bom7.vsnl.net.in

Textbook of Human Histology

First Edition: 1987
Second Edition: 1992
Third Edition: 1997
Fourth Edition: 2002
 Reprint: 2005

ISBN 81-7179-967-1

Layout design and composing by the author.
Printed at Gopsons Papers Ltd., Sector 60, Noida

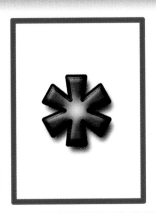

Preface
to the Fourth Edition

I have great pleasure in presenting the FOURTH EDITION of this book. Like previous editions, this edition seeks to be fairly complete, and user friendly. To this end the language has been kept simple so that students who have a limited knowledge of English should be able to follow it without difficulty; and the text is profusely illustrated.

The fourth edition represents a landmark as the book has been printed throughout in full colour. The Colour Atlas has been retained, but the short descriptions of each figure now appear alongside it. At the same time the atlas figures have been repeated in the text chapters wherever it was considered useful.

The text illustrations are now presented in full colour. As a result of this fact, and as a result of using better printing facilities readers should find the book much more attractive.

As before matters of detail are now clearly demarcated from the main text. They are printed in a smaller type-size; and are distinguished by a coloured band that runs along the left side of each such paragraph.

These improvements have been possible only because of the tremendous enthusiasm and initiative shown by Mr. J. P. Vij and I thank him warmly. Mr. Tarun Duneja has taken great interest in production of the book and his efforts have been invaluable.

It is a pleasure to thank all those who have written letters of encouragement and have made useful suggestions for improvement. I am most grateful to my young friend Sagar J. Adkar for pointing out errors.

Rohtak, April 2002   INDERBIR SINGH

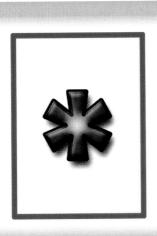

Contents

CONTENTS

CONTENTS

CONTENTS

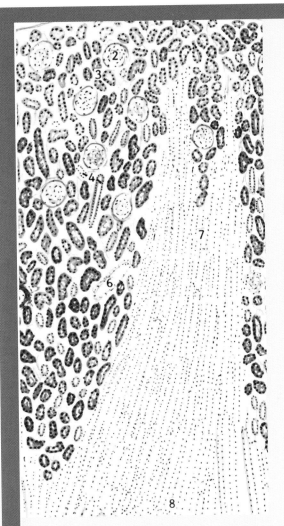

Colour Atlas

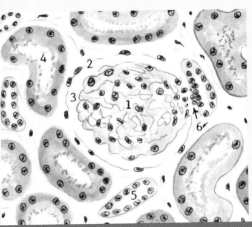

This section presents realistic colour drawings from histological preparations of tissues and organs that are commonly studied in classes. A brief description of each figure is given. Pages on which further descriptions are to be found are indicated. To distinguish atlas figures from those in the text chapters, they are numbered A1, A2 etc.

Figs. A1 to A10 illustrate some types of epithelia. Epithelia consist of one or more layers of cells that rest on a supporting layer of connective tissue called the lamina propria.

Epithelia may be simple, when they consist of only one layer of cells, or stratified when there are several layers of cells. Epithelial cells may be flat (or squamous), cuboidal, columnar etc.

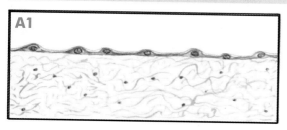

A1

Fig. A1. Simple squamous epithelium

Note that the cells are so thin that bulgings are produced by the nuclei.

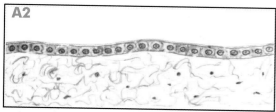

A2

Fig. A2. Simple cuboidal epithelium

The length and breadth of the cells are equal. Nuclei are rounded.

Figs. A3, A4. Simple columnar epithelium

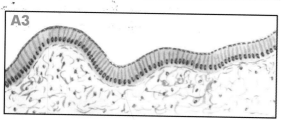

A3

The height of the cells is much greater than their width. The nuclei are oval being elongated in the same direction as the cells. They lie near the bases of the cells.

In Fig. A4 the epithelium is seen at higher magnification than in Fig. A3. In some regions the free surfaces of the cells show a thickening with vertical striations in it: this is called a striated border (See pages 25, 45 for details). In some situations simple columnar epithelium bears hair-like projections called cilia (See Fig. A6). Cilia are capable of movement (See page 23).

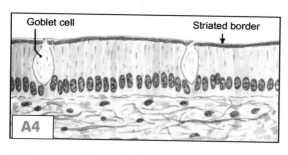

Goblet cell   Striated border

A4

Figs. A5. Pseudostratified columnar epithelium.

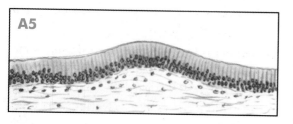

A5

This epithelium appears to be multi-layered. However, there is actually only one layer of cells. The multi-layered appearance is due to the fact that the nuclei lie at different levels in different cells. Note that there is a clear zone of cytoplasm between the nuclei and the free surfaces of the cells. As shown in Fig. A6 this kind of epithelium may be ciliated.

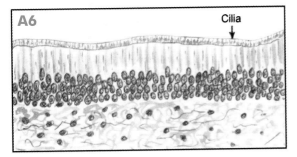

Fig. A6. Ciliated pseudostratified columnar epithelium.

This is similar to the epithelium shown in Fig. A5 except that it is ciliated.

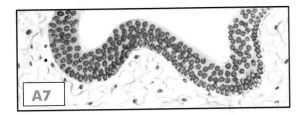

Figs. A7, A8. Transitional epithelium.

This is multi-layered. The cells in the deepest layer are columnar or cuboidal; in the middle layers they are polyhedral or pear shaped; and in the superficial layer the cells are large, and may be shaped like umbrellas. Note that the nuclei in all layers are round or oval.

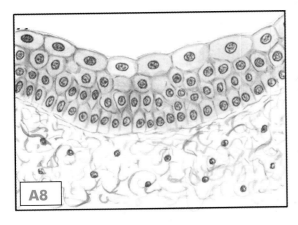

Fig. A9. Stratified squamous epithelium (Non-keratinized).

Although this is called stratified squamous epithelium, only the most superficail cells are squamous (flattened). The cells in the deepest (or basal) layer are columnar. In the middle layers they are polyhedral, while the more superficial layers show increasing degrees of flattening.

The nuclei are oval in the basal layer, rounded in the middle layer, and transversely elongated in the superficial layers.

This kind of epithelium is seen lining some internal organs like the oesophagus or the vagina.

A similar covers the skin (Fig. A10) but here the superficial layers are converted into non-living fibres.

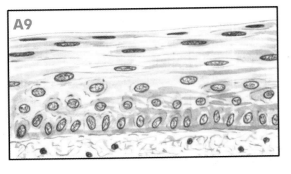

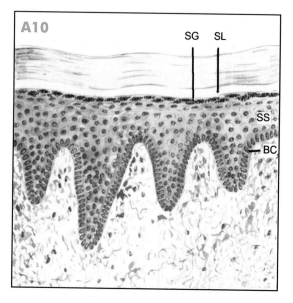

Fig. A10. *Stratified squamous epithelium (Keratinized)*

In Fig. A10 we see a type of epithelium that is characteristic of the epidermis of the skin. The deeper layers of the epithelium are similar to those shown in Fig. A9, but these are covered by additional layers that represent stages in the conversion of cells into non-living fibres: the process is called keratinization or cornification. Several such layers can be recognized. BC = basal cell layer; SS = stratum spinosum; SG = stratum granulosum; SL = stratum lucidum; SC = stratum corneum. See page 194 for details.

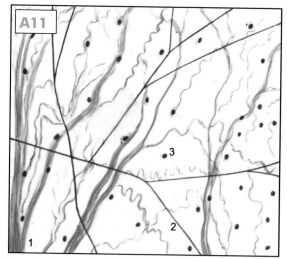

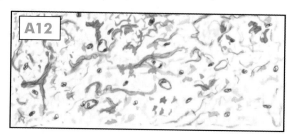

Figs. A11, A12. *Loose areolar tissue*

In Fig. A11 we see a stretch preparation of omentum. The light brown bundles (1) are of collagen fibres, many of which are seen to run a wavy course. The dark branching lines (2) are elastic fibres: these are seen only if a specific stain for them (e.g., orcein) is used. Note that the elastic fibres branch and anastomose with each other. The nuclei (3) belong to connective tissue cells, mostly fibroblasts.

In Fig. A12 we see the usual appearance of connective tissue as seen in sections. Collagen fibres stain pink. Elastic fibres are not seen unless special methods for them are used. Nuclei of cells of connective tissue can be made out, but cell outlines are not distinct. (Loose areolar tissue is described on page 55.)

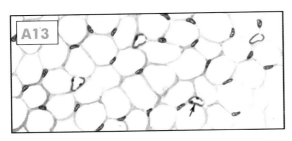

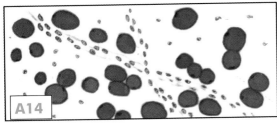

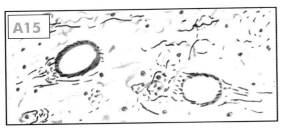

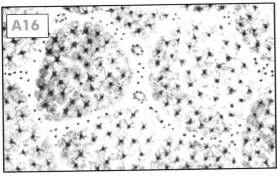

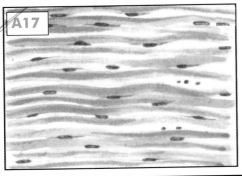

Figs. A13, A14. Adipose tissue

Adipose tissue is made up mainly of fat cells. In routine sections (Fig. A13) the cells appear empty as the fat in them gets dissolved during preparation of the section. The cytoplasm of each cell is seen as a pink 'rim'. The nucleus is flat and lies to one side. Some capillaries (arrow) lined by endothelium are seen.

In Fig. A14 we see fat cells in a piece of omentum that has been stretched and stained by a specific stain for fat (Sudan IV). Note the peripheral position of the nuclei. Two blood capillaries (seen as rows of nuclei) are present in the field. Some collagen fibres and nuclei of connective tissue are also present. (Adipose tissue is described on page 66).

Fig. A15. Reticular fibres

This section shows connective tissue that has been specifically stained for reticular fibres which are seen as black lines. Collagen fibres and nuclei are pink.

Figs. A16, A17. Tendon

Fig. A16 shows a transverse section across a tendon, and Fig. A17 shows a longitudinal section. Note the bundles of collagen fibres (pink) arranged parallel to each other. Fibroblasts are present in the intervals between the fibres. In Fig. A16 the cells appear to be star shaped, while in Fig. A17 they appear to be spindle shaped. The collagen bundles are separated by some loose connective tissue.

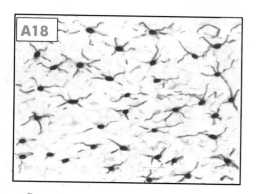

Fig. A18. Mucoid tissue

This tissue consists of star shaped cells embedded in a homogeneous (gelatinous) matrix. (See page 68).

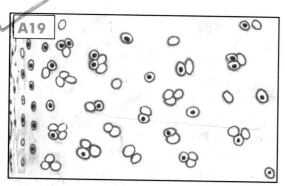

Fig. A19. Hyaline cartilage

Note groups of cartilage cells (chondrocytes) surrounded by a homogeneous matrix. Near the surface of the cartilage (to the left of the figure) the cells are flattened and merge with the cells of the overlying connective tissue. This connective tissue forms the perichondrium. (Hyaline cartilage is described on page 90).

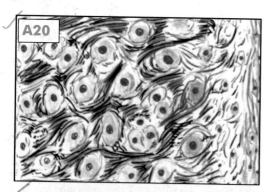

Fig. A20. Elastic cartilage

The section is stained by Verheoff's method for elastic fibres. Note the dense network of elastic fibres separating the cartilage cells. The perichondrium is seen at the right end of the figure. (Elastic cartilage is described on page 92).

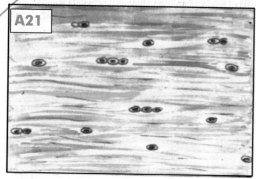

Fig. A21. Fibrocartilage

Fibrocartilage consists of rounded cartilage cells embedded amongst thick bundles of collagen fibres. Distinguish carefully from tendon (Fig. A17). (Fibrocartilage is described on page 91).

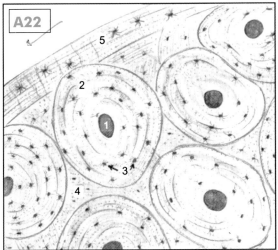

Fig. A22. Compact bone

This figure shows a transverse section through unstained compact bone. It is made up of ring-like osteons (or Haversian systems). At the centre of each osteon there is a Haversian canal (1). Around the canal there are concentric lamellae of bone (2) amongst which there are small spaces called lacunae (3). Delicate canaliculi radiate from the lacunae. Interstitial lamellae fill intervals between Haversian systems (4). Deep to the surface of the bone (upper left) there are circumferential lamellae (5) that run parallel to the surface. (For details see page 97).

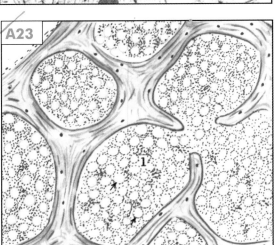

Fig. A23. Spongy (or cancellous) bone

This is made up of a network of bony trabeculae (pink) in which the nuclei of some osteocytes can be seen. The spaces of the network are filled in by bone marrow (1) in which numerous fat cells (arrow) are present. The spaces between the fat cells are occupied by numerous blood forming cells (only nuclei of which are seen).

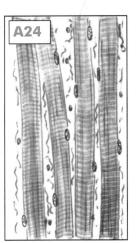
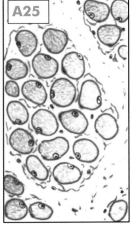

Figs. A24, A25. Skeletal muscle

In Fig. A24 we see a longitudinal section through skeletal muscle. The fibres show characteristic transverse striations, and peripherally placed nuclei. In Fig. A25 we see a transverse section in which the muscle fibres are seen as irregularly rounded structures with peripheral nuclei. The dots within the fibres are myofibrils. (For further details see page 119).

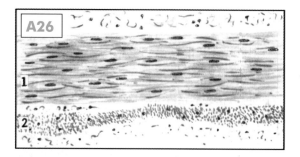

Fig. A26. Smooth muscle

This figure shows smooth muscle in a section stained by haematoxylin and eosin. The muscle is seen cut longitudinally (1) as well as transversely (2). (For description see page 130). Loose connective tissue is seen above and below the layers of muscle.

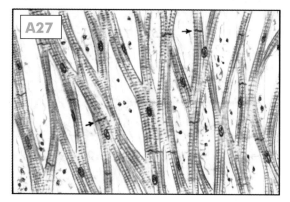

Fig. A27. Cardiac muscle

Note that the fibres branch and anastomose. They have striations that are faint. The fibres are made up of 'cells' each of which has a centrally placed nucleus. Adjacent 'cells' are separated from one another by transverse lines (arrows) called intercalated discs. (For details see page 128).

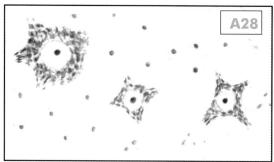

Fig. A28. Neurons

This figure shows large neurons from the anterior grey column of the spinal cord. Note the multipolar appearance of each neuron, the large lightly staining nucleus, and the prominent nucleolus. The cytoplasm contains clumps of dark staining Nissl substance. Nuclei seen in the rest of the field belong to neuroglial cells. (This section is stained by a special method that stains Nissl substance well). (Nervous tissue is described on page 135).

Fig. A29. Peripheral nerve T.S.

The nerve has been fixed in osmic acid which stains the myelin sheaths (around the nerve fibres) black. The myelin sheaths, therefore, appear as black rings. Note that the nerve fibres are arranged in bundles that are held together by connective tissue (called perineurium). In the insert we seen nerve fibres at higher magnification.

Note the varying size of the fibres. The connective tissue around individual nerve fibres is called endoneurium. (Also see page 147).

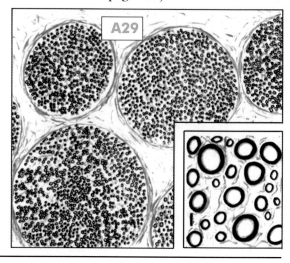

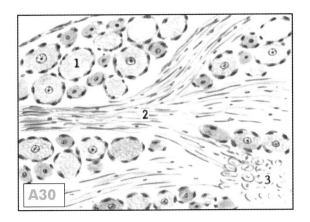

A30

Figs. A30, A31. Sensory ganglia.

Ganglia are of two types, sensory and autonomic. In Fig. A30 we see a sensory ganglion. Note the large neurons (1) arranged in groups, that are separated by bundles of nerve fibres (2). Nerve fibres are cut transversely at '3'. Each neuron has a vesicular nucleus with a prominent nucleolus. The neuron is surrounded by a ring of satellite cells.

A31

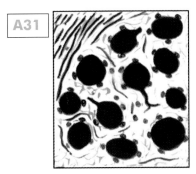

In Fig. A31 we see a similar ganglion stained by silver impregnation. Each neuron (stained dark brown) has only one process (i.e., it is unipolar). The process is not seen in some cells as it does not lie in the plane of section.

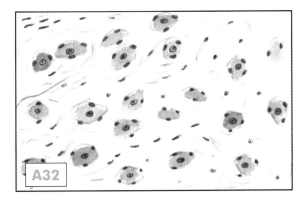

A32

Figs. A32. A33. Autonomic ganglia.

In Fig. A32 we see an autonomic ganglion. The neurons are not arranged in groups, but are scattered amongst nerve fibres. They are smaller than in sensory ganglia. Satellite cells are present, but are less prominent than in sensory ganglia.

A33

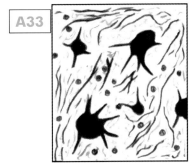

In Fig. A33 we see a similar ganglion stained by silver impregnation. The neurons are seen to be multipolar.

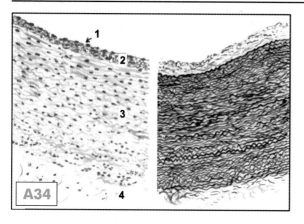

A34

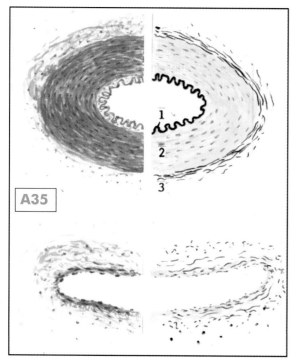

A35

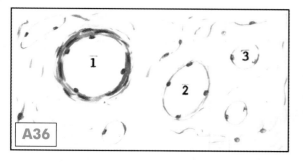

A36

BLOOD VESSELS

In Fig. A34 we see an *elastic artery*. The left half of the figure shows the appearance in a section stained with haematoxylin and eosin. The right half shows the appearance in a section stained by Verheoff's method. The elastic fibres are stained black, muscle fibres are yellow, and collagen is pink.

1 = endothelial lining; 2 = tunica intima; 3 = tunica media containing abundant elastic tissue arranged in the form of a number of membranes. Some muscle is also present. 4 = tunica adventitia.

In Fig. A35 we see a *medium sized artery* (above) *and vein* (below). Staining is as in Fig. A34. The tunica intima of the artery is sharply separated from the tunica media (2) by the internal elastic lamina (1). The media is composed mainly of smooth muscle. The adventitia (3) contains collagen fibres and several elastic fibres. (For details about arteries see page 169).

The vein has a thinner wall and a larger lumen than the artery. The tunica intima, media and adventitia can be made out, but they are not sharply demarcated. The media is thin and contains only a small quantity of muscle. The adventitia is relatively thick. Elastic fibres are present both in the media and in the adventitia. (For details about veins see page 172).

In Fig. A36 we see an *arteriole* (1), a *venule* (2), and *capillaries* (3). All vessels are lined by endothelium. The wall of the arteriole contains smooth muscle, but an internal elastic lamina is not present. The wall of the venule is thin, the endothelium being surrounded by collagen fibres. The walls of capillaries are formed mainly by endothelial cells. (For details see page 173).

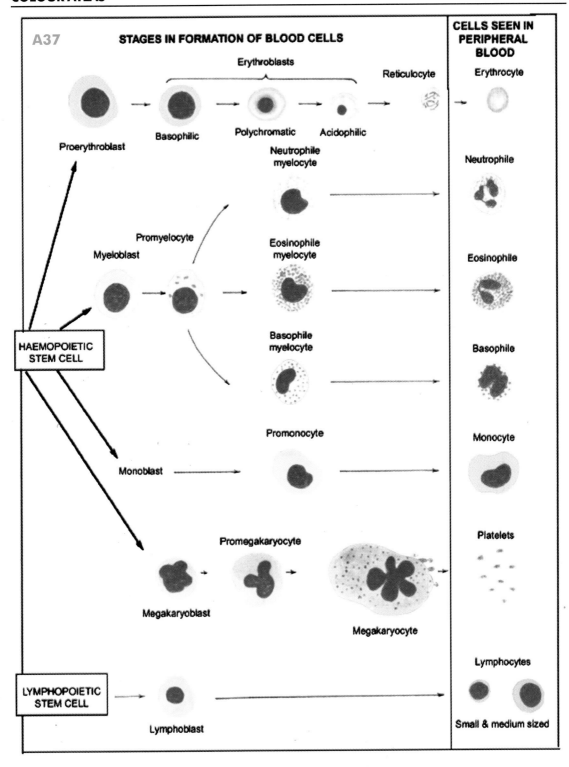

A37

STAGES IN FORMATION OF BLOOD CELLS

CELLS SEEN IN PERIPHERAL BLOOD

Erythroblasts

Reticulocyte

Erythrocyte

Proerythroblast

Basophilic

Polychromatic

Acidophilic

Neutrophile myelocyte

Neutrophile

Promyelocyte

Myeloblast

Eosinophile myelocyte

Eosinophile

HAEMOPOIETIC STEM CELL

Basophile myelocyte

Basophile

Promonocyte

Monocyte

Monoblast

Promegakaryocyte

Platelets

Megakaryoblast

Megakaryocyte

Lymphocytes

LYMPHOPOIETIC STEM CELL

Lymphoblast

Small & medium sized

Fig. A37. Formation of blood cells.

Ths figure (page Atlas 10) shows the various stages in the formation of different kinds of blood cells. Haemopoietic stem cells present in bone marrow give rise to all blood cells other than lymphocytes. Lymphocytes are derived from lymphopoietic stem cells that are present in bone marrow as well as in various lymphoid tissues.

Precursor cells of the erythrocyte series are called erythroblasts or normoblasts. The earliest precursors are large cells called proerythroblasts. They are succeeded (in that order) by basophilic, polychromatic, and acidophilic erythroblasts: the change in colour is due to gradual accumulation of haemoglobin in the cell. Acidophilic erythroblasts lose their nuclei and give rise to immature erythrocytes that are called reticulocytes, because a bluish network is seen in their cytoplasm. Reticulocytes enter the peripheral blood and soon become mature erythrocytes.

Precursors of granulocytes are called myeloblasts. These are transformed to promyelocytes and then to myelocytes. Characteristic granules (neutrophil, acidophil or basophil) appear in the cytoplasm so that three corresponding types of myelocytes can be distinguished. Each myelocyte has an indented nucleus. The myelocytes are transformed into corresponding leucocytes. Note the differences in appearances of nuclei of different granulocytes.

Precursors of monocytes are called monoblasts. These are transformed into promonocytes and then into monocytes.

Blood platelets are derived from large cells called megakaryocytes. The nuclei of these cells undergo repeated division, but do not separate, so that the nucleus comes to have several sets of chromosomes (i.e., it becomes polyploid), and appears to be made up of several lobes. Small masses of cytoplasm bud off from the parent cell to form blood platelets.

Precursors of lymphocytes are called lymphoblasts. They develop into lymphocytes that are predominantly small, but some are large and others are of medium size.

In the description given above no attempt has been made to describe the precise appearances of different stages in formation of blood cells. This is a highly specialized field of study well outside the scope of undergraduate students. However, the appearances of cells in peripheral blood are very important and should be studied along with the descriptions on page 70 onwards.

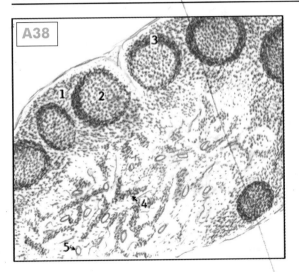

Fig. A38. Lymph node

The node consists of an outer cortex and an inner medulla. The cortex is packed with lymphocytes (1). A number of rounded lymphatic follicles (or nodules) are present. Each nodule has a pale staining germinal centre (2) surrounded by a zone of densely packed lymphocytes (3). Within the medulla the lymphocytes are arranged in the form of anastomosing cords (4). Several blood vessels (5) can be seen in the medulla. (For details see page 180).

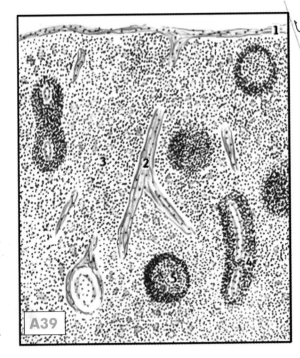

Fig. A39. Spleen

This section is stained by haematoxylin and eosin. Note the capsule (1) and the septa or trabeculae (2) extending into the organ from the capsule. The substance of the organ is divisible into the red pulp (3) in which there are diffusely distributed lymphocytes and numerous sinusoids; and the white pulp in which dense aggregations of lymphocytes are present. The latter are in the form of cords surrounding arterioles (4). When cut transversely (5) the cords resemble the lymphatic nodules of lymph nodes (Fig. A37), and like them they have germinal centres surrounded by rings of densely packed lymphocytes. However, the nodules of the spleen are easily distinguished from those of lymph nodes because of the presence of an arteriole in each nodule. The arteriole is placed eccentrically at the margin of the germinal centre. (For details see page 184).

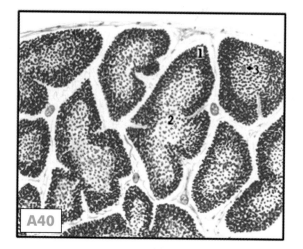

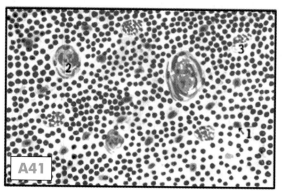

Figs. A40, A41. Thymus

This organ is made up of lymphoid tissue arranged in the form of distinct lobules. The presence of this lobulation enables easy distinction of the thymus from all other lymphoid organs. The lobules are partially separated from each other by connective tissue. Each lobule has an outer cortex (1) in which lymphocytes are densely packed; and an inner medulla (2) in which the cells are diffuse. The medulla contains pink staining rounded masses called the corpuscles of Hassall (3). These are better seen in Fig. A41 (which is a high power view of the medulla). In this figure the corpuscles (2) are seen as pink staining rounded masses. Their central parts appear homogeneous, but the peripheral parts are made up of concentrically arranged cells. In this figure also note the diffusely distributed lymphocytes. Scattered amongst them there are cells with a pink staining cytoplasm: these are epithelial cells (1). Some blood capillaries are also seen. (For details see page 186).

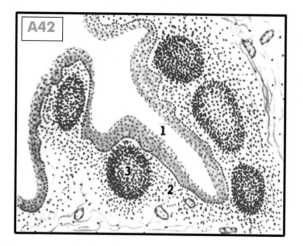

Fig. A42. Palatine tonsil

This is an aggregation of lymphoid tissue that is readily recognized by the fact that it is covered by a stratified squamous epithelium. At places the epithelium dips into the tonsil in the form of deep crypts (1). Deep to the epithelium there is diffuse lymphoid tissue (2) in which typical lymphatic nodules (3) can be seen. (For details see page 191).

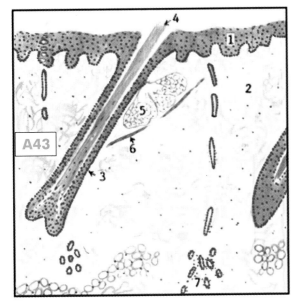

Fig. A43, A44. Skin

In Fig. A43 we see a low power view of the skin. Note the epidermis (1), the dermis (2), a hair follicle (3) with a hair (4) in it, a sebaceous gland (5), an arrector pili muscle (6) and parts of sweat glands (7). Some adipose tissue is present in the deeper part.

In Fig. A44, which is a high power view, we see parts of a sebaceous gland (1), of a hair follicle (2) and of an arrector pili muscle (3).

For a high power view of the epidermis see Fig. A10. (For description of the skin and its appendages see page 193 onwards).

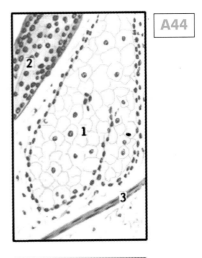

A44

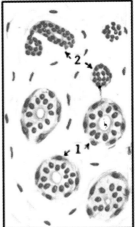

A45

Fig. A45. Sweat gland

In this figure we see a high power view of parts of a sweat gland. The secretory parts (1) are lined by a single layer of cubical or polyhedral cells. These are surrounded by a layer of myoepithelial cells (2). The ducts (3) are lined by two or more layers of cuboidal cells: this is an example of a stratified cuboidal epithelium.

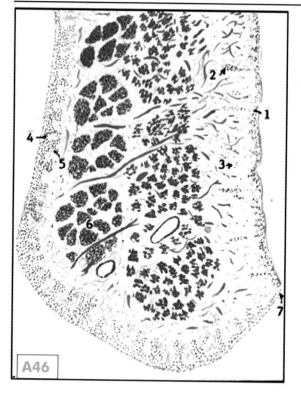

A46

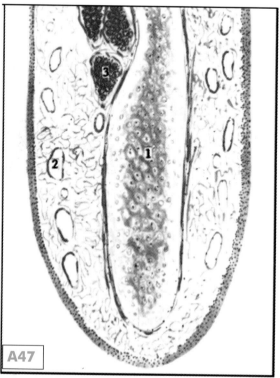

A47

Figs. A46 to A49 represent sections of four tissues that have a superficial resemblance to one another as each is a fold of tissue covered by stratified squamous epithelium. Figs. A46 and A48 are stained by Masson's trichrome method in which muscle stains red and collagen blue. Fig. A47 is stained by haematoxylin and eosin, while Fig. A49 is stained by Verheoff's method in which elastic fibres and nuclei are stained black and collagen is pink.

Fig. A46. Lip

The substance of the lip is occupied by a mass of skeletal muscle (cut transversely) and by connective tissue. The outer surface (1) of the lip is covered by true skin in which hair follicles (2) and sebaceous glands (3) can be made out. The inner surface is covered by mucous membrane which has a covering of thick stratified squamous epithelium (4), with deep papillae (5) extending into the underlying connective tissue. Numerous glands (6), some serous and some mucous, are present deep to the mucosa. The junction of skin and mucosa lies at '7'.

Fig. A47. Epiglottis

The core is made of a plate of elastic cartilage (1) covered by connective tissue in which there are numerous blood vessels (2) and glands (3). The surface is covered (on both sides) by stratified squamous epithelium. (Also see page 210).

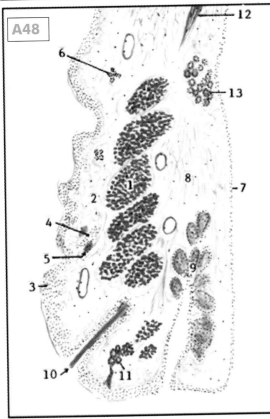

Fig. A48. Eyelid.

Like the lip the eyelid has a core of striated muscle (1) and dense connective tissue (2). Its external surface is covered by true skin (3) in which hair follicles (4), sebaceous glands (5), and sweat glands (6) are present. The inner surface is lined by palpebral conjunctiva (7): the epithelium here is stratified columnar (Also see page 317). The connective tissue intervening between the conjunctiva and the layer of muscle is dense and forms the tarsal plate (8) in which tarsal glands (9) are embedded. An eyelash is seen at 10, just behind which there are the ciliary glands (11) which are modified sweat glands. In the upper part of the figure we see fibres of the levator palpebrae superioris (12), and accessory lacrimal glands (13).

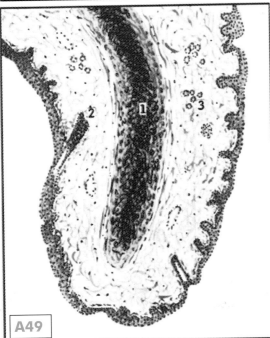

Fig. A49. Pinna

This has a core of elastic cartilage (1) lined on both sides by true skin in which hair follicles (2) and sweat glands (3) are seen.

Compare the appearance of elastic cartilage in Figs. A47 and A49, and also with Fig. A20. The differences are due to the differing staining methods used.

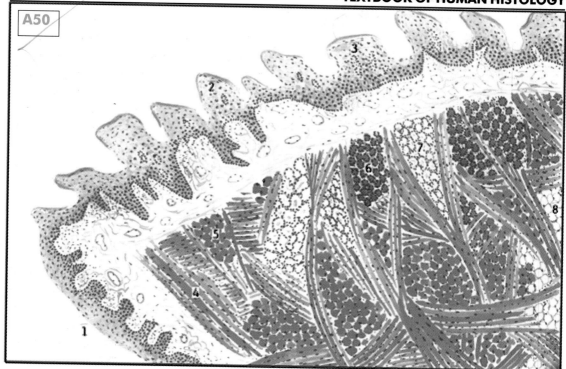

Figs. A50, A51. Tongue

Fig. A50 is a panoramic view of a section of the tongue near its tip. The surface is covered by stratified squamous epithelium. The undersurface of the tongue is smooth (1), but on the dorsum the surface shows numerous projections or papillae. Each papilla has a core of connective tissue covered by epithelium. Some papillae are pointed (filiform - 2), while others are broad at the top (fungiform - 3). A third type of papilla (circumvallate) is shown in Fig. A51. The top of this papilla is broad and lies at the same level as the surrounding mucosa. Going right round the papilla there is a deep groove (1). Taste buds (2) are present on both walls of the groove.

The main mass of the tongue is formed by skeletal muscle (Fig. A50): the fibres run in various directions so that some are cut longitudinally (4) and some transversely (5). Some of the muscle fibres extend into the circumvallate papillae (4 in Fig. A51). Some adipose tissue is present amongst the muscle fibres (Fig. A50, 8). Numerous serous glands (Fig. A50, 6) and mucous glands (7) are present amongst the muscle fibres. In Fig. A51 note the serous glands of Von Ebner (3) opening into the bottom of the sulcus around the circumvallate papilla. For details of the structure of the tongue see page 222.

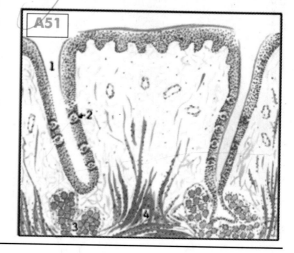

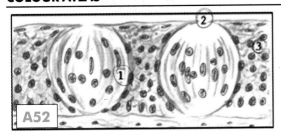

A52

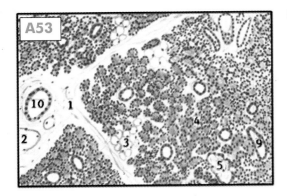

A53

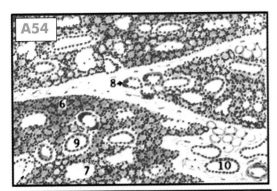

A54

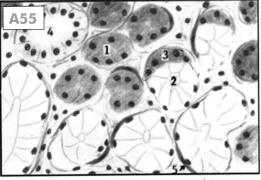

A55

Fig. A52. Tastebuds

In this figure we see a high power view of two taste buds. The buds are oval structures occupying the entire thickness of the epithelium. The cells in them are elongated and shaped like crescents (1). Each bud opens on to the surface through a pore (2). Normal stratified squamous epithelium (3) intervenes between the taste buds.

Figs. A53. Parotid gland

Figs. A53 to A56 depict the structure of salivary glands. There are three pairs of salivary glands: parotid, submandibular and sublingual.

In Fig. A53 we see a section through the parotid gland. Compare it with Fig. A54 which illustrates a section through the submandibular gland, and with Fig. A55 which shows a sublingual gland. All these are compound tubulo-alveolar glands. The gland is divided into lobules separated by interlobular connective tissue (1) in which some blood vessels (2) and adipose tissue (3) are present. The glandular tissue is made up of acini. Numerous intralobular (9) and interlobular (10) ducts can be seen.

In the parotid gland (Fig. A53) the acini are almost entirely serous (4), but a rare mucous acinus (5) may be seen.

Fig. A54. A55. Submandibular gland

In general the submandibular gland is similar to the parotid gland. However, both serous (6) and mucous (7) acini are seen. In some cases serous cells are present in relation to mucous acini forming demilunes (or crescents) (8).

In Fig. A55 we see a high power view of the submandibular gland to show the appearance of serous (1) and mucous (2) acini, and demilunes (3). A duct is also seen (4). Note the myoepithelial cells (5) present in relation to the acini. (See page 228).

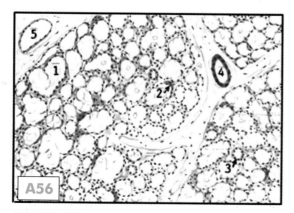

A56

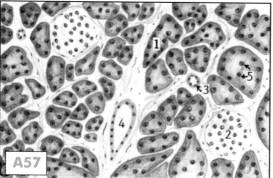

A57

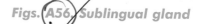

The general description of this gland is the same as given for the parotid and submandibular glands, but the acini are almost entirely mucous (1). An occasional serous demilune (2) may be seen. Intralobular ducts (3) are relatively few. An interlobular duct is seen at '4', and a blood vessel at '5'.

For further descriptions of the salivary glands see page 225.

Fig. A57. Pancreas

This is a compound tubulo-alveolar gland made up of serous acini (1) and, therefore, resembling the parotid gland. The two are, however, easily distinguished because of the presence (in the pancreas) of groups of cells that form the pancreatic islets (2): these islets are endocrine in function. Intralobular ducts (3) are few. An interlobular duct is shown at 4. The cells forming the acini of the pancreas are highly basophilic. The lumen of the acinus is seldom seen. The central parts of the acini are occupied by centroacinar cells (5).

Fig. A59. Lacrimal gland

This is a serous gland which can be distinguished by the distinct lumen of each acinus (1), and by its pink (rather than blue) staining. Myoepithelial cells (2) are present. A duct is seen at '3'.

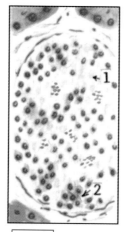

A58

Fig. A58. Pancreatic islet (of Langherhans)

In this figure we see a high power view of a pancreatic islet. The preparation has been specially stained to differentiate between alpha cells (1) that are stained pink, and beta cells (2) that are stained bluish. A number of capillaries (3) are seen. (For details see page 254).

A59

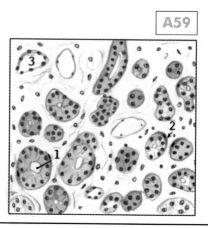

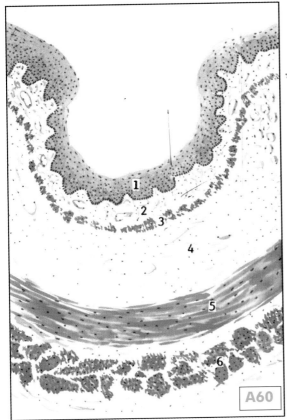

A60

Fig. A60. Oesophagus (T.S)

Note the lining of non-keratinized stratified squamous epithelium (1), the underlying connective tissue of the lamina propria (2), the muscularis mucosae (3) in which the muscle fibres are cut transversely, the submucosa (4), the layer of circular muscle (5), and the layer of longitudinal muscle (6).

The muscle is of the striated variety in the upper one third of the oesophagus, mixed in the middle one third, and smooth in the lower one third.

For details see page 233.

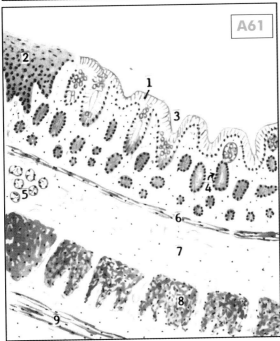

A61

Fig. A61. Stomach, cardiac end

The cardiac end of the stomach is lined by columnar cells (1). The epithelium is sharply demarcated from the stratified squamous epithelium lining the lower end of the oesophagus (2).

The mucosa of the stomach shows a number of shallow depressions called gastric pits (3) deep to which there are cardiac glands (4).

Some oesophageal (mucous) glands (5) are seen in the submucosa (7). A muscularis mucosae (6), and circular (8) and longitudinal (9) coats of muscle are present.

For further details see page 237.

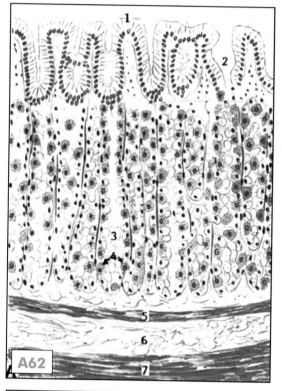

Fig. A62. Stomach, body

Note the thick mucosa, muscularis mucosae (5), submucosa (6) and part of circular muscle coat (7). The mucosa has a lining of columnar epithelium (1) which dips inwards to form numerous gastric pits (2) which occupy the superficial one fourth of the mucosa. The area between the pits and the muscularis mucosae is packed with tubular gastric glands (3). The glands are lined mainly by blue staining chief cells (3) or peptic cells. Amongst these there are pink staining oxyntic cells (4). These are large cells that are placed peripherally in the wall of the gland. They are more numerous in the upper parts of the gastric glands.

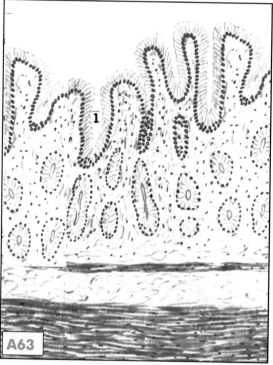

Fig. A63. Stomach, pylorus

Here the gastric pits (1) are much deeper than in the body (occupying upto two thirds of the depth of the mucosa). Deep to the pits there are pyloric glands (2) that are lined by mucous secreting cells. The muscularis mucosae (3), submucosa (4), and part of the muscle coat (5) are also seen.

For further details about the stomach see page 234).

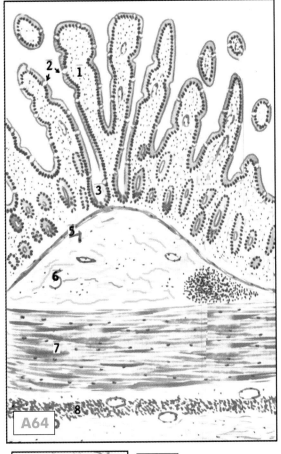

A64

Fig. A64. Jejunum

In this figure we see features of the typical structure of the small intestine. The mucosa shows numerous finger like projections or villi (1). Each villus has a covering of columnar epithelium that covers a core of delicate connective tissue. Some goblet cells (2) are also seen. Numerous tubular depressions, or crypts (3) dip into the lamina propria. These crypts are also lined by columnar cells. The mucosa is separated from the submucosa (5) by the muscularis mucosae (4). A solitary lymph nodule (6) is present in the submucosa. The intestine is surrounded by circular (7) and longitudinal (8) layers of smooth muscle.

Also see Figs. A65 and A66.

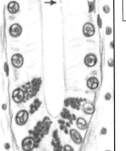

A65

Fig. A65. Paneth cells

In this figure we see the lower part of one crypt in the small intestine. Some of the cells contain red staining supranuclear granules: these are Paneth cells. A goblet cell (arrow) is seen in the upper part of the figure.

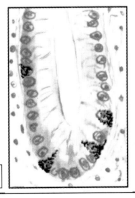

A66

Fig. A66. Argentaffin cells

In this figure we see an intestinal crypt stained by silver impregnation to demonstrate argentaffin cells having granules that are stained black. The granules are mainly infranuclear.

(For further details of the structure of the small intestine see page 238).

Fig. A67. Duodenum

The general structure of the duodenum is the same as that described for the jejunum, except that the submucosa is packed with mucous secreting glands of Brunner. Note that the intestinal crypts lie 'above' the muscularis mucosae while the glands of Brunner lie 'below' it. The presence of the glands of Brunner is a distinctive feature of the duodenum.

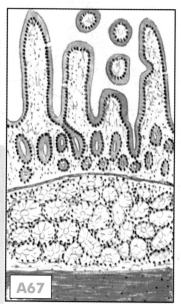

A67

Fig. A68. Ileum

The general structure of the ileum is similar to that of the jejunum (Fig. A64). This figure is a low power view showing an aggregated lymphatic follicle (or Peyer's patch). The entire thickness of the lamina propria is infiltrated with lymphocytes amongst which typical lymphatic follicles can be seen. Overlying the 'patch' villi may be rudimentary or absent. The muscularis mucosae is poorly developed in the region of the aggregated lymphatic follicle. Peyer's patches can also be seen in the distal jejunum, but they are much more numerous, and larger, in the ileum. For details see page 242.

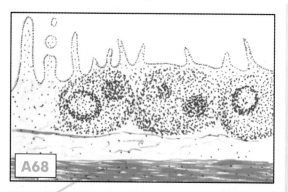

A68

Fig. A69. Large intestine

The mucosa shows numerous tubular glands or crypts (1). The surface of the mucosa, and the crypts, are lined by columnar cells amongst which there are numerous goblet cells. A section of the large intestine is easily distinguished from that of the small intestine because of the absence of villi; and from the stomach because of the presence of goblet cells (which are absent in the stomach). Crypts of the large intestine do not show Paneth cells, but argentaffin cells are present. A lymphatic nodule (2) is seen in the lamina propria. The muscularis mucosae (3), submucosa (4) and circular muscle coat (5) are similar to those in the small intestine. However, the longitudinal muscle coat is gathered into three thick bands called taenia coli, one of which is seen at '6'. The longitudinal muscle is thin in the intervals between the taenia (7).

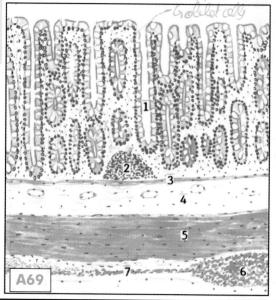

Goblet cell

A69

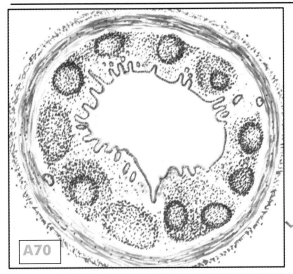

A70

Fig. A70. Vermiform appendix

The basic structure of the vermiform appendix is similar to that of the large intestine, but the mucosa is poorly developed. The lamina propria is infiltrated by lymphocytes, and numerous lymphatic nodules are present. For further details see page 245.

Fig. A71. Liver

In Fig. A71 we see a low power view. The substance of the liver is made up of liver cells (hepatocytes) arranged in the form of hexagonal areas called hepatic lobules. The lobules are partially separated by connective tissue. Each lobule has a central vein (1) from which numerous sinusoids (seen as empty spaces) pass radially. The spaces between the sinusoids are occupied by plates of liver cells; the plates look like cords when seen in section (2). Along the periphery of the lobules there are angular intervals filled by connective tissue. Each such area contains a branch of the portal vein (3), a branch of the hepatic artery (4), and an interlobular bile duct (5). These three constitute a portal triad.

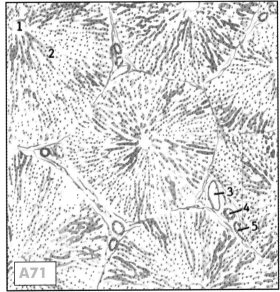

A71

In Figs. A72 and A73 we see parts of the liver at higher magnification. Polygonal liver cells arranged in a radial manner, separated by sinusoids, are seen. In Fig. A72 the tissue has been specially prepared to show phagocytic cells (of Kupffer) (arrows) in the walls of sinusoids. Particles of black ink injected into the circulation of the living animal have been taken up by these cells. In Fig. 73 the tissue has been prepared to demonstrate bile capillaries (arrows) present in the intervals between liver cells.

For further details of liver structure see page 248.

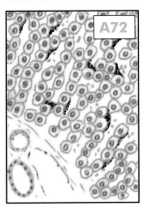

A72

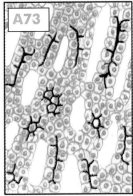

A73

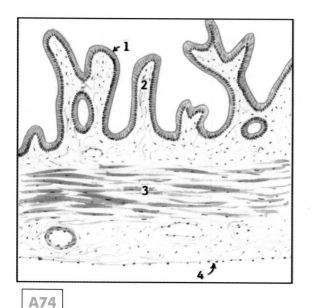

A74

Fig. A74. Gall bladder

The mucous membrane is lined by tall columnar cells (1). The mucosa is highly folded and some of the folds (2) might look like villi. Because of this beginners might confuse sections of the gall bladder with those of the small intestine. Distinction is easy if it is remembered that in the gall bladder there are no goblet cells, and no muscularis mucosae. The muscle coat (3) is poorly developed there being numerous connective tissue fibres amongst the muscle fibres. A serous covering (4) lined by flattened mesothelium is seen.

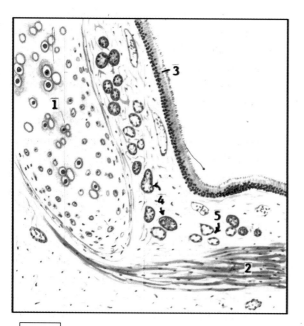

A75

Fig. A75. Trachea

A part of the wall of the trachea is seen. The tracheal wall has a 'skeleton' made up of C-shaped cartilages: one end of a cartilage is seen (1). The gap between the free ends of the cartilages are filled in by smooth muscle (2). The mucous membrane is lined by pseudostratified ciliated columnar epithelium (3). The subepithelial connective tissue contains serous glands (4) and mucous glands (5). For further details see page 211.

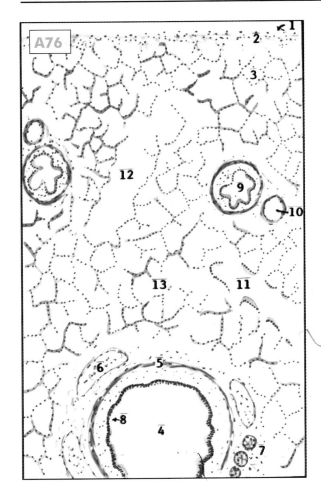

Fig. A76. Lung

The lung surface is covered by pleura which consists of a lining of mesothelium (1) resting on a layer of connective tissue (2).

The lung substance is made up of numerous thin-walled spaces or alveoli (3). The alveoli are filled with air that reaches them through a series of respiratory passages some of which are as follows.

A large bronchus (4) is seen in the lower part of the figure. Its structure is similar to that of the trachea in that smooth muscle (5), cartilage (6), and glands (7) are present in its wall; and it is lined by a similar epithelium (8). Two smaller, bronchioles (9) are seen: they are lined by a simple columnar epithelium, and have a wall of smooth muscle. There is no cartilage in their walls. Two arteries (10) are seen near the bronchioles. A respiratory bronchiole is seen at '11', an alveolar duct at '12', and an atrium at '13'.

For explanation of these terms and details of lung structure see page 212.

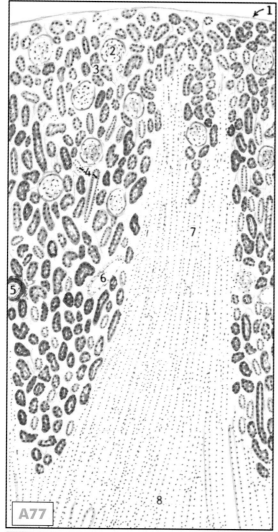

A77

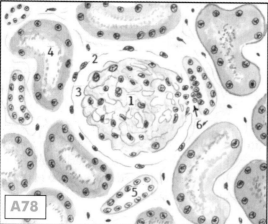

A78

Fig. A77. Kidney (low power view)

In Fig. A77 we see a section through part of a kidney at low magnification. The kidney is covered by a capsule (1). Deep to the capsule there is the cortex (occupying the upper 4/5 of the figure). In the cortex we see circular structures called renal corpuscles (2) surrounding which there are tubules cut in various shapes. The dark pink stained tubules are parts of the proximal convoluted tubules (3): their lumen is small and indistinct. Lighter staining tubules, each with a distinct lumen, are the distal convoluted tubules (4). An artery is seen at '5', and a vein at '6'. The very light staining, elongated, parallel running tubules seen in the medulla (8) are collecting ducts. Some of them extend into the cortex (7) forming a medullary ray.

Fig. A78. Renal cortex (high power view)

In this figure we see a high power view of the cortex. Note the large renal corpuscle consisting of a tuft of capillaries that form a rounded glomerulus (1), and an outer wall, the glomerular capsule (2). Note the urinary space (3) between the glomerulus and the capsule. Proximal convoluted tubules (4) are dark staining. They are lined by cuboidal cells with a prominent brush border. Distal convoluted tubules (5) are lighter staining. The cuboidal cells lining them do not have a brush border. Their lumen is distinct. At '6' we see a distal convoluted tubule closely related to the renal corpuscle. The nuclei in part of its wall are closely packed to form a structure called the macula densa: the macula is part of an important region called the juxtaglomerular apparatus. For a high power view of the renal medulla see Fig. A79.

For further details of renal structure see page 258 onwards.

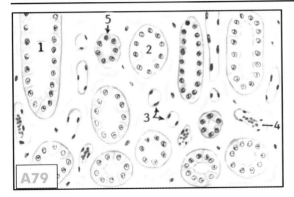

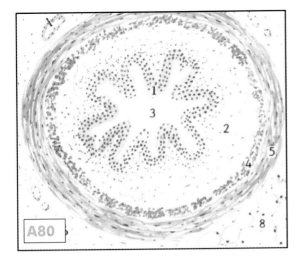

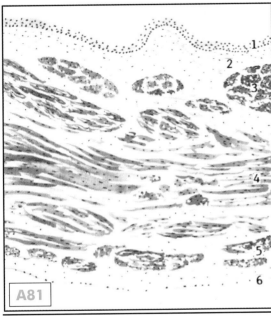

Fig. A79. Renal medulla (high power view)

This is a high power view of a part of the medulla. Note the following.

(a) A number of collecting ducts cut longitudinally (1) or transversely (2) are seen. They are lined by a cuboidal epithelium, the cells of which stain lightly. Cell boundaries are usually distinct. The lumen of the tubule is also distinct.

(b) Sections of the thin segment of the loop of Henle are seen at '3': they are lined by flattened cells, the walls being very similar in appearance to those of blood capillaries (4).

(c) Sections through the thick segments of loops of Henle are seen at '5': they are lined by cuboidal epithelium. (For details see page 258).

Fig. A80. Ureter (T.S)

The mucous membrane is lined by transitional epithelium (1) (Also see Figs. A7, A8) which rests on a layer of connective tissue (2). The mucosa shows folds that give the lumen a star shaped appearance (3). The muscle coat has an inner layer of longitudinal fibres (4) and an outer layer of circular fibres (5). Note that this arrangement is the reverse of that in the gut. The muscle coat is surrounded by connective tissue (6) in which blood vessels (7) and fat cells (8) are present.

Fig. A81. Urinary bladder

The mucous membrane is lined by transitional epithelium (1) that rests on a layer of connective tissue (2). The muscle layer is thick. It has inner and outer longitudinal layers (3,5) between which there is a layer of circular or oblique fibres (4). The layers are not clearly marked off from each other. The external surface is lined (in part) by a serous coat (6).

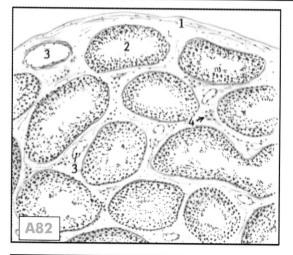

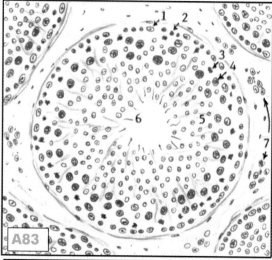

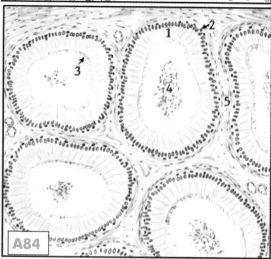

Fig. A82. A83 Testis

In Fig. A82 we see a low power view. The testis has an outer fibrous layer, the tunica albuginea (1) deep to which are seen a number of seminiferous tubules (2) cut in various directions.

The tubules are separated by connective tissue containing blood vessels (3) and groups of interstitial cells (4). Each seminiferous tubule is lined by several layers of cells.

Fig. A83 shows details of cells lining a seminiferous tubule seen at a high magnification. Note that the cell boundaries are indistinct, and nuclei are prominent.

The outermost row of nuclei belongs to sustentacular cells (1) and to spermatogonia (2), some of which are undergoing mitosis (3: note very dense nucleus of irregular shape). Passing inwards towards the centre of the tubule we have large darkly staining nuclei of spermatocytes (4), and many smaller nuclei of spermatids (5). Towards the centre of the tubule a number of developing spermatozoa are seen (6). Note groups of interstitial cells (7) in the connective tissue between the seminiferous tubules.

For significance of the various cells mentioned above see page 275.

Fig. A84. Epididymis

The section passes through the body of the epididymis which consists of a long convoluted duct which is cut up several times.

The duct is lined by pseudostratified columnar epithelium in which there are tall columnar cells (1) and shorter basal cells (2) that do not reach the lumen. The columnar cells bear stereocilia (3) that are non-motile (see page 23).

Clumps of spermatozoa (4) are present in the lumen. Note the smooth muscle (5) in the wall of the duct.

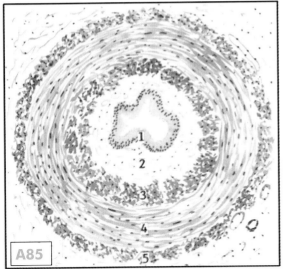

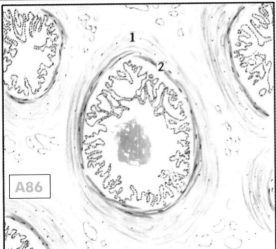

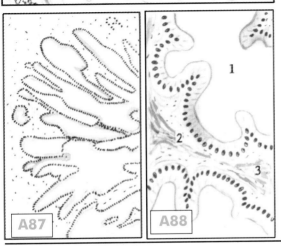

Fig. A85. Ductus deferens

The mucous membrane is lined by pseudostratified columnar epithelium (1) which rests on a lamina propria (2). The muscle coat is very thick. Three layers, inner longitudinal (3), middle circular (4) and outer longitudinal (5) are seen.

Figs. A86, A87. Seminal vesicle

It is made up of a convoluted tubule which is cut up several times in any section. The tube has an outer covering of connective tissue (1), a thin layer of smooth muscle (2) and an inner mucosa. The mucosal lining is thrown into numerous folds that branch and anastomose to form a network. The lining epithelium (See Fig. A87) is simple columnar or pseudostratified.

Figs. A88, A89. Prostate

Figs. A88 and A89 are high and low power views respectively. The prostate consists of glandular tissue embedded in prominent fibro-muscular tissue. The glandular tissue is in the form of follicles of irregular shape (1) that are lined by columnar epithelium. The lumen may contain amyloid bodies (2). The follicles are separated by broad bands of fibromuscular tissue (3): this tissue is a characteristic feature of the prostate. The prostate is traversed by the prostatic urethra (4) which is lined by transitional epithelium.

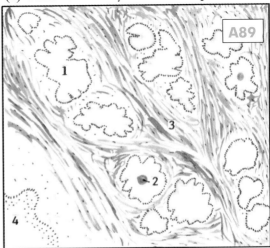

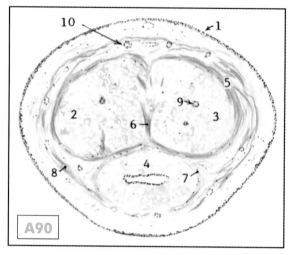

Fig. A90. Penis

This figure shows a transverse section through the body of the penis seen at very low magnification.

The penis has an outer covering of skin (1). The substance of the organ is made up of three masses of erectile tissue. Two masses, placed side by side, towards the dorsum, are the right and left corpora cavernosa (2,3). One mass lying in the midline, ventral to the corpora cavernosa is the corpus spongiosum (4). This is traversed by the penile urethra. Each corpus cavernosum is surrounded by a thick fibrous sheath (5) which also forms a median septum (6). The corpus spongiosum has a thinner sheath (7). There is an additional sheath (8) common to all three masses of erectile tissue. Note the artery in the centre of each corpus cavernosum (9), the two dorsal arteries (10), and numerous other vessels.

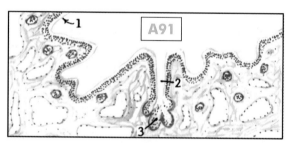

Fig. A91. Penile urethra

In this figure we see a high power view of part of the penis . Note the penile urethra lined by pseudostratified columnar epithelium (1). Diverticulae (2)(or crypts of Morgagni) arise from the urethra. A urethral gland (3) is seen opening into a crypt. Around the urethra there is erectile tissue of the corpus spongiosum.

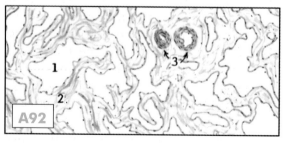

Fig. A92. Erectile tissue

This figure is a high power view of erectile tissue (present in the penis). This tissue consists of numerous spaces (1) that are lined by endothelium. The spaces are separated by a network of connective tissue (2). Two arteries (3) with thick muscular walls are seen.

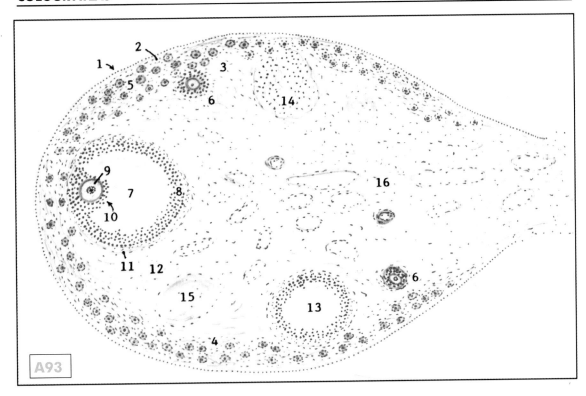

A93

Fig. A 93. Ovary (low power view)

In this figure we see a panoramic view of the ovary. The surface is covered by a cuboidal epithelium (1). Deep to the epithelium there is a layer of connective tissue that constitutes the tunica albuginea (2). The substance of the ovary shows an outer cortex in which follicles of various sizes are present (3,4); and an inner medulla consisting of connective tissue containing numerous blood vessels (16). Just deep to the tunica albuginea we see many primordial follicles (5) each of which contains a developing ovum surrounded by flattened follicular cells. Somewhat more developed ovarian follicles having several layers of follicular cells are seen at '6'. A large follicle is seen at '7'. It has a follicular cavity (7) surrounded by several layers of follicular cells (8). On one side within the follicle there is a developing ovum (9). The cells surrounding the ovum constitute the cumulus oophoricus (10). The follicle is surrounded by a condensation of connective tissue which forms a capsule (11) for it. The capsule consists of an inner cellular part (the theca interna), and an outer fibrous part (the theca externa). The follicle is surrounded by a stroma (12) made up of reticular fibres and fusiform cells. At '13' we have another follicle in which an ovum is not seen as the section does not pass through the plane in which the ovum lies. At '14' we see a structure called the corpus luteum. A high power view of the corpus luteum is seen in Fig. D. Note that it is made up of large polyhedral luteal cells. Also note the capillaries present amongst the cells. At '15' in Fig. A we see two rounded masses of fibrous tissue that represent remnants of degenerated or atretic follicles.

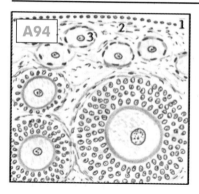

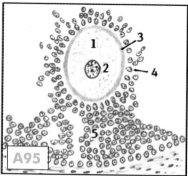

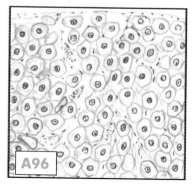

Fig. A94. Ovarian cortex

In Fig. A94 we see a high power view of a part of the ovarian cortex. Observe the germinal epithelium (1), the tunica albuginea (2), the primordial follicles (3), and three ovarian follicles at different stages of formation. Each follicle contains a developing ovum.

Fig. A95. Mature ovarian follicle

In this figure we see a high power view of part of a mature ovarian follicle to show the ovum. The ovum is a large cell with a granular cytoplasm (1) and a large vesicular nucleus (2). It is surrounded by a homogeneous membrane (3) called the zona pellucida. The ovum is surrounded by follicular cells that constitute the cumulus oophoricus (4). The follicular cells that connect the ovum to the wall of the follicle (5) constitute the discus proligerus.

(For further details of the structure of the ovary see page 286).

Fig. A96. Corpus luteum

The corpus luteum is made up of large polyhedral luteal cells. Also note the capillaries present amongst the cells.

Figs. A97, A98. Uterine tube

Figs. A97 and A98 are low power and high power views, respectively, of the uterine tube. The uterine tube has a muscular wall with an outer longitudinal (1) and inner circular (2) layer. The mucous membrane shows numerous branching folds which almost fill the lumen of the tube. The mucosa is lined by ciliated columnar epithelium. (Details on page 292).

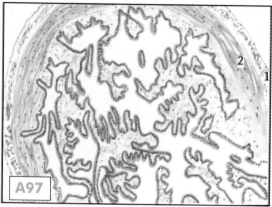

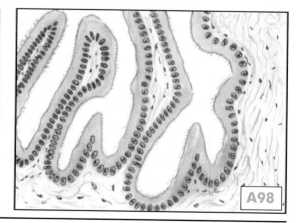

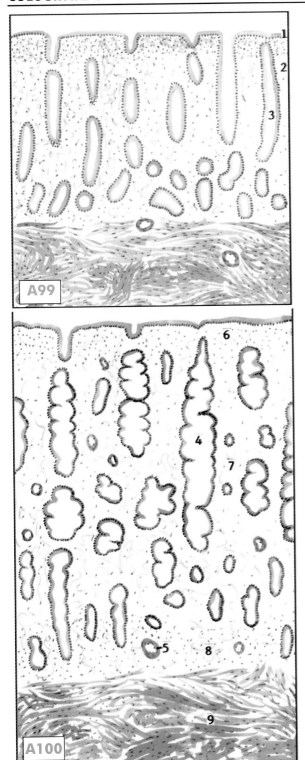

Figs. A99, A100. *Uterus*

The wall of the uterus consists of a mucous membrane (called the endometrium) and a very thick layer of muscle (the myometrium). Only a very small part of the myometrium is included in these figures.

The endometrium has a lining of columnar epithelium (1) that rests on a stroma of connective tissue (2). Numerous tubular uterine glands (3) dip into the stroma. The appearance of the endometrium varies considerably depending upon the phase of the menstrual cycle.

In Fig. A99 the endometrium is shown in the proliferative phase; while in Fig. A100 it is shown in the secretory phase. In the proliferative phase the endometrium is relatively thin, and the glands in it are straight (3). In the secretory phase the thickness of the endometrium is much increased. The uterine glands elongate, become dilated, and tortuous as a result of which they have saw-toothed margins in sections (4). Blood vessels become more conspicuous (5). The stroma becomes divisible into three parts: there is a superficial stratum compactum (6) in which the cells are closely packed, a middle stratum spongiosum (7) which is relatively loose, and a stratum basale (8) in which the cells are again densely packed (as indicated by density of nuclei).

The myometrium is described as having various layers, but these are difficult to make out as the fibres run in various directions (9). For further details of the structure of the uterus see page 293.

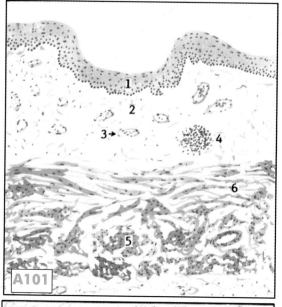

Fig. A101. Vagina

The vagina has a mucosa which is lined by stratified squamous epithelium (non-keratinized) (1) that rests on connective tissue (2) in which there are many blood vessels (3). Lymphoid follicles (4) are also present. There are no glands in the mucosa. The muscle coat has an outer layer of longitudinal fibres (5) and a thin inner layer of circular fibres (6).

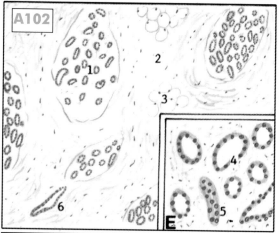

Fig. A102 . Mammary gland (resting)

In this figure we see a section of a mammary gland in the resting phase. It consists of lobules of glandular tissue (1) separated by considerable quantity of connective tissue (2) and fat (3). The glandular elements are lined by cuboidal epithelium (4) and have large lumina so that they look like ducts. Some of them may be in form of solid cords of cells (5). A duct (6) is seen: it is lined by an unusual epithelium made up of two layers of cuboidal or flattened cells (see inset).

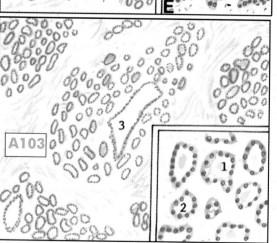

Fig. A103. Mammary gland (lactating)

In this figure we see sections through the lactating mammary gland. The glandular elements proliferate so that they become relatively more prominent than the connective tissue. Some of the alveoli are lined by large vacuolated cells and have an irregular lumen (1), while others that are depleted of secretion show a cuboidal lining (2). Secretion is present in several alveoli. Some ducts (3) are also seen.

For details of structure of the mammary gland see page 297.

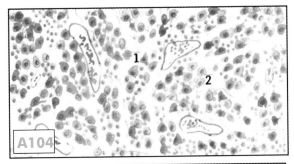

A104

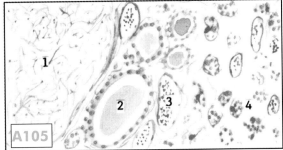

A105

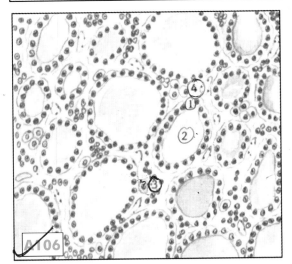

A106

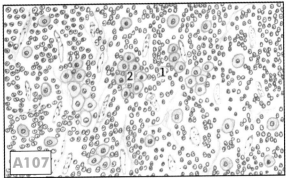

A107

Figs. A104, A105. Hypophysis cerebri

In Fig. A104 we see the pars anterior of the hypophysis cerebri. This part consists of groups or cords of cells with numerous sinusoids between them. The cells are of three types. The pink staining cells (1) are alpha cells or acidophils. The cells with bluish cytoplasm (2) are beta cells or basophils. Cells in which the cytoplasm is not conspicuous, and the nuclei are closely packed, are chromophobe cells. (For details see page 300).

In Fig. A105 we see the pars posterior (left) and the pars intermedia (right) of the hypophysis cerebri. The pars posterior (1) is made up of nerve fibres and neuroglial cells (details of which cannot be made out in routine sections). The pars intermedia contains some colloid filled vesicles (2), blood capillaries (3) and clumps of cells (4) in which some acidophil and basophil cells can be identified.

Fig. A106. Thyroid gland

It is made up of follicles lined by cuboidal epithelium (1). The follicles contain pink staining colloid (2). In the intervals between the follicles there is some connective tissue. Parafollicular cells (3) are present in relation to the follicle's and also as groups in the connective tissue (4). For details of the structure of the thyroid gland see page 306.

Fig. A107. Parathyroid glands

These are made up of masses of cells with numerous capillaries in between. Most of the cells (of which only nuclei are seen) are the chief cells (1). The large cells with pink cytoplasm are oxyphil cells (2). For details see page 308.

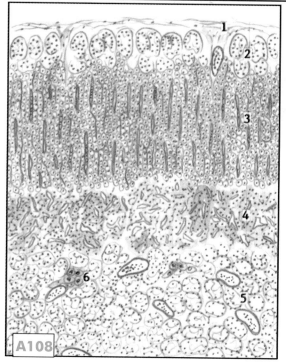

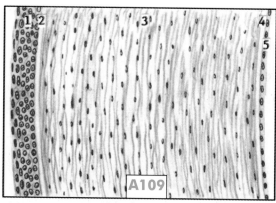

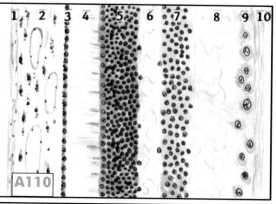

Fig. A108. Suprarenal gland

Note the connective tissue capsule (1) from which septa extend into the gland substance. The gland consists of an outer cortex (upper 2/3 of figure) and an inner medulla (lower 1/3). The cortex is divisible into three zones. The zona glomerulosa (2) is most superficial. Here the cells are arranged in the form of inverted U-shaped structures or acinus-like groups. In the zona fasciculata (3) the cells are arranged in straight columns (typically two cell thick). Sinusoids intervene between the columns. The zona reticularis (4) is made up of cords of cells that branch and form a network.

The medulla (5) is made up of groups of cells separated by wide sinusoids. Some sympathetic neurons (6) are also present.

Fig. A109. Cornea

The outermost layer (to the left)(1) is of non-keratinized stratified squamous epithelium. Next, there is the structureless anterior limiting membrane. Most of the thickness of the cornea is made up of several layers of collagen fibres embedded in a ground substance (3). These layers form the substantia propria. Deep to the substantia propria there is a thin homogeneous layer called the posterior limiting lamina (4). The posterior surface of the cornea is lined by a single layer of flattened or cuboidal cells (5).

Fig. A110. Eyeball

The various layers of the eyeball are as follows. 1 = Sclera, made up of collagen fibres. 2 = Choroid, containing blood vessels and pigment cells.

The remaining layers are subdivisions of the retina.

3 = Pigment cell layer. 4 = Layer of rods and cones. 5 = Outer nuclear layer. 6 = Outer plexiform layer. 7 = Inner nuclear layer. 8 = Inner plexiform layer. 9 = Layer of ganglion cells. 10 = Layer of optic nerve fibres.

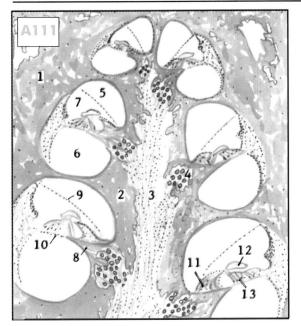

This is a low power view to show the general structure of the cochlea.

The cochlea is embedded in the petrous temporal bone (1). It is in the form of a spiral canal and is, therefore, cut up six times. The cone-shaped mass of bone surrounded by these turns of the cochlea is called the modiolus (2) which contains a canal through which fibres of the cochlear nerve (3) pass. A mass of neurons belonging to the spiral ganglion (4) lies to the inner side of each turn of the cochlea.

The parts to be identified in each turn of the cochlea are the scala vestibuli (5), the scala tympani (6), the duct of the cochlea (7), the spiral lamina (8), the vestibular membrane (9), the basilar membrane (10), the spiral limbus (11), the membrana tectoria (12), and the organ of Corti (13). (See page 336).

A high power view of the organ of Corti is shown in Fig. B.

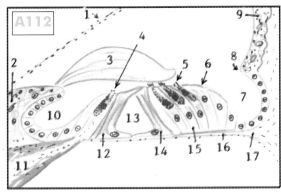

Identify the following parts. 1 = Vestibular membrane. 2 = Spiral limbus. 3 = Membrana tectoria. 4 = Inner hair cell. 5 = Outer hair cell. 6 = Supporting cells (of Henson). 7 = Outer spiral sulcus. 8 = Spiral prominence. 9 = Stria vasculosa. 10 = Inner spiral sulcus. 11 = Spiral lamina. 12 = Inner rod cell. 13 = Tunnel of Corti. 14 = Outer rod cell. 15 = Phalangeal cells. 16 = Basilar membrane. 17 = Spiral ligament.

(For description of these terms see page 341).

Description on page Atlas 40

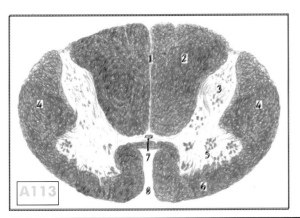

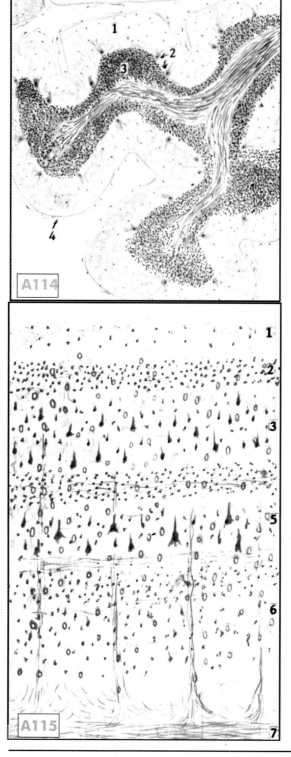

A114

A115

Fig. A113. Spinal cord (on p. Atlas39)

This section has been stained by a method that stains myelin sheaths blue and cell bodies of neurons red. As a result white matter (made up mainly of myelinated fibres) stains dark blue, while grey matter (containing neurons and unmyelinated fibres) stains lightly. 1 = Posterior median septum. 2 = Posterior white column. 3 = Posterior grey column. 4 = Lateral white column. 5 = Anterior grey column. 6 = Anterior white column. 7 = Central canal lying in grey commissure. The fibres in front of the grey commissure form the anterior white commissure. 8 = Anterior median sulcus.

Fig. A114. Cerebellum

Note the leaf like folia. The core of each folium is formed by blue staining fibres of the white matter. The layers overlying the white matter form the cerebellar cortex which consists of: 1 = Molecular layer; 2 = Purkinje cells; 3 = Granule cell layer. The cortex is covered by piamater (4).

Fig. A115. Cerebral cortex

Myelinated nerve fibres are stained blue. 1 = Molecular layer. 2 = External granular layer. 3 = Pyramidal cell layer. 4 = Internal granular layer. 5 = Ganglionic layer. 6 = Multiform layer. 7 = White matter.

For descriptions of the spinal cord, the cerebellum and the cerebral cortex see the author's Textbook of Human Neuroanatomy.

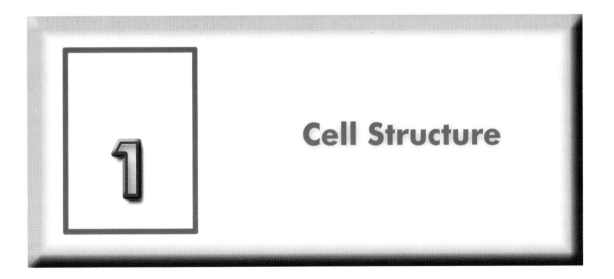

Cell Structure

Histology & Its Study

Histology is the study of cells, tissues and organs as seen with a microscope. The microscopes commonly used in class rooms and in laboratories are light microscopes. Magnified images of objects are seen through these microscopes by the use of glass lenses. The maximum magnification possible with a light microscope is about 1500 times.

Early histological observations were, of necessity, empirical. With the development, in recent years, of refined methods for preparation and study of tissues, and because of accompanying developments in our knowledge of the chemical composition of cells, and of constant chemical transformations within them, we now have a much better comprehension of the physiological and biochemical significance of microscopic structures. Some of the techniques that have contributed to the development of this knowledge are briefly summarized below.

Traditional Histological Methods

The earliest histological observations were made on unfixed tissue (usually teased to make a flat preparation). The first significant advance was the discovery of chemicals for *fixation* and for *staining* of tissues. The next major development was the invention of instruments (called *microtomes*) for cutting thin sections of tissue. These sections could be mounted on glass slides and stained.

The process of fixation preserves a tissue by denaturing its proteins. It also makes the handling of tissue, and the preparation and staining of sections, more efficient. Numerous fixatives are known, the most commonly used being formaldehyde. (Formaldehyde is a gas. This gas dissolved in water is called formalin).

Before a tissue can be sectioned it has to be given a firm consistency. One way of doing this is to freeze the tissue and cut sections while it is still frozen (such sections being called *frozen sections*). Techniques for the production of frozen sections have undergone great refinement and at present they are prepared using a microtome enclosed in a refrigerated chamber. Such an instrument is called a *cryostat*. Preparation of frozen sections is the fastest method of examining a tissue. The technique allows the examination of pieces of tissue removed by a surgeon, while the patient is still on the operating table, making it possible for the surgeon to plan his operation keeping in mind the nature of disease.

Apart from freezing a tissue, it can be made suitable for sectioning by embedding it in a suitable medium, the most common being paraffin wax. Such *paraffin sections* can be thinner than frozen sections, and reveal more details of structure. However, some materials (e.g., fat) are lost during the process of embedding tissues in paraffin wax.

The commonest staining procedure used in histology is *haematoxylin-eosin* staining. In sections stained with this procedure nuclei are stained blue, and most other components are seen in varying shades of pink. Numerous other staining methods are available for demonstrating specific tissue elements.

Electronmicroscopy

In the last few decades many new discoveries in the field of histology have become possible because of the development of the electron microscope (usually abbreviated to EM). This microscope uses an electron beam instead of light; and electromagnetic fields in place of lenses. With the EM magnifications in excess of 100,000 times can be achieved. The structure of a cell or tissue as seen with the EM is referred to as *ultrastructure*.

For electronmicroscopic studies small pieces of tissue are fixed very rapidly after removal from the animal body. Special fixatives are required (the most common being glutaraldehyde). Very thin sections are required, and for this purpose tissues have to be embedded in media that are harder than wax. Epoxy resins (e.g., araldite) are used. The microtomes used for cutting sections are much more sophisticated versions of traditional microtomes and are called *ultramicrotomes*. Thin sections prepared in

this way are also very useful in light microscopy. They reveal much more detail than can be seen in conventional paraffin sections.

Before sections are examined under an electronmicroscope they are often treated with solutions containing uranium or lead, to increase contrast of the image. Osmium tetroxide acts both as fixative and staining agent and has been extensively used for preparing tissues for electronmicroscopy.

In conventional EM studies (or *transmission electronmicroscopy*) images are formed by electrons passing through the section. Wide use is also made of *scanning electronmicroscopy* in which the images are produced by electrons reflected off the surface of a tissue. The surface appearances of tissue can be seen, and three dimensional images can also be obtained. Specially useful details of some tissues (e.g., membranes) can be obtained by freezing a tissue and then fracturing it to view the fractured surface.

Histochemistry

In many cases the chemical nature of cellular and intercellular constituents can be determined by the use of staining techniques. Lipids and carbohydrates (glycogen) present in cells are easily demonstrated. The presence of many enzymes can be determined by placing sections in solutions containing the substrate of the enzyme, and by observing the product formed by action of enzyme on substrate. The product is sometimes visible, or can be made visible using appropriate staining agents.

For enzyme studies, the use of frozen sections is essential. Good frozen sections can be obtained by using cryostats (mentioned above).

Immunocytochemistry

Specific molecules within cells can be identified by treating tissue sections with antibodies specific to the molecules. The technique enables chemical substances to be localized in cells with great precision. Such studies have greatly enhanced our knowledge of chemical transformations taking place within cells.

Autoradiography

Many molecules (e.g., aminoacids) injected into an animal become incorporated into the tissues of the animal. Sometimes it is possible to replace a normal aminoacid with a radioactive substitute. For example if a radioactive isotope of thymidine is injected, it becomes incorporated in proteins in place of normal thymidine. The sites of presence of the radioactive material can be determined by covering tissue sections with a photographic emulsion. Radiations emerging from radioactive material act on the emulsion.

After a suitable interval the emulsion is 'developed'. Grains of silver can be seen under the microscope at sites where the radioisotope was present.

Units of measurement used in histology

The study of histology frequently involves the measurement of microscopic distances. The units used for this purpose are as follows.

1 micrometer or micron (μm) = 1/1000 of a millimetre (mm).

1 nanometre (nm) = 1/1000 of a micrometer.

Cells, Tissues And Organs

The human body, like that of most other animals and plants, is made up of units called cells. Cells can differ greatly in their structure.

However, most of them have certain features in common. These are described in this chapter.

Aggregations of cells of a common type (or of common types) constitute tissues. Apart from the cells many tissues have varying intercellular substances that may separate the cells from one another. Organs (e.g., the heart, stomach or liver) are made up of combinations of various kinds of tissue.

CELL STRUCTURE

A cell is bounded by a **cell membrane** (or **plasma membrane**) within which is enclosed a complex material called **protoplasm**. The protoplasm consists of a central, more dense, part called the **nucleus**; and an outer less dense part called the **cytoplasm**. The nucleus is separated from the cytoplasm by a nuclear membrane. The cytoplasm has a fluid base (matrix) which is referred to as the **cytosol** or **hyaloplasm**. The cytosol contains a number of **organelles** which have distinctive structure and functions. Many of them are in the form of membranes that enclose spaces. These spaces are collectively referred to as the **vacuoplasm**.

From what has been said above it is evident that membranes play an important part in the constitution of the cell. The various membranes within the cell have a common basic structure which we will consider before going on to study cell structure in detail.

Basic Membrane Structure

When suitable preparations are examined by EM the average cell membrane is seen to be about 7.5 nm thick. It consists of two densely stained

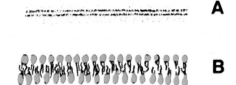

Fig. 1.1. A. Trilaminar structure of a cell membrane as revealed by high magnifications of EM.

B. Diagram showing the arrangement of phospholipid molecules forming the membrane.

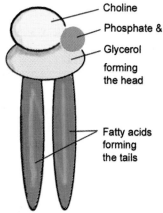

Fig. 1.2. Diagram showing the structure of a phospholipid molecule (phosphatidyl choline) seen in a cell membrane.

layers separated by a lighter zone, thus creating a trilaminar appearance (Fig. 1.1A).

Cell membranes are made up predominantly of lipids. Proteins and carbohydrates are also present.

Lipids in cell membranes

It is now known that the trilaminar structure of membranes is produced by the arrangement of lipid molecules (predominantly phospholipids) that constitute the basic framework of the membrane (Fig. 1.1B).

Each phospholipid molecule consists of an enlarged head in which the phosphate portion is located; and of two thin tails (Fig. 1.2). The

head end is also called the *polar end* while the tail end is the *non-polar end*. The head end is soluble in water and is said to be *hydrophilic*. The tail end is insoluble and is said to be *hydrophobic*.

When such molecules are suspended in an aqueous medium they arrange themselves so that the hydrophilic ends are in contact with the medium; but the hydrophilic ends are not. They do so by forming a bi-layer.

The dark staining parts of the membrane (seen by EM) are formed by the heads of the molecules, while the light staining intermediate zone is occupied by the tails, thus giving the membrane its trilaminar appearance.

Because of the manner of its formation, the membrane is to be regarded as a fluid structure that can readily reform when its continuity is disturbed. For the same reasons proteins present within the membrane (see below) can move freely within the membrane.

Some details regarding the lipid content of cell membranes are as follows.

1. As stated above phospholipids are the main constituents of cell membranes. They are of various types including phosphatidylcholine, sphingomyelin, phosphatidylserine, and phosphatidyl-ethanolamine.

2. Cholesterol provides stability to the membrane.

3. Glycolipids are present only over the outer surface of cell membranes. One glycolipid is galactocerebroside which is an important constituent of myelin. Another category of glycolipids seen are ganglionosides.

Proteins in cell membranes

In addition to molecules of lipids the cell membrane contains several proteins. It was initially thought that the proteins formed a layer on each side of the phospholipid molecules

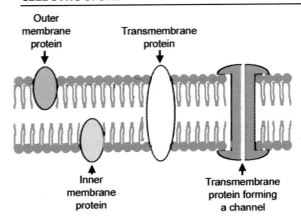

Fig. 1.3. Some varieties of membrane proteins.

(forming a protein-phospholipid sandwich). However, it is now known that this is not so. The proteins are present in the form of irregularly rounded masses. Most of them are embedded within the thickness of the membrane and partly project on one of its surfaces (either outer or inner). However, some proteins occupy the entire thickness of the membrane and may project out of both its surfaces (Fig. 1.3). These are called transmembrane proteins.

The proteins of the membrane are of great significance as follows.

(**a**) They may form an essential part of the structure of the membrane i.e., they may be structural proteins.

(**b**) Some proteins play a vital role in transport across the membrane and act as pumps. Ions get attached to the protein on one surface and move with the protein to the other surface.

(**c**) Some proteins are so shaped that they form passive channels through which substances can diffuse through the membrane. However, these channels can be closed by a change in the shape of the protein.

(**d**) Other proteins act as receptors for specific hormones or neurotransmitters.

(**e**) Some proteins act as enzymes.

Carbohydrates of cell membranes

In addition to the phospholipids and proteins, carbohydrates are present at the surface of the membrane. They are attached either to the proteins (forming glycoproteins) or to the lipids (forming glycolipids) (Fig. 1.4). The carbohydrate layer is specially well developed on the external surface of the plasma membrane forming the cell boundary. This layer is referred to as the cell coat or **glycocalyx**. *(Glycolipids + Glycoprotein*

Membranes in cells are highly permeable to water, and to oxygen, but charged ions (Na^+, K^+) do not pass through easily.

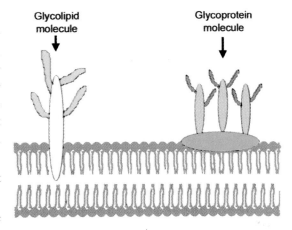

Fig. 1.4. Glycolipid and glycoprotein molecules attached to the outer aspect of cell membrane.

THE CELL MEMBRANE

The membrane separating the cytoplasm of the cell from surrounding structures is called the **cell membrane** or the **plasma membrane**. It has the basic structure described above. We have seen that the carbohydrate layer, or **glycocalyx**, is specially well formed on the external surface of this membrane.

The glycocalyx is made up of the carbohydrate portions or glycoproteins and glycolipids present in the cell membrane. Some functions attributed to the glycocalyx are as follows.

(a) Special adhesion molecules present in the layer enable the cell to adhere to specific types of cells, or to specific extracellular molecules.

(b) The layer contains antigens. These include major histocompatibility antigens (MHC). In erythrocytes the glycocalyx contains blood group antigens.

(c) Most molecules in the glycocalyx are negatively charged causing adjoining cells to repel one another. This force of repulsion maintains the 20 nm interval between cells. However, some molecules that are positively charged adhere to negatively charged molecules of adjoining cells, holding the cells together at these sites.

The cell membrane is of great importance in regulating the activities as follows.

(**a**) The membrane maintains the shape of the cell.

(**b**) It controls the passage of all substances into or out of the cell. Some substances (consisting of small molecules) pass through the passive channels already described: this does not involve deformation of the membrane. Larger molecules enter the cell by the process of endocytosis described below.

(**c**) The cell membrane forms a sensory surface. This function is most developed in nerve and muscle cells. The plasma membranes of such cells are normally polarized: the external surface bears a positive charge and the internal surface bears a negative charge, the potential difference being as much as 100 mv. When suitably stimulated there is a selective passage of sodium and potassium ions across the membrane reversing the charge. This is called *depolarisation*: it results in contraction in the case of muscle, or in generation of a nerve impulse in the case of neurons.

(**d**) The surface of the cell membrane bears *receptors* that may be specific for particular molecules (e.g., hormones or enzymes). Stimulation of such receptors (e.g., by the specific hormone) can produce profound effects on the activity of the cell. Receptors also play an important role in absorption of specific molecules into the cell as described below.

Enzymes present within the membrane may be activated when they come in contact with specific molecules. Activation of the enzymes can influence metabolism within the cell as explained below.

When a receptor on the cell surface is stimulated this often activates some substances within the cell that are referred to as *second messengers*. Important second messengers are as follows.

1. Adenylate cyclase: This enzyme changes the concentration of cyclic adenosine monophosphate (cyclic AMP) within the cell. In turn this can lead to alterations in many functions of the cell including protein synthesis and synthesis of DNA.

2. Enzymes controlling cyclic GMP have effects that are usually opposite to those controlling cyclic AMP.

3. Phosphoinositol (a phospholipid) affects calcium regulatory processes within the cell.

(**e**) Membrane proteins help to maintain the structural integrity of the cell by giving attachment to cytoskeletal filaments (page 20). They also help to provide adhesion between cells and extracellular materials.

(**f**) Cell membranes may show a high degree of specialisation in some cells. For example, the membranes of rod and cone cells (present in the retina) bear proteins that are sensitive to light.

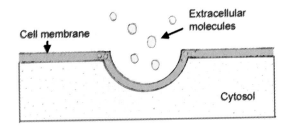

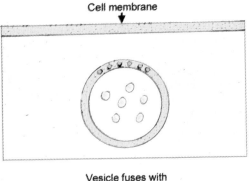

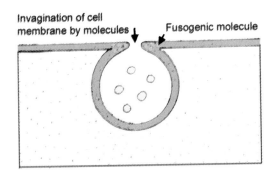

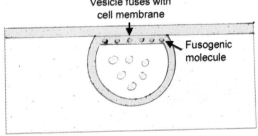

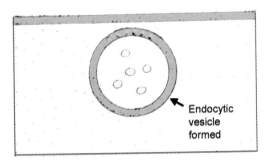

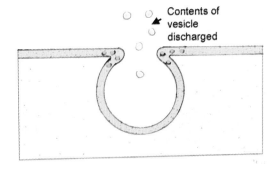

Fig. 1.5. Three stages in the absorption of extra-cellular molecules by endocytosis.

Fig. 1.6. Three stages in exocytosis. The fusogenic proteins facilitate adhesion of the vesicle to the cell membrane.

Role of cell membrane in transport of material into or out of the cell

We have seen, above, that some molecules can enter cells by passing through passive channels in the cell membrane. Large molecules enter the cell by the process of **endocytosis** (Fig. 1.5). In this process the molecule invaginates a part of the cell membrane, which first surrounds the molecule, and then separates (from the rest of the cell membrane) to form an **endocytic vesicle**. This vesicle can move through the cytosol to other parts of the cell.

The term **pinocytosis** is applied to a process similar to endocytosis when the vesicles (then called **pinocytotic vesicles**) formed are used for absorption of fluids (or other small molecules) into the cell.

Some cells use the process of endocytosis to engulf foreign matter (e.g., bacteria). The process is then referred to as **phagocytosis**.

Molecules produced within the cytoplasm (e.g.,

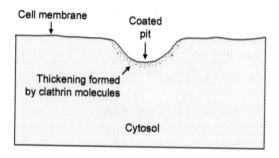

Fig. 1.7. Diagram to show a coated pit
as seen by EM.

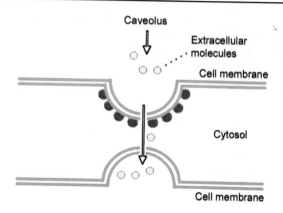

Fig. 1.8. Scheme to illustrate how extracellular
molecules can pass through the entire thickness of
a cell (transcytosis). Caveolae are involved.

secretions) may be enclosed in membranes to form vesicles that approach the cell membrane and fuse with its internal surface. The vesicle then ruptures releasing the molecule to the exterior. The vesicles in question are called *exocytic vesicles*, and the process is called *exocytosis* or *reverse pinocytosis* (Fig. 1.6).

We will now consider some further details about transfer of substances across cell membranes

1. As endocytic vesicles are derived from cell membrane, and as exocytic vesicles fuse with the latter, there is a constant transfer of membrane material between the surface of the cell and vesicles within the cell.

2. Areas of cell membrane which give origin to endocytic vesicles are marked by the presence of *fusogenic proteins* that aid the formation of endocytic vesicles. Fusogenic proteins also help in exocytosis by facilitating fusion of membrane surrounding vesicles with the cell membrane.

3. When viewed by EM areas of receptor mediated endocytosis are seen as depressed areas called *coated pits* (Fig. 1.7). The membrane lining the floor of the pits is thickened because of the presence of a protein called *clathrin*. This protein forms a scaffolding around the developing vesicle and facilitates its separation from the cell membrane. Thereafter, the clathrin molecules detach from the surface of the vesicle and return to the cell membrane.

4. The term *transcytosis* refers to a process

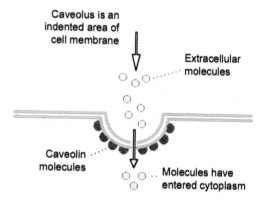

Fig. 1.9. Scheme to show how extracellular molecules enter the cytosol through caveolae. Endocytic vesicles are not formed. The process is called potocytosis.

where material is transferred right through the thickness of a cell. The process is seen mainly in flat cells (e.g., endothelium). The transport takes place through invaginations of cell membrane called *caveolae*. A protein *caveolin* is associated with caveolae (Fig. 1.8). Caveolae differ from coated pits in that they are not transformed into vesicles. Caveolae also play a role in transport of extracellular molecules to the cytosol (without formation of vesicles). (See Fig. 1.9).

Thickness of plasma membs = 7-8 nm
width of inter cellular gap = 20 nm

CONTACTS BETWEEN ADJOINING CELLS

In tissues in which cells are closely packed the cell membranes of adjoining cells are separated, over most of their extent by a narrow space (about 20 nm). This contact is sufficient to bind cells loosely together, and also allows some degree of movement of individual cells.

In some regions the cell membranes of adjoining cells come into more intimate contact: these areas can be classified as follows.

Classification Of Cell Contacts

Unspecialized contacts

These are contacts that do not show any specialized features on EM examination. At such sites adjoining cell membranes are held together as follows.

Some glycoprotein molelcules, present in the cell membrane, are called *cell adhesion molecules* (CAMs). These molecules occupy the entire thickness of the cell membrane (i.e., they are transmembrane proteins). At its cytosolic end each CAM is in contact with an *intermediate protein* (or *link protein*) (that appears to hold the CAM in place). Fibrous elements of the cytoskeleton are attached to this intermediate protein (and thus, indirectly, to CAMs). The other end of the CAM juts into the 20 nm intercellular space, and comes in contact with a similar molecule from the opposite cell membrane. In this way a path is established through which forces can be transmitted from the cytoskeleton of one cell to another (Fig. 1.10).

CAMs and intermediate proteins are of various types. Contacts between cells can be classified

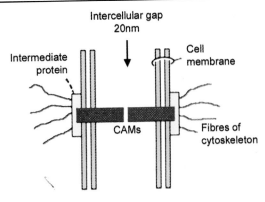

Fig. 1.10. Scheme to show the basic structure of an unspecialized contact between two cells.

on the basis of the type of CAMs proteins present. The adhesion of some CAMs is dependent on the presence of calcium ions; while some others are not dependent on them (Fig. 1.11). Intermediate proteins are also of various types (catenins, vinculin, α actinin).

Specialized junctional structures

These junctions can be recognized by EM. The basic mode of intercellular contact, in them, is similar to that described above and involves, CAMs, intermediate proteins, and cytoskeletal elements. Junctional areas that can be identified can be summarized as follows.

A. *Anchoring junctions* or *adhesive junctions* bind cells together, They can be of the following types.

1. *Adhesive spots* (also called *desmosomes*, or *maculae adherens*).

2. *Adhesive belts* or *zona adherens*.

3. *Adhesive strips* or *fascia adherens*.

Modified anchoring junctions attach cells to extracellular material. Such junctions are seen as *hemidesmosomes*, or as *focal spots*.

B. *Occluding junctions* (*zonula occludens* or *tight junctions*). Apart from holding cells

Fig. 1.11. Types of cell adhesion molecules		
Types of CAM	Subtypes	Present in
CALCIUM DEPENDENT	Cadherins (of various types)	Most cells including epithelia
	Selectins	Migrating cells e.g., leucocytes
	Integrins	Between cells and intercellular substances. About 20 types of integrins, each attaching to a special extracellular molecule.
CALCIUM INDEPENDENT	Neural cell adhesion molecule (NCAM)	Nerve cells
	Intercellular adhesion molecule (ICAM)	Leucocytes

together, these junctions form barriers to movement of material through intervals between cells.

C. Communicating junctions (or *gap junctions*). Such junctions allow direct transport of some substances from cell to cell.

The various types of cell contacts mentioned above are considered one by one below.

ANCHORING JUNCTIONS

Adhesion spots (Desmosomes, Maculae Adherens)

These are the most common type of junctions between adjoining cells. Desmosomes are present where strong anchorage between cells is needed e.g., between cells of the epidermis. As seen by EM a desmosome is a small

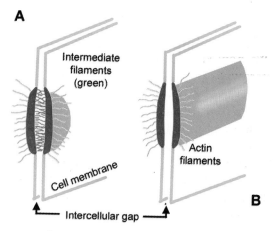

Fig. 1.12. A. EM appearance of a desmosome.
B. EM appearance of zonula adherens.

circumscribed area of attachment (Fig. 1.12A). At the site of a desmosome the plasma membrane (of each cell) is thickened because of the presence of a dense layer of proteins on its inner surface

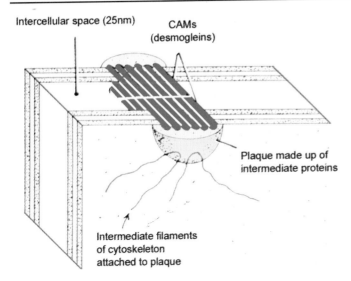

Intercellular space (25nm)

CAMs (desmogleins)

Plaque made up of intermediate proteins

Intermediate filaments of cytoskeleton attached to plaque

Fig. 1.13. Schematic diagram to show the detailed structure of a desmosome (in the epidermis).

(i.e., the surface towards the cytoplasm). The thickened areas of the two sides are separated by a gap of 25 nm. The region of the gap is rich in glycoproteins. The thickened areas of the two membranes are held together by fibrils that appear to pass from one membrane to the other across the gap.

We now know that the fibrils seen in the intercellular space represent CAMs (Fig. 1.13). The thickened area (or plaque) seen on the cytosolic aspect of the cell membrane is produced by the presence of intermediate (link) proteins. Cytoskeletal filaments attached to the thickened area are intermediate filaments (page 21). CAMs seen in desmosomes are integrins (desmogleins I, II). The link proteins are desmoplakins.

Adhesive Belts (Zonula Adherens)

In some situations, most typically near the apices of epithelial cells, we see a kind of junction called the zonula adherens, or adhesive belt (Fig. 1.12B). This is similar to a desmosome in being

marked by thickenings of the two plasma membranes, to the cytoplasmic aspects of which fibrils are attached. However, the junction differs from a desmosome in that:

(i) instead of being a small circumscribed area of attachment the junction is in the form of a continuous band passing all around the apical part of the epithelial cell; and

(ii) in that the gap between the thickenings of the plasma membranes of the two cells is not traversed by filaments.

The CAMs present are cadherins. In epithelial cells zona adherens are located immediately deep to occluding junctions (Fig. 1.16).

Adhesive Strips (Fascia adherens)

These are similar to adhesive belts. They differ from the latter in that the areas of attachment are in the form of short strips (and do not go all round the cell). These are seen in relation to smooth muscle, intercalated discs of cardiac muscle, and in junctions between glial cells and nerves.

Hemidesmosomes

These are similar to desmosomes, but the thickening of cell membrane is seen only on one side. As such junctions the 'external' ends of CAMs are attached to extracellular structures. Hemidesmosomes are common where basal epidermal cells lie against connective tissue.

The cytoskeletal elements attached to intermediate proteins are keratin filaments (as against intermediate filaments in desmosomes). As in desmosomes, the CAMs are integrins.

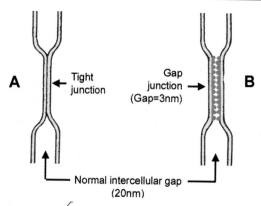

Fig. 1.14. A. Zonula occludens as seen by EM.
B. Gap junction as seen by EM.

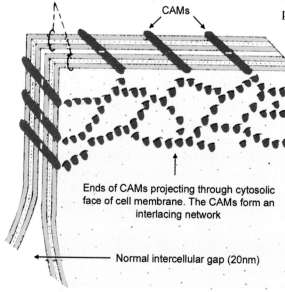

Fig. 1.15. Schematic diagram to show the detailed structure of part of an occluding junction.

Focal spots

These are also called *focal adhesion plaques*, or *focal contacts*. They represent areas of local adhesion of a cell to extracellular matrix. Such junctions are of a transient nature (e.g., between a leucocyte and a vessel wall). Such contacts may send signals to the cell and initiate cytoskeletal formation.

The CAMs in focal spots are integrins. The intermediate proteins (that bind integrins to actin filaments) are α actinin, vinculin and talin.

OCCLUDING JUNCTIONS (ZONULA OCCLUDENS)

Like the zonula adherens the zonula occludens is seen most typically near the apices of epithelial cells. At such a junction the two plasma membranes are in actual contact (Fig. 1.14A).

These junctions act as barriers that prevent the movement of molecules into the intercellular spaces. For example, intestinal contents are prevented by them from permeating into the intercellular spaces between the lining cells. Zonulae occludens are, therefore, also called *tight junctions*.

Recent studies have provided a clearer view of the structure of tight junctions (Fig. 1.15). Adjoining cell membranes are united by CAMs that are arranged in the form of a network that 'stiches' the two membranes together.

Other functions attributed to occluding junctions are as follows.

(a) These junctions separate areas of cell membrane that are specialized for absorption or secretion (and lie on the luminal side of the cell) from the rest of the cell membrane.

(b) Areas of cell membrane performing such functions bear specialized proteins. Occluding junctions prevent lateral migration of such proteins.

(c) In cells involved in active transport against a concentration gradient, occluding junctions prevent back diffusion of transported substances.

Sinusoids + Show big gaps more than 80 nm.
Continuous :-
Fenestrated :-

CELL STRUCTURE

13

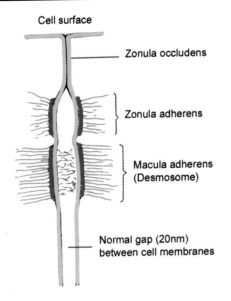

Fig. 1.16. Scheme to show a junctional complex.

Apart from epithelial cells, zonulae occludens are also present between endothelial cells.

In some situations occlusion of the gaps between the adjoining cells may be incomplete and the junction may allow slow diffusion of molecules across it. These are referred to as *leaky tight junctions*.

Junctional Complex

Near the apices of epithelial cells the three types of junctions described above, namely zonula occludens, zonula adherens and macula adherens are often seen arranged in that order (Fig. 1.16) They collectively form a junctional complex. In some complexes the zonula occludens may be replaced by a leaky tight junction, or a gap junction (see below).

COMMUNICATING JUNCTIONS (GAP JUNCTIONS)

At these junctions the plasma membranes are not in actual contact (as in a tight junction), but lie very close to each other, the gap being reduced (from the normal 20 nm) to 3 nm. In transmission electronmicrographs this gap is seen to contain bead-like structures (Fig. 1.14B). A minute canaliculus passing through each 'bead' connects the cytoplasm of the two cells thus allowing the free passage of some substances (sodium, potassium, calcium, metabolites) from one cell to the other (Also see below). Gap junctions are, therefore, also called *maculae communicantes*. They are widely distributed in the body.

Changes in pH or in calcium ion concentration can close the channels of gap junctions. By allowing passing of ions they lower transcellular electrical resistance. Gap junctions form electrical synapses between some neurons.

The number of channels present in a gap junction can vary considerably. Only a few may

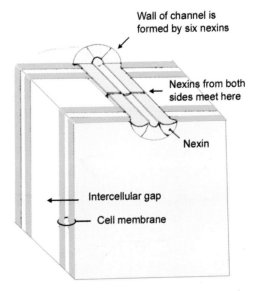

Fig. 1.17. Diagram to show the constitution of one channel of a communicating junction.

be present in which case the junctions would be difficult to identify. At the other extreme the junction may consist of an array of thousands of channels. Such channels are arranged in hexagonal groups.

The wall of each channel is made up of six protein elements (called *nexins*, or *connexons*). The 'inner' ends of these elements are attached to the cytosolic side of the cell membrane while the 'outer' ends project into the gap between the two cell membranes (Fig. 1.17). Here they come in contact with (and align perfectly with) similar nexins projecting into the space from the cell membrane of the opposite cell, to complete the channel.

CELL ORGANELLES

We have seen that (apart from the nucleus) the cytoplasm of a typical cell contains various structures that are referred to as organelles. They include the ER, ribosomes, mitochondria, the Golgi complex, and various types of vesicles (Fig. 1.18). The cytosol also contains a cytoskeleton made up of microtubules, microfilaments, and intermediate filaments. Centrioles are closely connected with microtubules. We shall deal with these entities one by one.

Endoplasmic Reticulum

The cytoplasm of most cells contains a system of membranes that constitute the endoplasmic reticulum (ER). The membranes form the boundaries of channels that may be arranged in the form of flattened sacs (or cisternae) or of tubules.

Because of the presence of the ER the cytoplasm

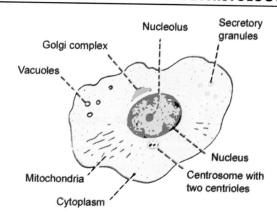

Fig. 1.18.Some features of a cell that can be seen with a light microscope.

is divided into two components, one within the channels and one outside them (Fig. 1.19). The cytoplasm within the channels is called the *vacuoplasm*, and that outside the channels is the *hyaloplasm* or *cytosol*.

In most places the membranes forming the ER are studded with minute particles of RNA (page 31) called *ribosomes*. The presence of these ribosomes gives the membrane a rough appearance. Membranes of this type form what is called the rough (or granular) ER. In contrast some membranes are devoid of ribosomes and constitute the smooth or agranular ER (Fig. 1.19).

Rough ER represents the site at which proteins are synthesized. The attached ribosomes play an important role in this process (page 34). The lumen of rough ER is continuous with the perinuclear space (between the inner and outer nuclear membranes). It is also continuous with the lumen of smooth ER.

Smooth ER is responsible for further processing of proteins synthesized in rough ER. It is also responsible for synthesis of lipids, specially that of membrane phospholipids (necessary for membrane formation). Most cells have very little smooth ER. It is a prominent feature of cells processing lipids.

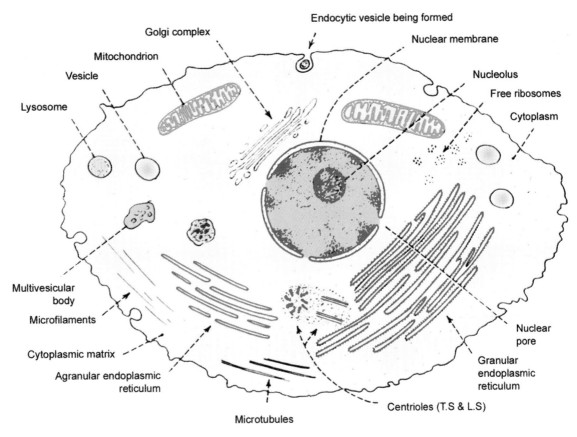

Fig. 1.19. Schematic diagram to show the various organelles to be found in a typical cell. The various structures shown are not drawn to scale.

Products synthesized by the ER are stored in the channels within the reticulum. Ribosomes, and enzymes, are present on the 'outer' surfaces of the membranes of the reticulum.

Ribosomes

We have seen above that ribosomes are present in relation to rough ER. They may also lie free in the cytoplasm. They may be present singly in which case they are called ***monosomes***; or in groups which are referred to as ***polyribosomes*** (or ***polysomes***). Each ribosome consists of proteins and RNA (ribonucleic acid) and is about 15 nm in diameter. The ribosome is made up of two subunits one of which is larger than the other. Ribosomes play an essential role in protein synthesis details of which are given on page 34.

Mitochondria

Mitochondria can be seen with the light microscope in specially stained preparations. They are so called because they appear either as granules or as rods (mitos = granule; chondrium = rod). The number of mitochondria varies from cell to cell being greatest in cells with high metabolic activity (e.g., in secretory cells). Mitochondria vary in size, most of them being 0.5 to 2 μm in length. Mitochondria are large in

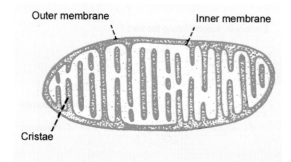

Fig. 1.20. Structure of a mitochondrion.

cells with a high oxidative metabolism.

A schematic presentation of some details of the structure of a mitochondrion (as seen by EM) is shown in Fig.1.20. The mitochondrion is bounded by a smooth *outer membrane* within which there is an *inner membrane*, the two being separated by an *intermembranous space*. The inner membrane is highly folded on itself forming incomplete partitions called *cristae*. The space bounded by the inner membrane is filled by a granular material called the *matrix*. This matrix contains numerous enzymes. It also contains some RNA and DNA: these are believed to carry information that enables mitochondria to duplicate themselves during cell division. An interesting fact, discovered recently, is that all mitochondria are derived from those in the fertilized ovum, and are entirely of maternal origin.

Mitochondria are of great functional importance. They contain many enzymes including some that play an important part in Kreb's cycle (TCA cycle). ATP and GTP are formed in mitochondria from where they pass to other parts of the cell and provide energy for various cellular functions. These facts can be correlated with the observation that within a cell mitochondria tend to concentrate in regions where energy requirements are greatest.

The enzymes of the TCA cycle are located in the matrix, while enzymes associated with the respiratory chain and ATP production are present

on the inner mitochondrial membrane. Enzymes for conversion of ADP to ATP are located in the intermembranous space. Enzymes for lipid synthesis and fatty acid metabolism are located in the outer membrane.

Mitochondrial abnormalities

Mitochondrial DNA can be abnormal. This interferes with mitochondrial and cell functions, resulting in disorders referred to as mitochondrial cytopathy syndromes. The features (which differ in intensity from patient to patient) include muscle weakness, degenerative lesions in the brain, and high levels of lactic acid. The condition can be diagnosed by EM examination of muscle biopsies. The mitochondria show characteristic para-crystalline inclusions.

Golgi Complex

The Golgi complex (Golgi apparatus, or merely Golgi) was known to microscopists long before the advent of electron microscopy. In light microscopic preparations suitably treated with silver salts the Golgi complex can be seen as a small structure of irregular shape, usually present near the nucleus (Fig. 1.18).

When examined with the EM the complex is seen to be made up of membranes similar to those of smooth ER. The membranes form the

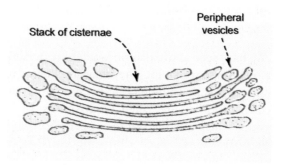

Fig. 1.21. Structure of the Golgi complex.

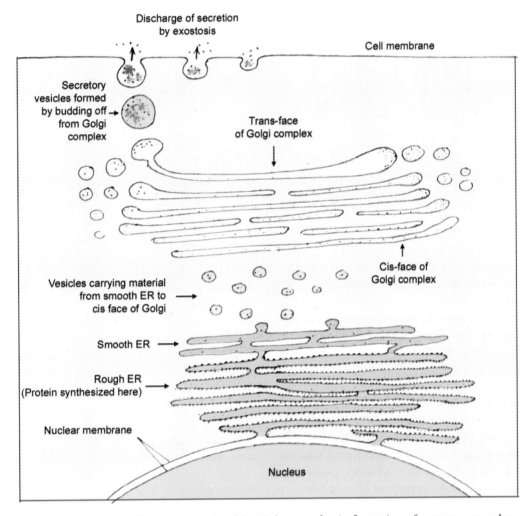

Fig. 1.22. Scheme to illustrate the role of the Golgi complex in formation of secretory vacuoles.

walls of a number of flattened sacs that are stacked over one another. Towards their margins the sacs are continuous with small rounded vesicles (Fig. 1.21). The cisternae of the Golgi complex form an independent system. Their lumen is not in communication with that of ER. Material from ER reaches the Golgi complex through vesicles.

From a functional point of view the Golgi complex is divisible into three regions (Fig. 1.22). The region nearest the nucleus is the *cis face* (or *cis Golgi*). The opposite face (nearest the cell membrane) is the *trans face* (also referred to as *trans Golgi*). The intermediate part (between the cis face and the trans face) is the *medial Golgi*.

Material synthesized in rough ER travels through the ER lumen into smooth ER. Vesicles budding off from smooth ER transport this material to the cis face of the Golgi complex. Some proteins are phosphorylated here. From the cis face all these materials pass into the medial Golgi. Here sugar residues are added to proteins to form protein-carbohydrate complexes.

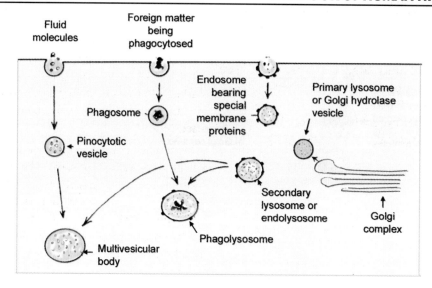

Fig. 1.23.Scheme to show how lysosomes, phagolysosomes and multivesicular bodies are formed.

Finally, all material passes to the trans face which performs the following functions.

(a) Proteolysis of some proteins converts them from inactive to active forms.

(b) Like the medial Golgi the trans face is also concerned in adding sugar residues to proteins.

(c) In the trans face various substances are sorted out and packed in appropriate vesicles. The latter may be secretory vesicles, lysosomes, or vesicles meant for transport of membrane to the cell surface.

The membranes of the Golgi complex contain appropriate enzymes for the functions performed by them. As proteins pass through successive sacs of Golgi they undergo a process of purification.

Membrane Bound Vesicles

The cytoplasm of a cell may contain several types of vesicles. The contents of any such vesicle are separated from the rest of the cytoplasm by a membrane which forms the wall of the vesicle.

Vesicles are formed by budding off from existing areas of membrane. Some vesicles serve to store material. Others transport material into or out of the cell, or from one part of a cell to another. Vesicles also allow exchange of membrane between different parts of the cell.

Details of the appearances of various types of vesicles will not be considered here. However, the student must be familiar with their terminology given below.

Phagosomes

Solid 'foreign' materials, including bacteria, may be engulfed by a cell by the process of **phagocytosis**. In this process the material is surrounded by a part of the cell membrane. This part of the cell membrane then separates from the rest of the plasma membrane and forms a free floating vesicle within the cytoplasm. Such membrane bound vesicles, containing solid ingested material are called **phagosomes**. (Also see lysosomes).

Pinocytotic vesicles

Some fluid may also be taken into the cytoplasm by a process similar to phagocytosis. In the case of fluids the process is called *pinocytosis* and the vesicles formed are called *pinocytotic vesicles*. (Also see page 7).

Exocytic vesicles

Just as material from outside the cell can be brought into the cytoplasm by phagocytosis or pinocytosis, materials from different parts of the cell can be transported to the outside by vesicles. Such vesicles are called *exocytic vesicles*, and the process of discharge of cell products in this way is referred to as *exocytosis* (or *reverse pinocytosis*).

Secretory Granules

The cytoplasm of secretory cells frequently contains what are called *secretory granules*. These can be seen with the light microscope. With the EM each 'granule' is seen to be a membrane bound vesicle containing secretion. The appearance, size and staining reactions of these secretory granules differ depending on the type of secretion. These vesicles are derived from the Golgi complex.

Other Storage Vesicles

Materials such as lipids, or carbohydrates, may also be stored within the cytoplasm in the form of membrane bound vesicles.

Lysosomes

These vesicles contain enzymes that can destroy unwanted material present within a cell. Such material may have been taken into the cell from outside (e.g., bacteria); or may represent organelles that are no longer of use to the cell. The enzymes present in lysosomes include (amongst others) proteases, lipases, carbohydrases, and acid phosphatase. (As many as 40 different lysosomal enzymes have been identified).

Lysosomes belong to what has been described as the *acid vesicle system*. The vesicles of this system are covered by membrane which contains H^+ATPase. This membrane acts as a H^+ pump creating a highly acid environment within the vesicle (up to pH5). The stages in the formation of a lysosome are as follows.

(**1**) Acid hydrolase enzymes synthesized in ER reach the Golgi complex where they are packed into vesicles (Fig. 1.23). The enzymes in these vesicles are inactive because of the lack of an acid medium. (These are called *primary lysosomes* or *Golgi hydrolase vesicles*).

(**2**) These vesicles fuse with other vesicles derived from cell membrane (*endosomes*). These endosomes possess the membrane proteins necessary for producing an acid medium. The product formed by fusion of the two vesicles is an *endolysosome* (or *secondary lysosome*).

(**3**) H^+ ions are pumped into the vesicle to create an acid environment. This activates the enzymes and a mature lysosome is formed.

Lysosomes help in 'digesting' the material within phagosomes (described above) as follows. A lysosome, containing appropriate enzymes, fuses with the phagosome so that the enzymes of the former can act on the material within the phagosome. These bodies consisting of fused phagosomes and lysosomes are referred to as *phagolysosomes* (Fig. 1.23).

In a similar manner lysosomes may also fuse with pinocytotic vesicles. The structures formed by such fusion often appear to have numerous small vesicles within them and are, therefore, called *multivesicular bodies*.

After the material in phagosomes or pinocytotic vesicles has been 'digested' by lysosomes, some waste material may be left. Some of it is thrown out of the cell by exocytosis. However, some material may remain within the cell in the form of membrane bound *residual bodies*.

Lysosomal enzymes play an important role in the destruction of bacteria phagocytosed by the cell. Lysosomal enzymes may also be discharged out of the cell and may influence adjoining structures.

Lysosomes are present in all cells except mature erythrocytes. They are a prominent feature in neutrophil leucocytes.

> Genetic defects can lead to absence of specific acid hydrolases that are normally present in lysosomes. As a result some molecules cannot be degraded, and accumulate in lysosomes. Examples of such disorders are *lysosomal glycogen storage disease* in which there is abnormal accumulation of glycogen, and *Tay-Sach's disease* in which lipids accumulate in lysosomes and lead to neuronal degeneration.

Peroxisomes

These are similar to lysosomes in that they are membrane bound vesicles containing enzymes. The enzymes in most of them react with other substances to form hydrogen peroxide which is used to detoxify various substances by oxidising them. The enzymes are involved in oxidation of very long chain fatty acids. Hydrogen peroxide resulting from the reactions is toxic to the cell. Other peroxisomes contain the enzyme catalase which destroys hydrogen peroxide, thus preventing the latter from accumulating in the cell. Peroxisomes are most prominent in cells of the liver and in cells of renal tubules.

> Defects in enzymes of peroxisomes can result in metabolic disorders associated with storage of abnormal lipids in some cells (brain, adrenal).

THE CYTOSKELETON

The cytoplasm is permeated by a number of fibrillar elements that collectively form a supporting network. This network is called the cytoskeleton. Apart from maintaining cellular architecture the cytoskeleton facilitates cell motility (e.g., by forming cilia), and helps to divide the cytosol into functionally discrete areas. It also facilitates transport of some constituents through the cytosol, and plays a role in anchoring cells to each other.

The elements that constitute the cytoskeleton consist of the following.

1. Microfilaments.

2. Microtubules.

3. Intermediate filaments.

These are considered below.

Microfilaments

These are about 5 nm in diameter. They are made up of the protein *actin*. Individual molecules of actin are globular (*G-actin*). These join together (polymerise) to form long chains called *F-actin, actin filaments,* or *microfilaments*.

Actin filaments form a meshwork just subjacent to the cell membrane. This meshwork is called the *cell cortex*. (The filaments forming the meshwork are held together by a protein called *filamin*). The cell cortex helps to maintain the shape of the cell. The meshwork of the cell cortex is labile. The filaments can separate (under the influence of actin severing proteins), and can reform in a different orientation. That is how the shape of a cell is altered.

Microvilli (see page 24) contain bundles of actin filaments, and that is how they are maintained. Filaments also extend into other protrusions from the cell surface.

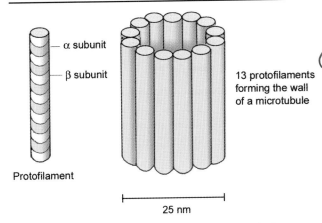

Fig. 1.24. Scheme to show how a microtubule is constituted.

Microtubules

Microtubules are about 25 nm in diameter (Fig. 1.24). The basic constituent of microtubules is the protein *tubulin* (composed of subunits α and β). Chains of tubulin form *protofilaments*. The wall of a microtubule is made up of thirteen protofilaments that run longitudinally (Fig. 1.24). The tubulin protofilaments are stabilized by *microtubule associated proteins* (MAPs).

Microtubules are formed in centrioles (see below) which constitute a *microtubule organising centre*.

The roles played by microtubules are as follows.

1. As part of the cytoskeleton, they provide stability to the cell. They prevent tubules of ER from collapsing.

2. Microtubules facilitate transport within the cell. Some proteins (dynein, kinesin) present in membranes of vesicles, and in organelles, attach these to microtubules, and facilitate movement along the tubules. Such transport is specially important in transport along axons.

3. In dividing cells microtubules form the mitotic spindle.

4. Cilia (page 22) are made up of microtubules (held together by other proteins).

Intermediate filaments

These are so called as their diameter (10 nm) is intermediate between that of microfilaments (5 nm) and of microtubules (25 nm). The proteins constituting these filaments vary in different types of cells.

They include *cytokeratin* (in epithelial cells), *neurofilament protein* (in neurons), *desmin* (in muscle), *glial fibrillary acidic protein* (in astrocytes); *lamin* (in the nuclear lamina of cells), and *vimentin* (in many types of cells).

The role played by intermediate filaments is as follows.

1. Intermediate filaments link cells together. They do so as they are attached to transmembrane proteins at desmosomes. The filaments also facilitate cell attachment to extracellular elements at hemidesmosomes.

2. In the epithelium of the skin the filaments undergo modification to form keratin. They also form the main constituent of hair and of nails.

3. The neurofilaments of neurons are intermediate filaments. Neurofibrils help to maintain the cylindrical shape of axons.

4. The nuclear lamina (page 26) consists of intermediate filaments.

Centrioles

All cells capable of division (and even some which do not divide) contain a pair of structures called centrioles. With the light microscope the two centrioles are seen as dots embedded in a region of dense cytoplasm which is called the *centrosome*. With the EM the centrioles are seen to be short cylinders that lie at right angles to each other. When we examine a transverse

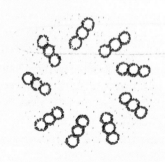

Fig. 1.25. Transverse section acros a centriole (near its base). Note nine groups of tubules, each group having three microtubules.

section across a centriole (by EM) it is seen to consist essentially of a series of microtubules arranged in a circle. There are nine groups of tubules, each group consisting of three tubules (Fig. 1.25).

Centrioles play an important role in the formation of various cellular structures that are made up of microtubules. These include the mitotic spindles of dividing cells, cilia, flagella, and some projections of specialized cells (e.g., the axial filaments of spermatozoa). It is of interest to note that cilia, flagella and the tails of spermatozoa all have the 9 + 2 configuration of microtubules that are seen in a centriole.

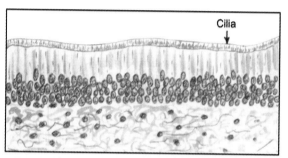

Fig. 1.26A. Pseudostratified columnar epithelium showing cilia.

PROJECTIONS FROM THE CELL SURFACE

Many cells show projections from the cell surface. The various types of projections are described below.

Cilia

These can be seen, with the light microscope, as minute hair-like projections from the free surfaces of some epithelial cells (Fig. 1.26A). In the living animal cilia can be seen to be motile. Details of their structure, described below, can be made out only by EM. A scanning EM view is shown in Fig. 1.26B.

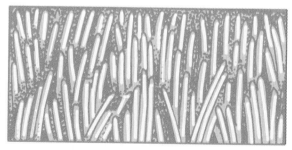

Fig. 1.26B. Drawing of cilia as seen by scanning electronmicroscopy.

The free part of each cilium is called the **shaft**. The region of attachment of the shaft to the cell surface is called the **base** (also called the **basal body**, **basal granule**, or **kinetosome**). The free end of the shaft tapers to a tip.

Each cilium is 0.25 μm in diameter. It consists of (a) an outer covering which is formed by an extension of the cell membrane; and (b) an inner core (**axoneme**) that is formed by microtubules arranged in a definite manner. The arrangement of these tubules, as seen in a transverse section

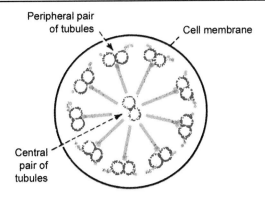

Fig. 1.27. Transverse section across a cilium.

across the shaft of a cilium is shown in Fig. 1.27. It has a striking similarity to the structure of a centriole (described above). There is a central pair of tubules which is surrounded by nine pairs of tubules. The outer tubules are connected to the inner pair by radial structures (which are like the spokes of a wheel). Other projections pass outwards from the outer tubules.

As the tubules of the shaft are traced towards the tip of the cilium it is seen that one tubule of each outer pair ends short of the tip so that near the tip each outer pair is represented by one tubule only. Just near the tip, only the central pair of tubules is seen (Fig. 1.28).

At the base of the cilium one additional tubule is added to each outer pair so that here the nine outer groups of tubules have three tubules each, exactly as in the centriole.

Microtubules in cilia are bound with proteins (dynein and nexin). Nexin holds the microtubules together. Dyenin molecules are responsible for bending of tubules, and thereby for movements of cilia.

Functional significance of cilia

The cilia lining an epithelial surface move in co-ordination with one another the total effect being that like a wave. As a result fluid, mucous, or small solid objects lying on the epithelium can be caused to move in a specific direction. Movements of cilia lining the respiratory epithelium help to move secretions in the trachea and bronchi towards the pharynx. Ciliary action helps in the movement of ova through the uterine tube, and of spermatozoa through the male genital tract.

In some situations there are cilia-like structures that perform a sensory function. They may be non-motile, but can be bent by external influences. Such 'cilia' present on the cells in the olfactory mucosa of the nose are called *olfactory cilia*; they are receptors for smell. Similar structures called *kinocilia* are present in some parts of the internal ear. In some regions there are hair-like projections called *stereocilia*; these are not cilia at all, but are large microvilli (see below). *Show bending movements in response to gravity.*

Abnormalities of cilia

Cilia can be abnormal in persons with genetic defects that interfere with synthesis of ciliary proteins. This leads to the *immotile cilia*

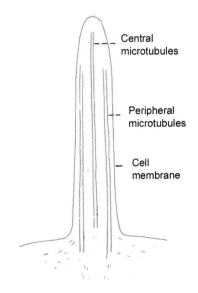

Fig. 1.28. Longitudinal section through a cilium.

A Show synchronic wave like rythmic movement propelling the surface film in a consistant direction.

syndrome. As secretions are not removed from respiratory passages the patient has repeated and severe chest infections. Women affected by the syndrome may be sterile as movement of ova along the uterine tube is affected. Ciliary proteins are present in the tails of spermatozoa, and an affected male may be sterile because of interference with the motility of spermatozoa.

Ciliary action is also necessary for normal development of tissues in embryonic life. Migration of cells during embryogenesis is dependent on ciliary action, and if the cilia are not motile various congenital abnormalities can result.

Flagella

These are somewhat larger processes having the same basic structure as cilia. In the human body the best example of a flagellum is the tail of the spermatozoon. The movements of flagella are different from those of cilia. In a flagellum, movement starts at its base. The segment nearest the base bends in one direction. This is followed by bending of succeeding segments in opposite directions so that a wave like motion passes down the flagellum. When a spermatozoon is suspended in a fluid medium this wave of movement propels the spermatozoon forwards (exactly in the way a snake moves forwards by a wavy movement of its body).

Microvilli & Basolateral folds

Microvilli are finger-like projections from the cell surface that can be seen by EM (Fig. 1.29). Each microvillus consists of an outer covering of plasma membrane and a cytoplasmic core in which there are numerous microfilaments (actin filaments). The filaments are continuous with actin filaments of the cell cortex (page 20). Numerous enzymes, and glycoproteins, concerned with absorption have been located

in microvilli.

With the light microscope the free borders of

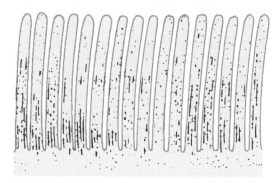

Fig. 1.29A. Microvilli as seen in longitudinal section. The regular arrangement of microvilli is characteristic of the striated border of intestinal abssorptive cells.

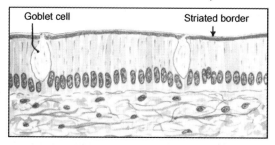

Fig. 1.29B. Light microscopic appearance of striated border formed by microvilli.

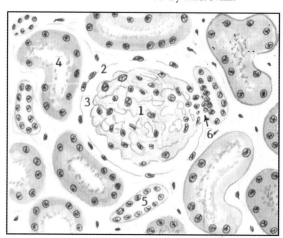

Fig. 1.29C. Light microscopic appearance of a brush border (at 4) in epithelium lining renal tubules.

ft: ↑se the surface area, not always absorptive.
Some times secretory as in renal tubules.

epithelial cells lining the small intestine appear to be thickened: the thickening has striations perpendicular to the surface. This **striated border** of light microscopy (Fig. 1.29B) has been shown by EM to be made up of long microvilli arranged parallel to one another.

In some cells the microvilli are not arranged so regularly. With the light microscope the microvilli of such cells give the appearance of a **brush border** (Fig. 1.29C).

Microvilli greatly increase the surface area of the cell and are, therefore, seen most typically at sites of active absorption e.g., the intestine, and the proximal and distal convoluted tubules of the kidneys. Modified microvilli called stereocilia are seen on receptor cells in the internal ear, and on the epithelium of the epididymis.

In some cells the cell membrane over the basal or lateral aspect of the cell shows deep folds (basolateral folds). Like microvilli basolateral folds are an adaptation to increase cell surface area.

Basal folds are seen in renal tubular cells, and in cells lining the ducts of some glands. Lateral folds are seen in absorptive cells lining the gut.

diff from cilia but big modified large micro villi

THE NUCLEUS

The nucleus constitutes the central, more dense part of the cell. It is usually rounded or ellipsoid. Occasionally it may be elongated, indented or lobed. It is usually 4-10 μm in diameter. The nucleus contains inherited information which is necessary for directing the activities of the cell as we shall see below.

In usual class room slides stained with

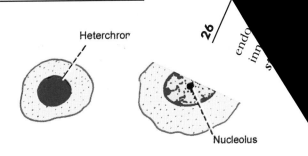

Fig. 1.30. Comparison of a heterochromatic nucleus (left), and a euchromatic nucleus (right).

haematoxylin and eosin, the nucleus stains dark purple or blue while the cytoplasm is usually stained pink. In some cells the nuclei are relatively large and light staining. Such nuclei appear to be made up of a delicate network of fibres: the material making up the fibres of the network is called **chromatin** (because of its affinity for dyes). At some places (in the nucleus) the chromatin is seen in the form of irregular dark masses that are called **heterochromatin**. At other places the network is loose and stains lightly: the chromatin of such areas is referred to as **euchromatin**. Nuclei which are large and in which relatively large areas of euchromatin can be seen are referred to as **open-face nuclei.** Nuclei which are made up mainly of heterochromatin are referred to as **closed-face nuclei** (Fig. 1.30).

In addition to the masses of heterochromatin (which are irregular in outline), the nucleus shows one or more rounded, dark staining bodies called **nucleoli** (See below). The nucleus also contains various small granules, fibres and vesicles (of obscure function). The spaces between the various constituents of the nucleus described above are filled by a base called the **nucleoplasm**.

With the EM the nucleus is seen to be surrounded by a double layered **nuclear membrane** or **nuclear envelope**. The outer nuclear membrane is continuous with plasmic reticulum. The space between the ...er and outer membranes is the ***perinuclear pace***. This is continuous with the lumen of rough ER. The inner layer of the nuclear membrane provides attachment to the ends of chromosomes (see below). Deep to the inner membrane there is a layer containing proteins and a network of filaments: this layer is called the ***nuclear lamina***. Specific proteins present in the inner nuclear membrane give attachment to filamentous proteins of the nuclear lamina. These proteins (called ***lamins***) form a scaffolding that maintains the spherical shape of the nucleus. At several points the inner and outer layers of the nuclear membrane fuse leaving gaps called ***nuclear pores***. Each pore is surrounded by dense protein arranged in the form of eight complexes. These proteins and the pore together form the ***pore complex***.

Nuclear pores represent sites at which substances can pass from the nucleus to the cytoplasm and vice versa (Fig. 1.19). The nuclear pore is about 80 nm across. It is partly covered by a diaphragm which allows passage only to particles less than 9 nm in diameter. A typical nucleus has 3000 to 4000 pores.

It is believed that pore complexes actively transport some proteins into the nucleus; and ribosomes out of the nucleus.

Nature and Significance of Chromatin

In recent years there has been a considerable advance in our knowledge of the structure and significance of chromatin. It is made up of a substance called ***deoxyribonucleic acid*** (usually abbreviated to DNA); and of proteins.

The structure of DNA is described on page 29. It is in the form of a long chain of nucleotides. Most of the proteins in chromatin are ***histones***. Some non-histone proteins are also present.

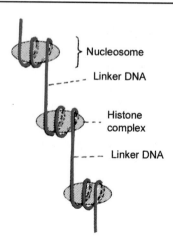

Fig. 1.31. Scheme to show the structure of a chromatin fibre. The DNA fibril makes two turns around a complex formed by histones to form a nucleosome. Nucleosomes give the chromatin fibre the appearance of a beaded string. The portion of the DNA fibre between the nucleosomes is called linker-DNA.

Filaments of DNA form coils around histone complexes. The structure formed by a histone complex and the DNA fibre coiled around it is called a ***nucleosome***. Nucleosomes are attached to one another forming long chains (Fig. 1.31). These chains are coiled on themselves (in a helical manner) to form filaments 30 nm in diameter. These filaments constitute chromatin.

Filaments of chromatin are again coiled on them selves (***supercoiling***), and this coiling is repeated several times. Each coiling produces a thicker filament. In this way a filament of DNA that is originally 50 mm long can be reduced to a chromosome only 5 μm in length. (A little calculation will show that this represents a reduction in length of 10,000 times!).

Some details of the formation of a histone complex are shown in Fig. 1.32. Five types of histones are recognized. These are H1, H2A, H2B, H3 and H4. Two molecules each of H2A, H2B, H3 and H4 join to form a granular mass, the ***nucleosome core***. The DNA filament is wound ***twice*** around this core, the whole complex forming a nucleosome. The length of the DNA filament in one nucleosome contains 146

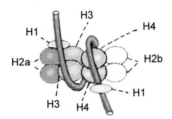

Fig. 1.32. Diagram showing detailed composition of a histone complex forming the nucleosome core.

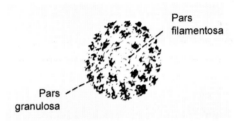

Fig. 1.33. EM structure of a nucleolus.

nucleotide pairs. One nucleosome is connected to the next by a short length of *linker DNA*. Linker DNA is made up of about 50 nucleotide pairs.

Heterochromatin represents areas where chromatin fibres are tightly coiled on themselves forming 'solid' masses. In contrast euchromatin represents areas where coiling is not so marked. During cell division the entire chromatin within the nucleus becomes very tightly coiled and takes on the appearance of a number of short, thick, rod-like structures called *chromosomes*. Chromosomes are made up of DNA and proteins. Proteins stabilize the structure of chromosomes.

Chromosomes are considered in detail on page 28. The structure of DNA is considered on page 29. Also see sex-chromatin (page 42).

Nucleoli

We have seen that nuclei contain one or more nucleoli. These are spherical and about 1-3 μm in diameter. They stain intensely both with haematoxylin and eosin, the latter giving them a slight reddish tinge. In ordinary preparations they can be distinguished from heterochromatin by their rounded shape. (In contrast masses of heterochromatin are very irregular). Nucleoli are larger and more distinct in cells that are metabolically active.

Using histochemical procedures that distinguish between DNA and RNA (page 31) it is seen that the nucleoli have a high RNA content. With the EM nucleoli are seen to have a central filamentous zone (*pars filamentosa*) and an outer granular zone (*pars granulosa*) both of which are embedded in an amorphous material (*pars amorphosa*) (Fig. 1.33).

Nucleoli are formed in relationship to the secondary constrictions of specific chromosomes (page 35). These regions are considered to be nucleolar organizing centres. Parts of the chromosomes located within nucleoli constitute the *pars chromosoma* of nucleoli.

Nucleoli are sites where ribosomal RNA is synthesized. The templates for this synthesis are located on the related chromosomes. Ribosomal RNA is at first in the form of long fibres that constitute the fibrous zone of nucleoli. It is then broken up into smaller pieces (ribosomal subunits) that constitute the granular zone. Finally, this RNA leaves the nucleolus, passes through a nuclear pore, and enters the cytoplasm where it takes part in protein synthesis as described on page 32.

(Note: Some parts of the above description of nucleoli may be confusing: they will become clear after the following section on chromosomes is read).

CHROMOSOMES

Haploid and Diploid Chromosomes

We have seen that during cell division the chromatin network in the nucleus becomes condensed into a number of thread-like or rod-like structures called chromosomes. The number of chromosomes in each cell is fixed for a given species, and in man it is 46. This is referred to as the *diploid number* (diploid = double). However, in spermatozoa and in ova the number is only half the diploid number i.e., 23: this is called the *haploid number* (haploid = half).

Autosomes and Sex Chromosomes

The 46 chromosomes in each cell can again be divided into 44 *autosomes* and two *sex chromosomes*. The sex chromosomes may be of two kinds, X or Y. In a man there are 44 autosomes, one X chromosome, and one Y chromosome; while in a woman there are 44 autosomes and two X chromosomes in each cell. When we study the 44 autosomes we find that they really consist of 22 pairs, the two chromosomes forming a pair being exactly alike (*homologous chromosomes*). In a woman the two X chromosomes form another such pair; but in a man this pair is represented by one X and one Y chromosome. We shall see later that one chromosome of each pair is obtained (by each individual) from the mother, and one from the father.

As the two sex chromosomes of a female are similar the female sex is described as *homogametic*; in contrast the male sex is *heterogametic*.

Significance of Chromosomes

Each cell of the body contains within itself a store of information that has been inherited from precursor cells. This information (which is necessary for the proper functioning of the cell) is stored in chromatin. Each chromosome bears on itself a very large number of functional segments that are called *genes*. Genes represent 'units' of stored information which guide the performance of particular cellular functions, which may in turn lead to the development of particular features of an individual or of a species. Recent researches have told us a great deal about the way in which chromosomes and genes store and use information.

The nature and functions of a cell depend on the proteins synthesized by it. Proteins are the most important constituents of our body. They make up the greater part of each cell and of intercellular substances. Enzymes, hormones, and antibodies are also proteins.

It is, therefore, not surprising that one cell differs from another because of the differences in the proteins that constitute it. Individuals and species also owe their distinctive characters to their proteins. We now know that chromosomes control the development and functioning of cells by determining what type of proteins will be synthesized within them.

Chromosomes are made up predominantly of a nucleic acid called *deoxyribonucleic acid* (or *DNA*), and all information is stored in molecules of this substance. When the need arises this information is used to direct the activities of the cell by synthesizing appropriate proteins. To understand how this becomes possible we must consider the structure of DNA in some detail.

Basic Structure of DNA

DNA in a chromosome is in the form of very fine fibres. If we look at one such fibre it has the appearance shown in Fig. 1.34. It is seen that each fibre consists of two strands that are twisted spirally to form what is called a **double helix**. The two strands are linked to each other at regular intervals. (Note the dimensions shown in Fig. 1.34).

Each strand of the DNA fibre consists of a chain of **nucleotides**. Each nucleotide consists of a sugar, deoxyribose, a molecule of phosphate and a base (Fig. 1.35). The phosphate of one

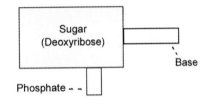

Fig. 1.35. Composition of a nucleotide. The base may be adenine, cytosine, guanine or thymine.

nucleotide is linked to the sugar of the next nucleotide (Fig. 1.36). The base which is attached to the sugar molecule may be **adenine, guanine, cytosine** or **thymine**. The two strands of a DNA fibre are joined together by the linkage of a base on one strand with a base on the opposite strand (Fig. 1.37).

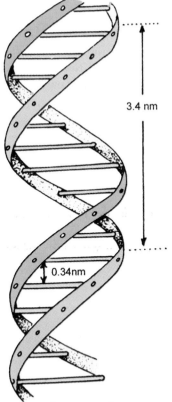

Fig. 1.34. Diagram showing part of a DNA molecule aranged in the form of a double helix.

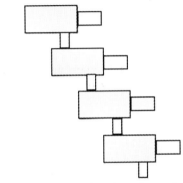

Fig. 1.36. Linkage of nucleotides to form one strand of a DNA molecule.

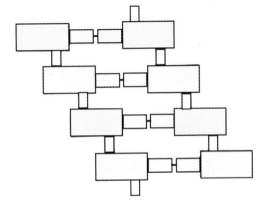

Fig. 1.37. Linkage of two chains of nucleotides to form part of a DNA molecule.

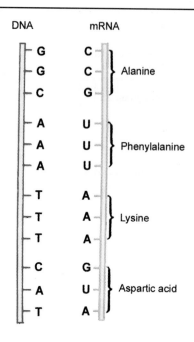

Fig. 1.38. Codes for some amino acids made up of the bases adenine (A), cytosine (C), guanine (G), and thymine (T) on a DNA molecule. When this code is transferred to messenger RNA, cytosine is formed opposite guanine (and vice versa), adenine is formed opposite thymine, while uracil (U)is formed opposite adenine.

This linkage is peculiar in that adenine on one strand is always linked to thymine on the other strand, while cytosine is always linked to guanine. Thus the two strands are complementary and the arrangement of bases on one strand can be predicted from the other.

The order in which these four bases are arranged along the length of a strand of DNA determines the nature of the protein that can be synthesized under its influence. Every protein is made up of a series of amino acids; the nature of the protein depending upon the amino acids present, and the sequence in which they are arranged. Amino acids may be obtained from food or may be synthesized within the cell. Under the influence of DNA these amino acids are linked together in a particular sequence to form proteins.

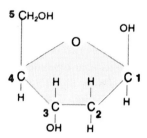

Fig. 1.39. Diagram to show the structure of deoxyribose. Note the numbering of carbon atoms. From Fig. 1.40 you can see that C3 of one molecule is attached to C5 of the next molecule through a phosphate bond.

Further Details of DNA Structure

In the preceding paragraphs the structure of DNA has been described in the simplest possible terms. We will now consider some details.

1. The structure of the sugar deoxyribose is shown in Fig. 1.39. Note that there are five carbon atoms; and also note how they are numbered.

2. Next observe, in Fig. 1.40, that C-3 of one sugar molecule is linked to C-5 of the next molecule through a phosphate linkage (P). It follows that each strand of DNA has a 5' end and a 3' end.

3. Next observe that although the two chains forming DNA are similar they are arranged in opposite directions. In Fig. 1.40 the 5' end of the left chain, and the 3' end of the right chain lie at the upper end of the figure. The two chains of nucleotides are, therefore, said to be *antiparallel*.

4. The C-1 carbon of deoxyribose give attachment to a base. This base is attached to a base of the opposite chain as already described.

5. The reason why adenine on one strand is always linked to thymine on the other strand is that the structure of these two molecules is complementary and hydrogen bonds are easily formed between them. The same is true for cytosine and guanine.

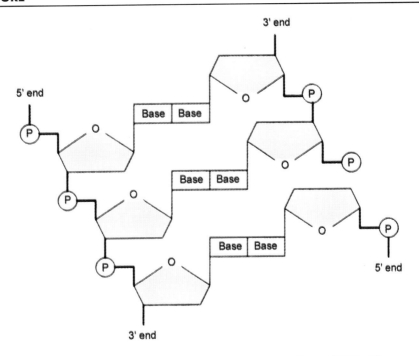

Fig. 1.40. Diagram to show how nucleotides are linked to form a chain of DNA. The asymmetric placing of bonds gives a helical shape to the chain.

Ribonucleic Acid (RNA)

In addition to DNA, cells contain another important nucleic acid called *ribonucleic acid* or *RNA*. The structure of a molecule of RNA corresponds fairly closely to that of one strand of a DNA molecule, with the following important differences.

(a) RNA contains the sugar ribose instead of deoxyribose.

(b) Instead of the base thymine it contains uracil.

RNA is present both in the nucleus and in the cytoplasm of a cell. It is present in three main forms namely *messenger RNA (mRNA)*, *transfer RNA (tRNA)* and *ribosomal RNA*. Messenger RNA acts as an intermediary between the DNA of the chromosome and the amino acids present in the cytoplasm and plays a vital role in the synthesis of proteins from amino acids.

Some forms of RNA are confined to nuclei. The small nuclear RNAs (SnRNA) are concerned with RNA splicing (page 33).

Synthesis of Protein

We have seen that a protein is made up of amino acids that are linked together in a definite sequence. This sequence is determined by the order in which the bases are arranged in a strand of DNA. Each amino acid is represented in the DNA molecule by a sequence of three bases (*triplet code*). It has been mentioned earlier that there are four bases in all in DNA, namely adenine, cytosine, thymine and guanine. These are like letters in a word. They can be arranged in various combinations so that as many as sixty four code 'words' can be formed from these four bases. There are only about twenty amino acids that have to be coded for so that each amino acid has more than one code. The code words for

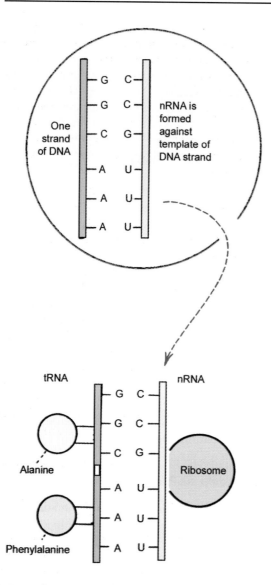

Fig. 1.41. Simplified scheme to show how proteins are synthesized under the influence of DNA. The process is actually more complex as explained in the text.

structural gene or *cistron*.

At this stage it must be emphasized that a chromosome is very long and thread-like. Only short lengths of the fibre are involved in protein synthesis at a particular time.

The main steps in the synthesis of a protein may now be summarized as follows (Fig.1.41).

1. The two strands of a DNA fibre separate from each other (over the area bearing a particular cistron) so that the ends of the bases that were linked to the opposite strand are now free.

2. A molecule of messenger RNA is synthesized using one DNA strand as a guide (or *template*), in such a way that one guanine base is formed opposite each cytosine base of the DNA strand, cytosine is formed opposite guanine, adenine is formed opposite thymine, and uracil is formed opposite adenine. In this way the code for the sequence in which amino acids are to be linked is passed on from DNA of the chromosome to messenger RNA. This process is called *transcription*. [Transcription takes place under the influence of the enzyme RNA polymerase.] That part of the messenger RNA strand that bears the code for one amino acid is called a *codon*.

3. This molecule of messenger RNA now separates from the DNA strand and moves from the nucleus to the cytoplasm (passing through a nuclear pore).

4. In the cytoplasm the messenger RNA becomes attached to a ribosome.

5. As mentioned earlier the cytoplasm also contains another form of RNA called transfer RNA. In fact there are about twenty different types of transfer RNA each corresponding to one amino acid. On one side transfer RNA becomes attached to an amino acid. On the other side it bears a code of three bases (*anticodon*) that are complementary to the bases coding for its amino acid on messenger RNA. Under the influence of the ribosome several units of transfer RNA, along

some amino acids are shown in Fig. 1.38. The code for a complete polypeptide chain is formed when the codes for its constituent amino acids are arranged in proper sequence. That part of the DNA molecule that bears the code for a complete polypeptide chain constitutes a

with their amino acids, become arranged along side the strand of messenger RNA in the sequence determined by the code on messenger RNA. This process is called *translation*.

6. The amino acids now become linked to each other to form a polypeptide chain. From the above it will be clear that the amino acids are linked up exactly in the order in which their codes are arranged on messenger RNA, which in turn is based on the code on the DNA molecule (but also see below). Chains of amino acids formed in this way constitute polypeptide chains. Proteins are formed by union of polypeptide chains.

The flow of information from DNA to RNA and finally to protein has been described as the "central dogma of molecular biology".

Some Further Details About Genes and Protein Synthesis

In addition to the protein coding sequences (of bases) DNA also bears other regions that have a controlling function. These regions provide signals for initiation and termination of the process of transcription, or for the control of the process in other ways. The DNA sequence that provides the signal for initiation of transcription is called the *promoter*. Binding of RNA polymerase to the promoter causes the DNA fibre to uncoil, and thus makes it possible for RNA polymerase to reach the fibre and to begin the process of transcription. Transcription continues up to the region of the DNA fibre which bears a code that gives a signal for termination of transcription.

Apart from initiating the process of transcription, the promoter also determines the rate of transcription.

Although all cells contain a complete complement of DNA all of it is not used for transcription in every cell. The region of DNA that is to be transcribed (in a particular cell) is determined by *gene regulatory proteins* present in the nucleus. These proteins bind to sites on DNA which are called *enhancers*. This binding is necessary before transcription can take place. Enhancers also control the rate of transcription by determining the number of RNA polymerase molecules that are engaged in transcription of the same length of DNA. Apart from sites on DNA that act that act as enhancers, there are others that act as *repressors*.

Messenger RNA formed as described above is modified before it is used for protein synthesis. Long chains of mRNA are broken up into short lengths. This process is called *splicing*. Some of the pieces formed by splicing again join together (in modified sequence) to form a new chain which is used for protein synthesis. Other short lengths are destroyed. Combination of the short lengths in different ways can enable formation of different proteins under the influence of the same DNA sequences. It will be obvious that only some of the DNA sequences used for transcription will actually be used for protein synthesis. These sequences are referred to as *exons*. Those not used are called *introns*. The process of RNA splicing may be regarded as a method to get rid of introns. Why introns are created in the first place is not clear, but they probably perform some regulatory function.

The initially formed mRNA (or *primary transcript*) is modified as follows.

(a) The mRNA has two ends. The end at which transcription begins is the 5' end (the other being the 3' end). A molecule of methylguanine gets attached to the 5' end (and is called the *methylguanine cap*). The cap is responsible for protecting mRNA from degradation.

The opposite (3') end is referred to as the *poly(A) tail*. This tail is also concerned with stability of mRNA.

(b) As mentioned above, the process of removal of introns from the primary transcript is called splicing. Splicing takes place while mRNA is still within the nucleus. The mechanism of splicing is complex and we will not consider it here. Apart from removal of introns splicing allows exons to be united in sequences different from the original.

(c) After entry into cytoplasm most mRNAs have a short life (a few minutes to a day) after which they are destroyed. The first region to undergo destruction is the poly(A) tail and this exposes the rest of mRNA to the action of ribonuclease (which is responsible for destruction of mRNA).

Formation of proteins by translation of mRNA is controlled by various factors. Newly synthesized protein often needs modification before it is in its final form. The modifications may include:

(a) A process of folding which may require the presence of accessory proteins.

(b) Addition of other molecules (sugar, phosphate).

(c) Cleavage of the originally formed protein to generate an active form.

Role of Ribosomes in Protein Synthesis

Ribosomes play an essential part in protein synthesis. They 'read' the code on mRNA and help to arrange units of tRNA in proper sequence. The two subunits of ribosomes (large and small) play different roles in protein synthesis. The smaller unit (40s unit) is concerned with the process of translation. The larger unit (60s unit) is responsible for release of new protein into the vacuoplasm within the cisternae of endoplasmic reticulum.

Messenger RNA entering the cytosol meets a free ribosome. Messenger RNA has an initial part that bears the code for a signal sequence. This signal sequence tells the ribosome about the nature of the protein to be formed, and determines how the ribosome will behave.

(a) If the signal is for a protein that is to remain in the cytosol, the ribosome does not get attached to ER. The protein synthesized is released into the cytosol.

(b) If the signal is for a membrane protein, or for a protein to be secreted, the ribosome attaches to the surface of ER. Membrane proteins synthesized get incorporated into ER membrane. They are transferred from rough ER to smooth ER and, thereafter, to the Golgi complex, and then to the cell surface.

Proteins that are to form secretions enter the lumen of rough ER. They pass into the lumen of smooth ER, and then (through vesicles) to the cis face of the Golgi complex. After being appropriately processed in the Golgi complex they are packaged into vesicles and are discharged from the cell by exocytosis.

Duplication of Chromosomes

One of the most remarkable properties of chromosomes is that they are able to duplicate themselves. From the foregoing discussion on the structure of chromosomes it is clear that duplication of chromosomes involves the duplication (or replication) of DNA. This takes place as follows (Fig. 1.42).

1. The two strands of the DNA molecule to be duplicated unwind and separate from each other so that their bases are 'free'.

2. A new strand is now synthesized opposite each original strand of DNA in such a way that adenine is formed opposite thymine, guanine is formed opposite cytosine, and vice versa. This new strand becomes linked to the original strand of DNA to form a new molecule. As the same process has taken place in relation to each of the two original strands, we now have two complete molecules of DNA. It will be noted that each molecule has one strand that belonged to the original molecule and one strand that is new. It will also be noted that the two molecules formed are identical to the original molecule.

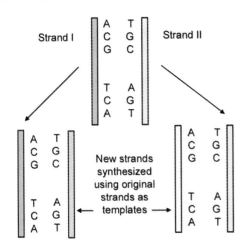

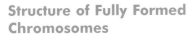

Fig. 1.42. Scheme to show how a DNA molecule is duplicated.

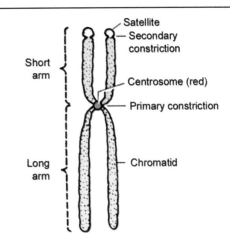

Fig. 1.43. Diagram to show the terms applied to some parts of a typical chromosome. Note that this chromosome is submetacentric.

Structure of Fully Formed Chromosomes

Each chromosome consists of two parallel rod-like elements that are called **chromatids** (Fig. 1.43). The two chromatids are joined to each other at a narrow area which is light staining and is called the **centromere** (or **kinetochore**). In this region the chromatin of each chromatid is most highly coiled and, therefore, appears to be thinnest. The chromatids appear to the 'constricted' here and this region is called the **primary constriction**. Typically the centromere is not midway between the two ends of the chromatids, but somewhat towards one end. As a result each chromatid can be said to have a **long arm** and a **short arm**. Such chromosomes are described as being **submetacentric** (when the two arms are only slightly different in length); or as **acrocentric** (when the difference is marked) (Fig. 1.44). In some chromosomes the two arms are of equal length: such chromosomes are described as **metacentric**. Finally, in some chromosomes the centromere may lie at one end: such a chromosome is described as **telocentric**.

Differences in the total length of chromosomes,

and in the position of the centromere are important factors in distinguishing individual chromosomes from each other. Additional help in identification is obtained by the presence in some chromosomes of **secondary constrictions**. Such constrictions lie near one end of the chromatid. The part of the chromatid 'distal' to the constriction may appear to be a rounded body almost separate from the rest of the chromatid: such regions are called **satellite bodies**. (Secondary constrictions are concerned with the formation of nucleoli and are, therefore, called **nucleolar organizing centres**). Considerable help in identification of individual chromosomes is also obtained by the use of special staining procedures by which each chromatid can be seen to consist of a number of dark and light staining transverse bands.

We have noted that chromosomes are distinguishable only during mitosis. In the interphase (between successive mitoses) the chromosomes elongate and assume the form of long threads. These threads are called **chromonemata** (Singular = **chromonema**).

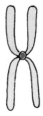

METACENTRIC CHROSOME

The two arms are of equal length

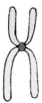

SUBMETACENTRIC CHROMOSOME

One arm is somewhat shorter than the other

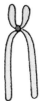

ACROCENTRIC CHROMOSOME

One arm is much shorter than the other

TELECENTRIC CHROMOSOME

Each chromatid has only one arm. The centromere is at one end of the chromosome

Fig. 1.44. Nomenclature used for different types of chromosomes, based on differences in lengths of the two arms of each chromatid.

Karyotyping

Using the criteria described above it is now possible to identify each chromosome individually and to map out the chromosomes of an individual. This procedure is called karyotyping. For this purpose a sample of blood from the individual is put into a suitable medium in which lymphocytes can multiply. After a few hours a drug (colchicin, colcemide) that arrests cell division at a stage when chromosomes are most distinct is added to the medium. The dividing cells are then treated with hypotonic saline so that they swell up. This facilitates the proper spreading out of chromosomes. A suspension containing the dividing cells is spread out on a slide and suitably stained. Cells in which the chromosomes are well spread out (without overlap) are photographed. The photographs are cut up and the chromosomes arranged in proper sequence. In this way a map of chromosomes is obtained, and abnormalities in their number or form can be identified. In many cases specific chromosomal abnormalities can be correlated with specific diseases.

(For details of chromosomal abnormalities see the author's HUMAN EMBRYOLOGY).

In recent years greater accuracy in karyotyping has been achieved by use of several different banding techniques, and by use of computerized analysis.

It has been estimated that the total DNA content of a cell (in all chromosomes put together) is represented by about 6×10^9 nucleotide pairs. Of these 2.5×10^8 are present in chromosome 1 (which is the largest chromosome). The Y-chromosome (which is the smallest chromosome) contains 5×10^7 nucleotide pairs.

In the region of the centromere the DNA molecule is specialized for attachment to the spindle. This region is surrounded by proteins that form a mass. This mass is the *kinetochore*. The ends of each DNA molecule are also specialized. They are called *telomeres*.

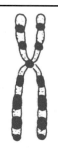

Fig. 1.45. Chromosome showing dark and light bands revealed by staining with the Giemza method. The pattern of banding is specific for each chromosome, but different patterns are obtained with different staining methods.

CELL DIVISION

Multiplication of cells takes place by division of preexisting cells. Such multiplication constitutes an essential feature of embryonic development. Cell multiplication is equally necessary after birth of the individual for growth and for replacement of dead cells.

We have seen that the chromosomes within the nuclei of cells carry genetic information that controls the development and functioning of various cells and tissues and, therefore, of the

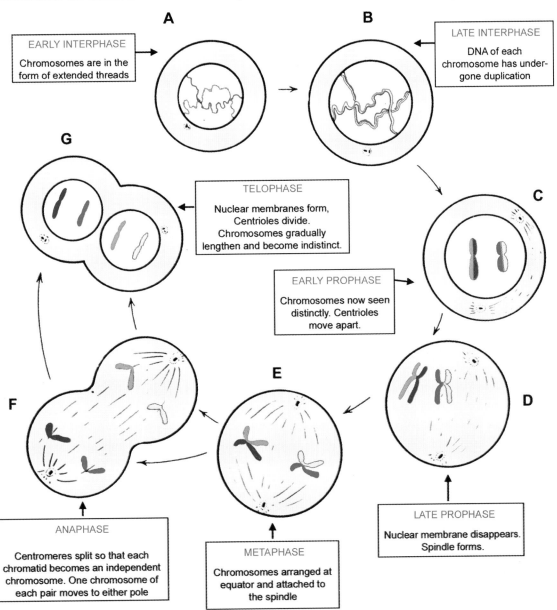

A

EARLY INTERPHASE

Chromosomes are in the form of extended threads

B

LATE INTERPHASE

DNA of each chromosome has undergone duplication

G

TELOPHASE

Nuclear membranes form, Centrioles divide. Chromosomes gradually lengthen and become indistinct.

C

EARLY PROPHASE

Chromosomes now seen distinctly. Centrioles move apart.

E

F

D

ANAPHASE

Centromeres split so that each chromatid becomes an independent chromosome. One chromosome of each pair moves to either pole

METAPHASE

Chromosomes arranged at equator and attached to the spindle

LATE PROPHASE

Nuclear membrane disappears. Spindle forms.

Fig. 1.46. Scheme to show the main steps in mitosis.

body as a whole. When a cell divides it is essential that the whole of the genetic information within it be passed on to both the daughter cells resulting from the division.

In other words the daughter cells must have chromosomes identical in number and in genetic content to those in the mother cell. This type of cell division is called *mitosis*.

A different kind of cell division called *meiosis* occurs during the formation of gametes. This consists of two successive divisions called the first and second meiotic divisions. The cells resulting from these divisions (i.e., the gametes) differ from other cells in the body in that:

(**a**) the number of chromosomes is reduced to half the normal number, and

(**b**) the genetic information in the various gametes produced is not identical.

Mitosis

Many cells of the body have a limited span of functional activity at the end of which they undergo division into two daughter cells. The daughter cells in turn have their own span of activity followed by another division. The period during which the cell is actively dividing is the phase of mitosis. The period between two successive divisions is called the *interphase*.

The greater part of interphase is called the *G1 stage*, which may last from a few hours to many years. During this period the cell carries out its 'normal' functions. About 12 hours before the onset of mitosis the synthesis of DNA takes place and is completed in about 7 hours: this period is called the *S stage* (S for synthesis). The last five hours before mitosis are utilized for synthesis of proteins required for cell division. This is called the *G2 stage* of interphase. Cells at G2 stage have a double complement of DNA.

Mitosis is conventionally divided into a number of stages called *prophase, metaphase, anaphase* and *telophase*. The later part of prophase is also called *prometaphase*. The sequence of events of the mitotic cycle is best understood by starting with a cell in telophase. At this stage each chromosome consists of a single chromatid (Fig.1.46G). With the progress of telophase the chromatin of the chromosome uncoils and elongates and the chromosome can no longer be identified as such. However, it is believed to retain its identity during the interphase (which follows telophase). This is shown diagrammatically in Fig.1.46A. During the S stage of interphase the DNA content of the chromosome is duplicated (as described on page 34) so that another chromatid identical to the original one is formed: the chromosome is now made up of two chromatids (Fig.1.46B). When mitosis begins (i.e., during the prophase) the chromatin of the chromosome becomes gradually more and more coiled so that the chromosome become recognizable as a thread-like structure that gradually acquires a rod-like appearance (Fig.1.46C). Towards the end of prophase the two chromatids constituting the chromosome become distinct (Fig.1.46D) and the chromosome now has the typical structure described above.

While the changes described above are occurring in the chromosomes a number of other events are taking place. The two centrioles separate and move to opposite poles of the cell. They produce a number of microtubules that pass from one centriole to the other and form a *spindle*. Tubules radiating from each centriole create a star like appearance or *aster*. The spindle and the two asters collectively form the *diaster* (also called *amphiaster* or *achromatic spindle*). Meanwhile the nuclear membrane breaks down and the nucleoli disappear (Fig. 1.46D). With the formation of the spindle the chromosomes move to a position midway between the two centrioles (i.e., at the equator of the cell) where each chromosome becomes attached to microtubules of the spindle by its centromere. This stage is referred to as metaphase (Fig.1.46E). The plane along which the chromosomes lie during metaphase is the *equatorial plate*.

In the anaphase the centromere of each chromosome splits longitudinally into two so that the chromatids now become independent chromosomes. At this stage the cell can be said to contain 46 pairs of chromosomes. One chromosome of each such pair now moves along the spindle to either pole of the cell (Fig. 1.46F). This is followed by telophase in which two daughter nuclei are formed by appearance of nuclear membranes around them. The chromosomes gradually elongate and become indistinct. Nucleoli reappear. The centriole is duplicated at this stage or in early interphase (Fig.1.46G).

The division of the nucleus is accompanied by the division of the cytoplasm. In this process the organelles are presumably duplicated and each daughter cell comes to have a full complement of them. The cleavage into two separate cells is referred to as *cytokinesis*.

The rate of cell division varies from tissue to tissue, being greatest in those epithelia which lose cells because of friction (e.g., the epidermis and the lining cells of the intestine). The rate varies with demand becoming much greater during repair after injury. The rate is precisely controlled to correlate with demand. Failure of such control results in uncontrolled growth leading to formation of tumours. Abnormalities in mitosis may be produced by exposure to various radiations, the most important being nuclear radiation. Mitosis can be arrested by chemicals. One of them is colchicin (or colcemide). It stops mitosis at metaphase and allows us to study chromosomes at this stage (page 36).

Some cells do not undergo mitosis (neurons, cardiac muscle cells). They are said to be in the Go phase. Some cells (e.g., those of the liver) do not normally divide. This may divide to replace cell damage by disease.

Meiosis

As already stated meiosis consists of two successive divisions called the first and second meiotic divisions. During the interphase preceding the first division duplication of the DNA content of the chromosomes takes place as in mitosis.

First Meiotic Division

The prophase of the first meiotic division is prolonged and is usually divided into a number of stages as follows.

(a) *Leptotene*: The chromosomes become visible (as in mitosis). Although each chromosome consists of two chromatids these cannot be distinguished at this stage (Fig.1.47A). At first the chromosomes are seen as threads bearing bead-like thickenings (*chromomeres*) along their length. One end of the thread is attached to the nuclear membrane. During leptotene the chromosomes gradually become thicker and shorter.

(b) *Zygotene*: We have seen (page 28) that the 46 chromosomes in each cell consist of 23 pairs (the X and Y chromosomes of the male being taken as a pair). The two chromosomes of each pair come to lie parallel to each other, and are closely apposed. This pairing of chromosomes is also referred to as *synapsis* or *conjugation*. The two chromosomes together constitute a *bivalent* (Fig. 1.47B).

(c) *Pachytene*: The two chromatids of each

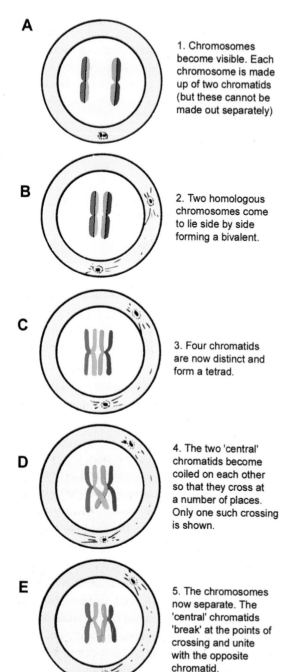

A

1. Chromosomes become visible. Each chromosome is made up of two chromatids (but these cannot be made out separately)

B

2. Two homologous chromosomes come to lie side by side forming a bivalent.

C

3. Four chromatids are now distinct and form a tetrad.

D

4. The two 'central' chromatids become coiled on each other so that they cross at a number of places. Only one such crossing is shown.

E

5. The chromosomes now separate. The 'central' chromatids 'break' at the points of crossing and unite with the opposite chromatid.

Fig. 1.47. Stages in the prophase of the first meiotic division.

chromosome become distinct. The bivalent now has four chromatids in it and is called a *tetrad*. There are two central and two peripheral chromatids, one from each chromosome (Fig. 1.47C). An important event now takes place. The two central chromatids (one belonging to each chromosome of the bivalent) become coiled over each other so that they cross at a number of points. This is called *crossing over*. For sake of simplicity only one such crossing is shown in Fig.1.47D. At the site where the chromatids cross they become adherent: the points of adhesion are called *chiasmata*.

(d) *Diplotene*: The two chromosomes of a bivalent now try to move apart. As they do so the chromatids 'break' at the points of crossing and the 'loose' pieces become attached to the opposite chromatid. This results in exchange of genetic material between these chromatids. A study of Fig. 1.47E will show that as a result of this *crossing over* of genetic material each of the four chromatids of the tetrad now has a distinctive genetic content.

The metaphase follows. As in mitosis the 46 chromosomes become attached to the spindle at the equator, the two chromosomes of a pair being close to each other (Fig.1.48A).

The anaphase differs from that in mitosis in that there is no splitting of the centromeres. One entire chromosome of each pair moves to each pole of the spindle (Fig.1.48B). The resulting daughter cells, therefore, have 23 chromosomes, each made up of two chromatids (Fig.1.48C).

The telophase is similar to that in mitosis.

The first meiotic division is followed by a short interphase. This differs from the usual interphase in that there is no duplication of DNA. Such duplication is unnecessary as the chromosomes of the cells resulting from the first meiotic division already possess two chromatids each (Fig.1.48C).

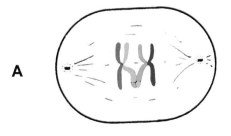

METAPHASE

The nuclear membrane disappears. Spindle forms and chromosomes are attached to it by their centromeres.

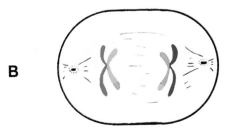

ANAPHASE

One entire chromosome of the pair moves to either pole. Note that the centromeres do not divide.

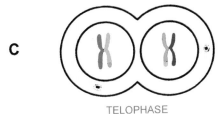

TELOPHASE

Note that the chromosomes in each cell have been reduced to the haploid number

Fig. 1.48. Metaphase (A), anaphase (B), and telophase (C) of the first meiotic division.

Second Meiotic Division

The second meiotic division is usually said to be similar to mitosis, as there is no reduction in chromosome number. However, as explained in Chapter 18, the DNA content of the daughter cells

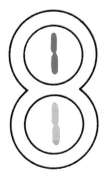
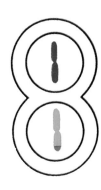

Fig. 1.49. Daughter cells resulting from the second meiotic division. The daughter cells are not alike because of the crossing over during the first division.

is reduced to half. Because of the crossing over that has occurred during the first division, the daughter cells are not identical in genetic content (Fig. 1.49). These reasons make the second meiotic division different from a typical mitosis.

At this stage it may be repeated that the 46 chromosomes of a cell consist of 23 pairs, one chromosome of each pair being derived from the mother and one from the father.

During the first meiotic division the chromosomes derived from the father and those derived from the mother are distributed between the daughter cells entirely at random. This, along with the phenomenon of crossing over, results in thorough shuffling of the genetic material so that the cells produced as a result of various meiotic divisions (i.e., ova and spermatozoa) all have a distinct genetic content. A third step in this process of genetic shuffling takes place at fertilization when there is a combination of randomly selected spermatozoa and ova. It is, therefore, not surprising that no two persons (except identical twins) are alike.

CHROMOSOMAL SEX AND SEX CHROMATIN

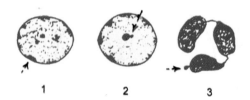

Fig. 1.50. Sex chromatin. 1. Typical possition deep to the nuclear membrane. 2. As a nucleolar satellite in neurons. 3. As an appendage shaped like a drum stick in neutrophil leucocytes. Only the nuclei are drawn.

On page 28 we have seen that each cell of a human male has 44+X+Y chromosomes, and that each cell of a female has 44+X+X chromosomes. We have also seen that during the formation of gametes by meiosis the chromosome number is reduced to half. As a result all ova contain 22+X chromosomes. Spermatozoa are of two types. Some have the chromosomal constitution 22+X and the others have the constitution 22+Y. If an ovum is fertilized by a sperm bearing an X-chromosome the resulting child has (22+X)+(22+X) = 44+X+X chromosomes and is a girl. On the other hand if an ovum is fertilized by a sperm bearing a Y-chromosome the child has (22+X) +(22+Y) = 44+X +Y chromosomes and is a boy.

Of the two X-chromosomes in a female only one is functionally active. The other (inactive) X-chromosome forms a mass of hetero-chromatin that lies just under the nuclear membrane. This mass of heterochromatin can be identified in suitable preparations and can be useful in determining whether a particular tissue belongs to a male or a female. Because of this association with sex this mass of heterochromatin is called the *sex chromatin*. It is also called a *Barr-body* after the name of the scientist who discovered it. In some cells the sex chromatin occupies a different position from that described above. In neurons it forms a rounded mass lying very close to the nucleolus and is, therefore, called a *nucleolar satellite*. In neutrophil leucocytes it may appear as an isolated round mass attached to the rest of the nucleus by a narrow band, thus resembling the appearance of a *drumstick*.

Rarely, some individuals may have more than two X-chromosomes. In these cases, only one X-chromosome is active (and hence euchromatic) while others are represented by masses of heterochromatin. Thus in a person with three X-chromosomes two masses of sex chromatin are seen.

In some cases the sex of an individual may not be clear (at birth) because of abnormalities in the genital organs. In such cases the true sex of the individual may be determined by looking for the sex chromatin. Methods are also available for identifying the Y-chromosome in cells. However, the best thing to do is to make a karyotype (page 36).

For a description of common chromosomal abnormalities see the author's HUMAN EMBRYOLOGY.

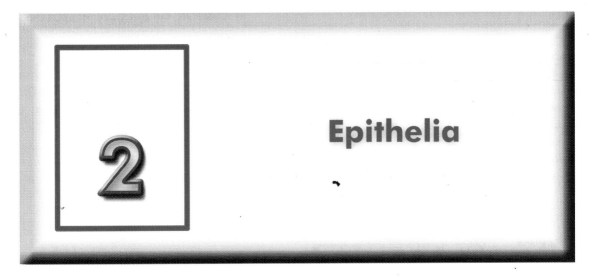

Epithelia

The outer surface of the body and the luminal surfaces of cavities within the body are lined by one or more layers of cells that completely cover them. Such layers of cells are called *epithelia* (singular=epithelium). Epithelia also line the ducts and secretory elements of glands (which develop as outgrowths from epithelium lined surfaces).

CLASSIFICATION OF EPITHELIA

An epithelium may consist of only one layer of cells when it is called a *unilayered* or *simple* epithelium. Alternatively, it may be *multi-layered* or *stratified*.

Simple epithelia may be further classified according to the shape of the cells constituting them.

(1) In some epithelia the cells are flattened, their height being very little as compared to their width. Such an epithelium is called a *squamous epithelium* (Figs. 2.1 A, B).

(2) When the height and width of the cells of the epithelium are more or less equal (i.e., they look like squares in section) it is described as a *cuboidal epithelium* (Fig. 2.5 A,B).

(3) When the height of the cells of the epithelium is distinctly greater than their width, it is described as a *columnar epithelium* (Figs. 2.2 A,B).

Multilayered epithelia are of two main types. In the most common type the deeper layers are columnar, but in proceeding towards the surface of the epithelium the cells become increasingly flattened (or squamous). Such an epithelium is described as *stratified squamous* (Fig. 2.8A). It may be noted that all cells in this kind of epithelium are not squamous. In the other type of multilayered epithelium all layers are made up of cuboidal, polygonal or rounded cells. The cells towards the surface of the epithelium are not flattened. This type of epithelium is called *transitional epithelium* (being transitional between unilayered epithelia and stratified squamous epithelium) (Fig. 2.9). As transitional epithelium is confined to the urinary tract it is also called *urothelium*.

A third, rather rare type of multilayered epithelium is made up of two or more layers of cuboidal or columnar cells (***stratified cuboidal***, or ***stratified columnar*** epithelium) (Fig. 2.10). Lastly, in some situations a columnar epithelium which is really single layered may give the appearance of a stratified epithelium: such an epithelium is referred to as ***pseudostratified columnar epithelium***.

The various types of epithelia named above are considered further below. All epithelia rest on a very thin ***basement membrane*** (See page 49).

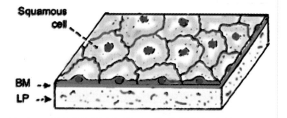

Fig. 2.1 A. Simple squamous epithelium (diagrammatic). BM= Basement membrane; LP= Lamina propria.

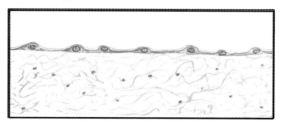

Fig. 2.1 B. Simple squamous epithelium as seen in a section.

Squamous Epithelium

The cytoplasm of cells in this kind of epithelium forms only a thin layer. The nuclei produce bulgings of the cell surface (Fig. 2.1 A, B). In surface view the cells have polygonal outlines that interlock with those of adjoining cells. With the EM the junctions between cells are marked by occluding junctions(see page 12): the junctions are thus tightly sealed and any substance passing through the epithelium has to pass through the cells, and not between them.

Squamous epithelium lines the alveoli of the lungs. It lines the free surface of the serous pericardium, of the pleura, and of the peritoneum: here it is called ***mesothelium***. It lines the inside of the heart, where it is called ***endocardium***; and of blood vessels and lymphatics, where it is called ***endothelium***. Squamous epithelium is also found lining some parts of the renal tubules, and in some parts of the internal ear.

Columnar Epithelium

We have seen that in vertical section the cells of this epithelium are rectangular. On surface view (or in transverse section) the cells are polygonal. In keeping with the elongated shape of the cells, the nuclei are also frequently elongated (Figs 2.2 A, B).

Columnar epithelium can be further classified

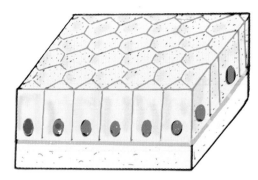

Fig. 2.2 A. Simple columnar epithelium (diagrammatic). Note the basally placed oval nuclei. The cells appear hexagonal in surface view.

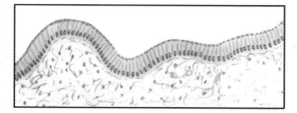

Fig. 2.2 B. Simple columnar epithelium as seen in a section.

according to the nature of the free surfaces of the cells as follows.

(**a**) In some situations the cell surface has no particular specialization: this is *simple columnar epithelium*.

(**b**) In some situations the cell surface bears cilia (described on page 22). This is *ciliated columnar epithelium* (Fig. 2.3 A).

(**c**) In other situations the surface is covered with microvilli. Although the microvilli are visible only with the EM, with the light microscope the region of the microvilli is seen as a *striated border* (when the microvilli are arranged regularly) (Fig. 2.4) or as a *brush border* (when the microvilli are irregularly placed) (Fig. 1.29C).

Some columnar cells have a secretory function. The apical parts of their cytoplasm contain secretory vacuoles.

Simple columnar epithelium (without cilia or microvilli) is present over the mucous membrane of the stomach and the large intestine.

Columnar epithelium with a striated border is

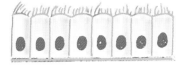

Fig. 2.3 A. Columnar epithelium showing cilia (diagrammatic). For structure of a cilium see Figs. 1.27, 1.28.

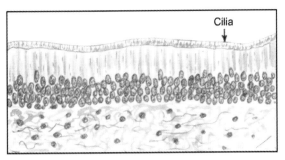

Fig. 2.3 B. Ciliated epithelium (pseudostratified columnar) as seen in a section.

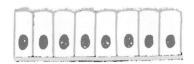

Fig. 2.4 A. Columnar epithelium showing a striated border made up of microvilli (diagrammatic).

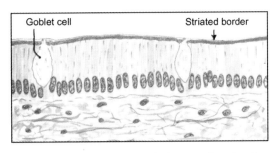

Fig. 2.4 B. Columnar epithelium with striated border as seen in a section.

seen most typically in the small intestine, and with a brush border in the gall bladder.

Ciliated columnar epithelium lines most of the respiratory tract, the uterus, and the uterine tubes. It is also seen in the efferent ductules of

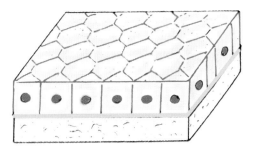

Fig. 2.5 A. Simple cuboidal epithelium (diagrammatic). Note that the cells appear cuboidal in section and hexagonal in surface view.

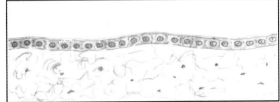

Fig. 2.5 B. Simple cuboidal epithelium as seen in a section.

the testis, parts of the middle ear and auditory tube; and in the ependyma lining the central canal of the spinal cord and the ventricles of the brain. In the respiratory tract the cilia move mucous accumulating in the bronchi (and containing trapped dust particles) towards the larynx and pharynx. When excessive this mucous is brought out as sputum during coughing. In the uterine tubes the movements of the cilia help in the passage of ova towards the uterus.

Secretory columnar cells are scattered in the mucosa of the stomach and intestines. In the intestines many of them secrete mucous which accumulates in the apical part of the cell making it very light staining. These cells acquire a characteristic shape (Fig. 2.4B) and are called *goblet cells*. Some columnar cells secrete enzymes.

Cuboidal Epithelium

Cuboidal epithelium is similar to columnar epithelium, but for the fact that the height of the cells is about the same as their width. The nuclei are usually rounded (Fig. 2.5).

A typical cuboidal epithelium may be seen in the follicles of the thyroid gland, in the ducts of many glands, and on the surface of the ovary (where it is called *germinal epithelium*). Other sites are the choroid plexuses, the inner surface of the lens, and the pigment cell layer of the retina.

An epithelium that is basically cuboidal (or columnar) lines the secretory elements of many glands. In this situation, however, the parts of the cells nearest the lumen are more compressed (against neighbouring cells) than at their bases, giving them a triangular shape (Fig. 2.6).

A cuboidal epithelium with a prominent brush border is seen in the proximal convoluted tubules of the kidneys (Fig. 1.29C).

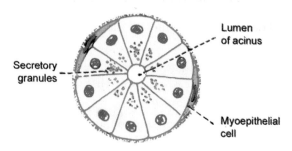

Fig. 2.6 A. Modified columnar cells in the wall of an acinus (of a gland) (diagrammatic). Note the triangular shape of the cells, the presence of secretory granules, and the myoepithelial cells lying between the gland cells and the basement membrane.

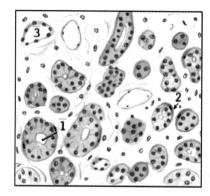

Fig. 2.6 B. Section through lacrimal gland showing acini of the kind described in Fig. 2.6 A.

Pseudostratified Columnar Epithelium

In usual class room slides the boundaries between epithelial cells are often not clearly seen. In spite of this we can make out what type of epithelium it is. This is because the shape and spacing of the nuclei gives a good idea of where the cell boundaries must lie.

Normally, in columnar epithelium the nuclei lie in a row, towards the bases of the cells. Sometimes, however, the nuclei appear to be arranged in two or more layers giving the impression that the epithelium is more than one cell thick (Fig. 2.7B). The reason for this will be understood easily from Fig.2.7A. It is seen that

[handwritten notes at top:] Cornea is rich in sensory cells. Organ of corti - the area fusern where endolymph. it is rich in mitra epithelial capillaries.

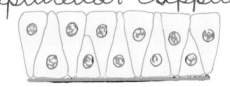

Fig. 2.7 A. Pseudostratified columnar epithelium (diagrammatic). This figure explains why the nuclei lie at various levels.

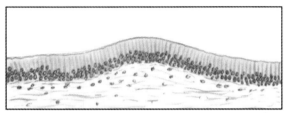

Fig. 2.7 B. Realistic appearance of pseudostratified columnar epithelium as seen in a section.

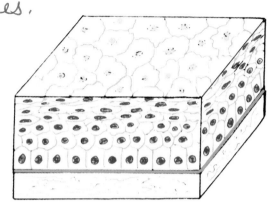

Fig. 2.8 A. Stratified squasmous epithelium. There is a basal layer of columnar cells that rests on the basement membrane. Overlying the columnar cells of this layer there are a few layers of polygonal cells or rounded cells. Still more superficially, the cells undergo progressive flattening, becoming squasmous.

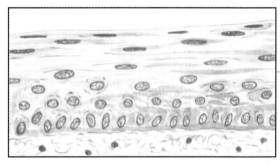

Fig. 2.8 B. Stratified squamous epithelium (non-keratinized) as seen in a section.

there is actually only one layer of cells, but some cells are broader near the base, and others near the apex. The nuclei lie in the broader part of each cell and are, therefore, not in one layer. To distinguish this kind of epithelium from a true stratified epithelium, it is referred to as *pseudostratified columnar epithelium*.

A pseudostratified columnar epithelium is found in some parts of the auditory tube, the ductus deferens, and the male urethra (membranous and penile parts). A ciliated pseudostratified columnar epithelium is seen in the trachea and in large bronchi (Fig. 2.3B).

Stratified Squamous Epithelium

This type of epithelium is made up of several layers of cells. The cells of the deepest (or basal) layer rest on the basement membrane: they are usually columnar in shape. Lying over the columnar cells there are polyhedral or cuboidal cells. As we pass towards the surface of the epithelium these cells become progressively more flat, so that the most superficial cells consist of flattened squamous cells (Fig. 2.8).

Stratified squamous epithelium can be divided into two types: *non-keratinized* and *keratinized*. In situations where the surface of the epithelium remains moist, the most superficial cells are living and nuclei can be seen in them. This kind of epithelium is described as non-keratinized. In contrast, at places where the epithelial surface is dry (as in the skin) the most superficial cells die and lose their nuclei. These cells contain a substance called *keratin*, which forms a non-living covering over the epithelium. This kind of epithelium constitutes keratinized stratified squamous epithelium.

Stratified squamous epithelium (both keratinized and non-keratinized) is found over those surfaces of the body that are subject to friction. As a result of friction the most superficial layers are constantly being removed and are replaced by proliferation of cells from the basal (or germinal) layer. This layer, therefore, shows frequent mitoses.

Keratinized stratified squamous epithelium covers the skin of the whole of the body and forms the epidermis. Non-keratinized stratified squamous epithelium is seen lining the mouth, the tongue, the pharynx, the oesophagus, the vagina and the cornea. Under pathological conditions the epithelium in any of these situations may become keratinized.

Transitional Epithelium

This is a multi-layered epithelium and is 4 to 6 cells thick. It differs from stratified squamous epithelium in that the cells at the surface are not squamous. The deepest cells are columnar or cuboidal. The middle layers are made up of polyhedral or pear-shaped cells. The cells of the surface layer are large and often shaped like an umbrella (Fig. 2.9).

Transitional epithelium is found in the renal pelvis and calyces, the ureter, the urinary bladder, and part of the urethra. Because of this distribution it is also called *urothelium*. In the urinary bladder it is seen that transitional epithelium can be stretched considerably without being damaged. When stretched it appears to be thinner and the cells become flattened or rounded.

> With the EM the cells of transitional epithelium are seen to be firmly connected to one another by numerous desmosomes. Because of these connections the cells retain their relative position when the epithelium is stretched or relaxed. At the surface of the epithelium the plasma membranes are unusual: embedded in the lipid

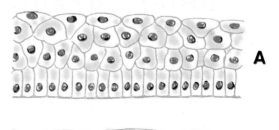
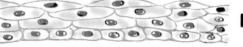

Fig. 2.9 A & B. Transitional epithelium (diagrammatic) in unstretched (A), and in stretched (B) conditions.

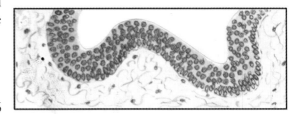

Fig. 2.9 C. Realistic appearance of transitional epithelium as seen in a section.

layer of the membranes (page 4) there are special glycoproteins. It is believed that these glycoproteins make the membrane impervious and resistant to the toxic effects of substances present in urine, and thus afford protection to adjacent tissues.

The cells in the basal layer of transitional epithelium show occasional mitoses, but these are much less frequent than those in stratified squamous epithelium, as there is normally little erosion of the surface. Many cells of the superficial (luminal) layers of the epithelium may contain two nuclei. In some cells the nucleus is single, but contains multiples of the normal number of chromosomes (i.e., it may be polyploid).

According to some workers. all cells of transitional epithelium reach the basal lamina through thin processes. If this observation is proved to be correct transitional epithelium would have to be classified as a pseudo-stratified epithelium (rather than as a stratified one).

Stable cells !(neuron) nerve cells of nervous system have no regenerative property. once they are dead they do not regenerate (except neuroglia); cartilage cells

EPITHELIA   49

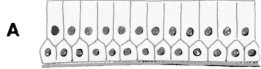

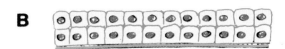

Fig. 2.10. A. Stratified columnar epithelium. B. Stratified cuboidal epithelium. These are rare epithelial seen in the ducts of some glands.

Diffusion thru,

Basement Membranes of Epithelia

We have seen that epithelial cells rest on a thin basement membrane. In multi-layered epithelia, the deepest cells lie on this membrane. Basement membranes are formed by thin layers of amorphous material and of reticular fibres.

A distinct basement membrane cannot be seen in H & E preparations, but can be well demonstrated using the PAS (periodic acid Schiff) method. The latter stains the glycoproteins present in the membrane.

Under the EM a basement membrane is seen to have a **basal lamina** (nearest the epithelial cells) and a **reticular lamina** or **fibroreticular lamina** (consisting of reticular tissue and merging into surrounding connective tissue). The basal lamina is divisible into the **lamina densa** containing fibrils; and the **lamina lucida** which appears to be transparent. The lamina lucida lies against the cell membranes of epithelial cells.

Some details of the chemical composition of basement membranes are given on page 57.

Membranes similar in structure and composition to basement membranes are also seen in relation to smooth muscle cells, Schwann cells, the glomerular membrane of the kidney, and in membranes covering the cornea and lens of the eye.

Several important functions have been ascribed to basement membranes as follows.

(a) They provide adhesion on one side to epithelial cells (or parenchyma); and on the other side to connective tissue (mainly collagen fibres).

(b) They act as barriers to the diffusion of mocelules. The barrier function varies with location (because of variations in pore size). Large proteins are prevented from passing out of blood vessels, but (in the lung) diffusion of gases is allowed.

(c) Recent work suggests that basement membranes may play a role in cell organization, as molecules within the membrane interact with receptors on cell surfaces. Substances present in the membrane may influence morphogenesis of cells to which they are attached.

(d) The membranes may influence the regeneration of peripheral nerves after injury, and may play a role in re-establishment of neuromuscular junctions.

Further Comments on Epithelia

(1) The shape of epithelial cells is related to the amount of contained cytoplasm and organelles. These are in turn related to metabolic activity. Squamous cells are least active. Columnar cells contain abundant mitochondria and endoplasmic reticulum and are highly active.

(2) Laterally, epithelial cells are in contact with other epithelial cells. The contact between adjoining cells is generally an intimate one because of the presence of desmosomes, zonulae adherens, and zonulae occludens (page 9). The intimate contact ensures that materials passing through the epithelium have to pass through the cells, rather than between them.

(3) We have seen that cilia are present on the free surfaces of some epithelial cells. Cilia have been described on page 22. The surface area of an epithelial cell may be greatly increased by the presence of microvilli (page 24), or of basolateral folds (page 24).

(4) Some epithelial cells contain pigment. Such

Permanent cells → liver cell. Do not regenerate
In case of Jaundice & Yellow fever [Renal & Gland
to some eset end
Protein & fat is not included
In diet

cells are present in the skin, the retina and the iris.

(5) Epithelia are generally devoid of blood vessels. Their cells obtain nutrition by diffusion from blood vessels in underlying tissues. In contrast, delicate nerve fibres frequently penetrate into the intervals between epithelial cells.

(6) Epithelia have considerable capacity for repair after damage. They grow rapidly after injury to repair the defect.

(7) It should be remembered that epithelial cells that look alike (on superficial examination) may have very different functions. For example, cuboidal cells lining follicles of the thyroid gland have very little in common with cuboidal cells covering the surface of the ovary.

(8) Epithelia in secretory portions of glands show specializations of structure that depend on the nature of the secretion produced by them (page 53).

(9) Epithelial cells in which transport of ions is an important function (e.g., renal tubules) are marked by the presence of basolateral folds, and the presence of large numbers of mitochondria. The mitochondria provide ATP which is the source of energy for ion transport. Tight junctions between the cells prevent passive diffusion of ions.

(10) Epithelial cells contain some proteins not present in non-epithelial cells. These include cytokeratin (present in intermediate filaments). Such proteins can be localized using immunohistochemical techniques (See below).

Mucous Membranes

We have seen that epithelia line many tubular structures within the body. In such structures the epithelium rests (with its basement membrane) on a layer of connective tissue called the *lamina*

propria (or *corium*). The layer of epithelium along with its lamina propria is referred to as the *mucous membrane* or *mucosa* (as its surface is kept moist by secretions of mucous glands).

In the intestines the mucous membrane has a third layer formed by a thin stratum of smooth muscle. This smooth muscle is called the *muscularis mucosae* (= muscle of the mucous membrane).

Tumours arising from epithelia

A tumour (or neoplasm) can arise from any tissue if there is uncontrolled growth of cells. Such a tumour may be benign, when it remains localized; or may be malignant. A malignant growth invades surrounding tissues. Cells of the tumour can spread to distant sites (through lymphatics or through the blood stream) and can start growing there producing what are called *secondaries* or *metastases*.

A malignant tumour arising from an epithelium is called a *carcinoma*. If it arises from a squamous epithelium it is a *squamous cell carcinoma*; and if it arises from glandular epithelium it is called an *adenoma*.

Quite commonly cells in tumours resemble those of the tissue from which they are derived, and this is useful in pathological diagnosis. However, in metastases of fast growing tumours the cells may show not show the characteristics of the tissue of origin (undifferentiated tumour), and it may be difficult to find out the location of the primary growth. In such cases diagnosis can be aided by localization of proteins that are present only in epithelia. As mentioned above this can be done by using immuno-histochemical techniques.

eg of Labile cells
basal cells of Stratified, epithelium. Squamous.
transverse epithelium
Crypts of Lieberkuhn
osteoblast,

Haemopoietic Cells :- (Labile Cell.)

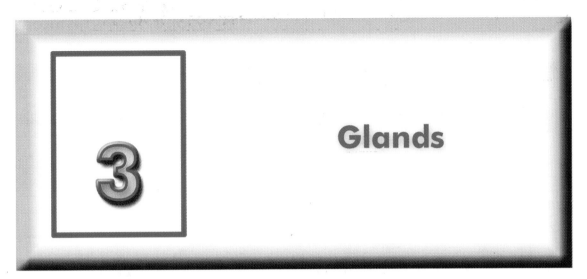

Glands

3

We have seen that some epithelial cells may be specialized to perform a secretory function. Such cells, present singly or in groups, constitute glands.

From this it is obvious that some glands are **unicellular**. Unicellular glands are interspersed amongst other (non-secretory) epithelial cells. They can be found, for example, in the epithelium lining the intestines.

Most glands are, however, **multicellular**. Such glands develop as diverticula from epithelial surfaces. The 'distal' parts of the diverticulae develop into secretory elements, while the 'proximal' parts form ducts through which secretions reach the epithelial surface.

Those glands that pour their secretions on to an epithelial surface, directly or through ducts are called **exocrine glands** (or **externally secreting glands**). Some glands lose all contact with the epithelial surface from which they develop: they pour their secretions into blood. Such glands are called **endocrine glands**, **internally secreting glands**, or **duct-less glands**.

When all the secretory cells of an exocrine gland discharge into one duct the gland is said to be a **simple gland**. Sometimes there are a number of groups of secretory cells, each group

discharging into its own duct. These ducts unite to form larger ducts which ultimately drain on to an epithelial surface. Such a gland is said to be a **compound gland**.

Both in simple and in compound glands the secretory cells may be arranged in various ways.

(a) The secretory element may be **tubular**. The tube may be straight, coiled, or branched.

(b) The cells may form rounded sacs or **acini**.

(c) They may form flask shaped structures called **alveoli**. However, it may be noted that the terms acini and alveoli are often used as if they were synonymous. Glands in which the secretory elements are greatly distended are called **saccular glands**.

(d) Combinations of the above may be present in a single gland. From what has been said above it will be seen that an exocrine gland may be:

1. Unicellular. — paneth cells, goblet cells.
2. Simple tubular. Crypts of Leiberkuhn.
3. Simple alveolar (or acinar). Mucous Secretory
4. Compound tubular. — Stomach, Brunner, Gland of duodenum
5. Compound alveolar. pancreatic gland.
6. Compound tubulo-alveolar (or racemose).

Some further subdivisions of these are shown in Fig. 3.1.

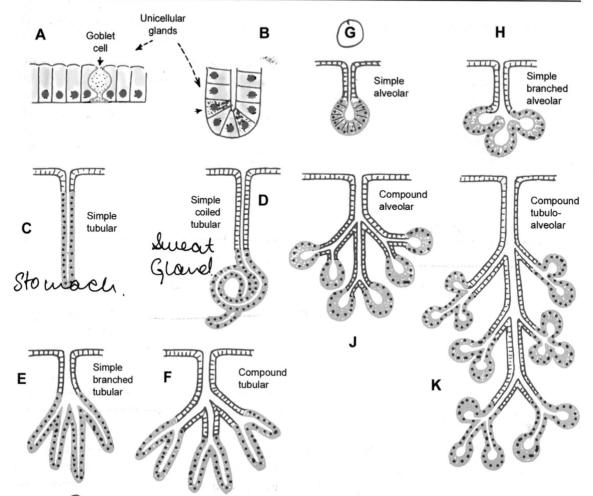

Fig. 3.1. Scheme to show various ways in which the secretory elements of a gland may be organized. A and B are examples of unicellular glands. All others are multicellular. Glands with a single duct are simple glands, while those with a branching duct system are compound glands.

Exocrine glands may also be classified on the basis of the nature of their secretions into **mucous glands** and **serous glands**. In mucous glands the secretion contains mucopolysaccharides. The secretion collects in the apical parts of the cells. As a result nuclei are pushed to the base of the cell, and may be flattened.

In class room slides stained with haematoxylin and eosin the secretion within mucous cells remains unstained so that they have an 'empty' look (Fig. A55).

However, the stored secretion can be brightly stained using a special procedure called the periodic acid Schiff (PAS) method. Unicellular cells secreting mucous are numerous in the intestines: they are called **goblet cells** because of their peculiar shape. (See Fig. 3.1A and Fig. 2.4B).

The secretions of serous glands are protein in nature. The cytoplasm of these cells is granular and often stains bluish with haematoxylin and eosin. Their nuclei are centrally placed. Some glands contain both serous and mucous elements.

Epithelia in secretory portions of glands show specializations of structure depending upon the nature of secretion as follows.

(1) Cells that are protein secreting (e.g., hormone producing cells) have a well developed rough ER, and a supranuclear Golgi complex. Secretory granules often fill the apical portions of the cells. The staining characters of the granules differ in cells producing different secretions (the cells being described as acidophile, basophile etc).

(2) Mucin secreting cells have a well developed rough ER (where the protein component of mucin is synthesized), and a very well developed Golgi complex (where proteins are glycosylated).

(3) Steroid producing cells are characterized by the presence of extensive smooth endoplasmic reticulum, and prominent mitochondria.

In addition to their classification on the basis of structure, and on the basis of the nature of their secretion, exocrine glands can also be classified on the basis of the manner in which their secretions are poured out of the cells. In most exocrine glands secretions are thrown out of the cells by a process of exocytosis (page 8) the cell remaining intact: this manner of secretion is described as merocrine (sometimes also called *eccrine* or *epicrine*). In some glands the apical parts of the cells are shed off to discharge the secretion: this manner of secretion is described as *apocrine*. An example of apocrine secretion is seen in some atypical sweat glands, and in mammary glands (but also see page 298). Finally, in some glands the entire cell disintegrates while discharging its secretion. This manner of discharging secretion is described as *holocrine*, and is seen typically in sebaceous glands (page 190). Depending on the mode of secretion glands may, therefore, be described as merocrine, apocrine or holocrine.

The secretory elements of exocrine glands are held together by connective tissue (mainly reticular fibres). The glandular tissue is often divisible into lobules separated by connective tissue septa. Aggregations of lobules may form distinct lobes. The connective tissue covering the entire gland forms a *capsule* for it.

When a gland is divided into lobes the ducts draining it may be *intralobular* (lying within a lobule), *interlobular* (lying in the intervals between lobules), or *interlobar* (lying between adjacent lobes), in increasing order of size.

Blood vessels and nerves pass along connective tissue septa to reach the secretory elements. As a rule exocrine glands have a rich blood supply. Their activity is under nervous or hormonal control.

The secretory cells of a gland constitute its *parenchyma*, while the connective tissue in which the former lie is called the *stroma*.

Endocrine glands are usually arranged in cords or in clumps that are intimately related to a rich network of blood capillaries or of sinusoids. In some cases (for example the thyroid gland) the cells may form rounded follicles.

Endocrine cells and their blood vessels are supported by delicate connective tissue, and are usually surrounded by a capsule.

As mentioned on page 50, neoplasms can arise from the epithelium lining a gland. A benign growth arising in a gland is an *adenoma*; and a malignant growth is an *adenocarcinoma*.

In this chapter we have considered the general features of glands. Further details of the structure of exocrine and endocrine glands will be considered while studying individual glands.

* modified Sweat Gland.

General Connective Tissue

Mechanical & nutritional.

INTRODUCTORY REMARKS

What is Connective Tissue?

The term ***connective tissue*** is applied to a tissue which fills the interstices between more specialized elements; and serves to hold them together and support them. For the latter reason some authorities prefer to call it ***support tissue***. A few examples will help the reader to get some idea of what connective tissue is like.

1. When an area of skin is lifted off from underlying tissues (during dissection) the two are seen to be connected by a delicate network of fibres. This network, which is referred to as ***superficial fascia,*** is an example of connective tissue.

2. Examine Fig. A55 (atlas). This figure shows a section across a salivary gland. Some epithelium lined acini and one duct are seen. Filling the interstices between these elements there is connective tissue, similar to that in superficial fascia. The tissue provides support to the delicate epithelial cells.

3. Next, examine Fig. A60 (oesophagus). We see an epithelial lined mucosa separated by a short distance from thick layers of muscle. The interval between the two is filled in by connective tissue (which constitutes the submucosa). This connective tissue holds the various layers in the walls of hollow organs together.

The three examples cited above show us that connective tissue serves to hold together, and to support, different elements within an organ. Such connective tissue is to be found in almost every part of the body. It is conspicuous in some regions and scanty in others. This kind of connective tissue is referred to as ***general connective tissue*** to distinguish it from more specialized connective tissues that we will consider separately. It is also called ***fibro-collagenous tissue***.

Basic Components of General Connective Tissue

Many tissues and organs of the body are made up mainly of aggregations of closely packed cells e.g., epithelia, and solid organs like the liver. In contrast, cells are relatively few in connective tissue, and are widely separated by a prominent ***intercellular substance***. The intercellular substance is in the form of a ***ground substance*** within which there are numerous ***fibres*** (Fig. 4.1). Connective tissue can assume various forms depending upon the nature of the ground

Nervous tissues, neuron structure
wrapping of area by Schwann cells
GENERAL CONNECTIVE TISSUE Protein is MAP-2 **55**

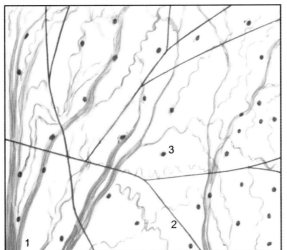

Fig. 4.1. Stretch preparation of omentum showing loose areolar tissue.

substance, and of the type of fibres and cells present.

Fibres in connective tissue

The most conspicuous components of connective tissue are the fibres within it. These are of three main types.

(a) *Collagen fibres* <u>are most numerous</u>. They can be classified into various types (page 59).

(b) *Reticular fibres* were once described as a distinct variety of fibres, <u>but they are now regarded as one variety of collagen fibre</u>.

(c) *Elastic fibres*.

We have seen that the fibres are embedded in an amorphous <u>ground substance</u> or *matrix*. (Some authors use the term matrix for the ground substance only, but others include fibres under the term). We will consider each type of fibre, and the ground substance in detail in subsequent sections.

Cells in general connective tissue

Various types of cells are present in connective tissue. These can be classed into two distinct categories.

(a) Cells that are intrinsic components of connective tissue:

In typical connective tissue the most important cells are *fibroblasts*. Others present are *undifferentiated mesenchymal cells*, *pigment cells*, and *fat cells*. Other varieties of cells are present in more specialized forms of connective tissues.

(b) Cells that belong to the immune system and are identical or closely related with certain cells present in blood and in lymphoid tissues:

These include *macrophage cells* (or *histiocytes*), *mast cells*, *lymphocytes, plasma cells*, *monocytes* and *eosinophils*.

We will consider each of the components named above in paragraphs that follow.

Different forms of Connective Tissue

Loose Connective Tissue

If we examine a small quantity of superficial fascia under a microscope, at low magnification, it is seen to be made up mainly of bundles of loosely arranged fibres that appear to enclose large spaces. This is *loose connective tissue*. Spaces are also called *areolae*, and such tissue is also referred to as *areolar tissue* (Fig. 4.1).

Fibrous tissue

We have seen that in loose areolar tissue the fibre bundles are loosely arranged with wide spaces in between them. In many situations the fibre bundles are much more conspicuous, and form a dense mass. This kind of tissue is referred

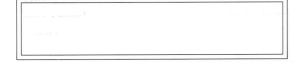

to as *fibrous tissue*. It appears white in colour and is sometimes called *white fibrous tissue*.

In some situations the bundles of collagen are arranged parallel to one another in a very orderly manner. This kind of tissue is called *regular fibrous tissue* (or regular connective tissue), and the best example of it is to be seen in tendons (Figs. A16, 17). Many ligaments are also made up of similar tissue, but in them there may be different layers in which fibres run in somewhat different directions. A similar arrangement is also seen in sheets of deep fascia, intermuscular septa, aponeuroses, the central tendon of the diaphragm, the fibrous pericardium and dura mater.

In other situations the collagen bundles do not show such a regular arrangement, but interlace in various directions forming dense irregular tissue. Such tissue is found in the dermis, connective tissue sheaths of muscles and nerves, capsules of glands, the sclera, the periosteum, and the adventitia of blood vessels.

Irrespective of whether connective tissue is regular or irregular the fibre bundles are so arranged as to be best suited to resist forces that tend to stretch the tissue. Where such forces are unidirectional (e.g., in tendons) the arrangement is more regular; but as the forces become more complex (as in deep fascia) the fibres are not so regularly arranged. In the case of membranes some interweaving of fibres is also a necessity for maintaining the integrity of the membrane.

The cornea is made up mainly of collagen fibres (Fig. A 109). Its transparency is made possible by the highly precise pattern in which the collagen fibres are arranged.

Elastic Tissue

We have seen that some elastic fibres can be seen in loose areolar tissue (Fig. 4.1). Some elastic fibres may also be present in any other variety of connective tissue. However, in some situations the bulk of the connective tissue is formed by elastic fibres: this is called *elastic tissue*. In contrast to white fibrous tissue, elastic tissue is yellow in colour. Some ligaments are made up of elastic tissue. These include the ligamentum nuchae (on the back of the neck); and the ligamenta flava (which connect the laminae of adjoining vertebrae). The vocal ligaments (of the larynx) are also made up of elastic fibres. Elastic fibres are numerous in membranes that are required to stretch periodically. For example the deeper layer of superficial fascia covering the anterior abdominal wall has a high proportion of elastic fibres to allow for distension of the abdomen.

Elastic fibres may fuse with each other to form sheets (usually fenestrated). Such sheets form the main support for the walls of large arteries (e.g., the aorta). In smaller arteries they form the internal elastic lamina (Figs. A34, A35).

Reticular Tissue

This is made up of reticular fibres. In many situations (e.g., lymph nodes, glands) these fibres form supporting networks for the cells (Fig. 4.3). In some situations (bone marrow, spleen, lymph nodes) the reticular network is closely associated with *reticular cells*. Most of these cells are fibroblasts, but some may be macrophages.

Other connective tissues

Bone and cartilage are regarded as forms of connective tissue as the cells in them are widely separated by intercellular substance. The firmness of cartilage, and the hardness of bone, are because of the nature of the ground substance in them. Cartilage and bone will be considered in Chapters 6 and 7 respectively. Blood is also

4.2 GLYCOSAMINOGLYCANS PRESENT IN VARIOUS TISSUES						
TISSUE	Chondroitin sulphate	Dermatan sulphate	Heparan sulphate	Heparin	Keratan sulphate	Hyaluronic acid
Typical connective tissue	+					+
Cartilage	+				+	+
Bone	+					
Skin	+	+		+		+
Basement membrane			+			
Others		Blood vessels Heart	Lung arteries	Mast cells Lungs Liver	Cornea Intervertebral discs	Synovial fluid

included amongst connective tissues as the cells are widely dispersed in a fluid intercellular substance, the plasma. Blood is considered in Chapter 5.

Two other varieties of connective tissue, namely, adipose tissue, and mucoid tissue will be considered later in this chapter.

In the above paragraphs the constituents of various types of connective tissue have been mentioned in the simplest possible terms. We will now go on to study the various components of these tissues in some detail.

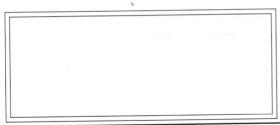

INTERCELLULAR GROUND SUBSTANCE OF CONNECTIVE TISSUE

If a small quantity of fresh areolar tissue is spread out on a slide, and is examined under a microscope, the spaces between the fibre bundles appear to be empty. If such a preparation is treated with silver nitrate the spaces are seen to be filled with a brown staining material.

By the use of a technique called freeze drying tissue can be prepared for sectioning without the use of extraneous chemicals. In areolar tissue prepared in this way the ground substance stains metachromatically (See page 64) with toluidine blue. It can also be stained with the PAS method (pages 49, 52). These early observations tell us that the ground substance is rich in protein-carbohydrate complexes or **proteoglycans**.

Various types of proteoglycans are known. Each of them is a complex formed by protein and long chained polysaccharides called **glycosaminoglycans**. The glycosaminoglycans, and the tissues in which each type is present are given in Table 4.2.

With the exception of hyaluronic acid, all other glycosaminoglycans listed in the table have the following features.

1. They are linked with protein (to form proteoglycans).

2. They carry sulphate groups (SO$_3^-$) and carboxyl groups (COO$^-$) which give them a strong negative charge.

3. The proteoglycans formed by them are in the form of long chains that do not fold. Because of this they occupy a large space (or **domain**), and hold a large amount of water. They also hold Na$^+$ ions.

Retained water and proteoglycans form a gell that gives a certain degree of stiffness to connective tissue; and helps it to resist compressive forces.

4. Because of the arrangement of molecules within it, ground substance acts like a sieve. The size of the pores of the sieve can be altered (by change in orientation of molecules, and by change in the charges on them). In this way ground substance forms a selective barrier. This barrier function is specially important in basement membranes. In the kidney this barrier prevents large protein molecules from passing (from blood) into urine. However, exchange of gases is permitted in the lungs.

In addition to proteoglycans the ground substance also contains **structural glycoproteins**. Their main function is to facilitate adhesion between various elements of connective tissue.

Intercellular ground substance is synthesized by fibroblasts. Osteoblasts, chondroblasts, and even smooth muscle cells can also produce ground substance.

FIBRES OF CONNECTIVE TISSUE

Collagen Fibres

With the light microscope collagen fibres are seen in bundles (Fig. 4.1). The bundles may be straight or wavy depending upon how much they are stretched. The bundles are made up of collections of individual collagen fibres which are 1-12 μm in diameter. The bundles often branch, or anastomose with adjacent bundles, but the individual fibres do not branch.

With the EM each collagen fibre is seen to be made of fibrils that are 20-200 nm in diameter. Each fibril consists of a number of microfibrils, 3.5 nm in diameter. At high magnifications of the EM each fibril shows characteristic cross striations (or periods) after every 67 nm (in unfixed tissue).

Staining Characters

Bundles of collagen fibres appear white with the naked eye. In sections stained with haematoxylin and eosin collagen fibres are stained light pink. With special methods they assume different colours depending upon the dye used. Two commonly used methods are **Masson's trichrome** with which the fibres stain blue (Fig. A46); and the **Van Gieson** method with which they stain pink (Fig. A49). After silver impregnation the fibres are stained brown.

Physical Properties

Collagen fibres can resist considerable tensile forces (i.e., stretching) without significant increase in their length. At the same time they are pliable and can bend easily.

When polarized light is thrown on the fibres the light is split into two beams that are refracted in different directions. This is called **birefringence**: it is an indication of the fact that each collagen fibre is made up of finer fibrils.

Collagen fibres swell and become soft when treated with a weak acid or alkali. They are destroyed by strong acids. (This fact is sometimes made use of to soften collagen fibres to facilitate preparation of anatomical specimens). On boiling, collagen is converted into gelatine.

Chemical Nature

Collagen fibres are so called because they are made up mainly of a protein called **collagen**. Carbohydrates are also present. Collagen is made up of molecules of **tropocollagen**.

Microfibrils of collagen are chains of tropocollagen molecules. Each molecule of tropocollagen is 300 nm in length. Within a fibre, the molecules of tropocollagen are arranged in a regular overlapping pattern which is responsible for producing the cross striated appearance of the fibres.

Each molecule of tropocollagen is made up of three polypeptide chains. The chains are arranged in the form of a triple helix. The polypeptide chains are referred to as **procollagen**. Each procollagen chain consists of a long chain of amino acids that are arranged in groups of three (triplets). Each triplet contains the amino acid glycine. The other two amino acids in each triplet are variable. Most commonly these are hydroxyproline and hydroxylysine. Variations in the amino acid pattern give rise to several types of collagen as described below.

Varieties of Collagen and their Distribution

Several types of collagen are recognized depending upon the diameter of fibres, the prominence of cross striations, and other features.

Type I: These are collagen fibres of classical description having the properties described above. They are found in connective tissue, tendons, ligaments, fasciae, aponeuroses etc. They are also present in the dermis of the skin, and in meninges.

They form the fibrous basis of bone and of fibrocartilage. Type I fibres are of large diameter (about 250 nm) and have prominent cross striations.

Type II: These are of two subtypes. The larger of these are about 100 nm in diameter, while the narrower fibres are about 20 nm in diameter. In type II collagen striations are less prominent than in type I.

Type II collagen fibres form the fibrous basis of hyaline cartilage. Fine type II fibres are also present in the vitreous body.

Type III: These form the reticular fibres described below.

Type IV: This type of collagen consists of short filaments that form sheets. It is present in the basal laminae of basement membranes (page 49). It is also seen in the lens capsule.

Various other types of collagen are also recognized (so that we have more than 20 types). The quantity of carbohydrate associated with different types of collagen is variable.

Production of Collagen Fibres

See page 62.

Reticular Fibres

These fibres are a variety of collagen fibre (type III). They show periodicity (striations) of 67 nm. They differ from typical (Type I) collagen fibres as follows.

(1) They are much finer.

(2) They are uneven in thickness.

(3) They form a network (or reticulum) by branching, and by anastomosing with each other. They do not run in bundles.

(4) They can be stained specifically by silver impregnation, which renders them black. They can thus be easily distinguished from type I collagen fibres which are stained brown. Because

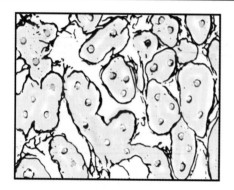

Fig. 4.3. Reticular fibres (black) forming a network in the liver. The white spaces represent sinusoids.

of their affinity for silver salts reticular fibres are sometimes called *argentophil fibres* (Fig. 4.3 and Fig. A15).

(5) Reticular fibres contain more carbohydrates than Type I fibres (which is probably the reason why they are argentophil).

Reticular fibres provide a supporting network in many situations. These include the spleen, lymph nodes and bone marrow; most glands, including the liver(Fig. 4.3); and the kidneys. Reticular fibres form an essential component of all basement membranes. They are also found in relation to smooth muscle and nerve fibres.

Elastic Fibres

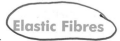

In areolar tissue, elastic fibres are much fewer than those of collagen. They run singly (not in bundles), branch and anastomose with other fibres. Elastic fibres are thinner than those of collagen (0.1-0.2 μm)(Fig. 4.1).

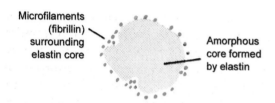

Microfilaments
(fibrillin)
surrounding
elastin core

Amorphous
core formed
by elastin

Fig. 4.4. EM appearance of an elastic fibre as seen in transverse section.

In some situations elastic fibres are thick (e.g., in the ligamenta flava). In other situations (as in walls of large arteries) they form fenestrated membranes.

With the EM each elastic fibre is seen to have a central amorphous core and an outer layer of fibrils (Fig. 4.4). The outer fibrils are made up of a glycoprotein called *fibrillin* (see below). (Periodic striations are not present in elastic fibres.

Staining Characters

Elastic fibres do not stain with the usual stains for collagen. They can be demonstrated by staining with orcein, with aldehyde fuchsin, and by Verheoff's method. (Figs. 4.1 and A49).

Physical Properties

As their name implies elastic fibres can be stretched (like a rubber band) and return to their original length when tension is released. They are highly refractile and are, therefore, seen as shining lines in unstained preparations. Relaxed elastic fibres do not show birefringence, but when stretched the fibres become highly birefringent.

Unlike collagen, elastic fibres are not affected by weak acids or alkalies, or by boiling. However, they are digested by the enzyme elastase.

Chemical Nature

Elastic fibres are composed mainly of a protein called *elastin* which forms their central amorphous core. Elastin is made up of smaller units called *tropoelastin*. Elastin contains a high quantity of the amino acids valine and alanine. Another amino acid called desmosine is found exclusively in elastic tissue. We have seen, above, that the outer fibrils of elastic fibres are composed of the glycoprotein fibrillin (see below).

Elastic fibres of connective tissue are produced by fibroblasts. In some situations elastic tissue can be formed by smooth muscle cells.

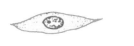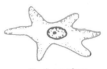

Profile   Surface view

Fig. 4.5. Structure of a fibroblast.

Some Recently Identified Glycoproteins present in connective tissue

1. *Fibrillin* is a glycoprotein that forms microfilaments. We have seen that these filaments are an essential part of elastic fibres (Fig. 4.4). Microfilaments are also present in the mesangium of renal glomeruli, and in the suspensory fibres of the lens. Fibrillin is believed to be responsible for adhesion of different extracellular components to one another. (Also see page 69).

2. *Fibronectin* is present in connective tissue (in the form of fibres). It binds with collagen fibres, and also to cells (through cell adhesion molecules or CAMs, page 9). In this way fibronectin connects collagen fibres to cells of connective tissue. It will be recalled that CAMs are attached (on their cytosolic side) to actin filaments of the cytoskeleton. Fibronectin therefore helps to bring the cytoskeleton into continuity with extracellular fibres.

3. *Laminin* and ***entactin*** are present in basement membranes.

4. *Tenascin* is seen in embryonic tissues. It is believed to play a role in cell migration specially within the developing nervous system.

CELLS OF CONNECTIVE TISSUE

As mentioned earlier, the cells of connective tissue can be divided into those that are intrinsic components of the tissue, and those that belong to the immune system but are commonly seen in connective tissues. In the first group we include fibroblasts, undifferentiated

mesenchymal cells, and pigment cells. Fat cells are commonly seen.

Cells of the immune system to be seen are some varieties of leucocytes and their derivatives. They include the following.

1. Lymphocytes, and plasma cells which are derived from lymphocytes.

2. Monocytes, and macrophages that are derived from monocytes.

3. Mast cells that are related to basophils.

4. Neutrophils and eosinophils are occasionally seen.

Fibroblasts

These are the most numerous cells of connective tissue. They are called fibroblasts because they are concerned with the production of collagen fibres. They also produce reticular and elastic fibres. Where associated with reticular fibres they are usually called ***reticular cells***.

Fibroblasts are present in close relationship to collagen fibres. They are 'fixed' cells i.e., they are not mobile. In tissue sections these cells appear to be spindle shaped, and the nucleus appears to be flattened. When seen from the surface the cells show branching processes (Fig. 4.5).

The nucleus is large, euchromatic, and has prominent nucleoli. The amount of cytoplasm and of organelles varies depending upon activity. In fibroblasts that are inactive the cytoplasm is scanty, organelles are few, and the nucleus may become heterochromatic. Inactive fibroblasts are often called ***fibrocytes***. In contrast to fibrocytes active fibroblasts have abundant cytoplasm (characteristic of cells actively engaged in protein synthesis). The endoplasmic reticulum, the Golgi complex and mitochondria become much more conspicuous. Fibroblasts become very active when there is need to lay down collagen fibres. This occurs, for example, in wound repair. When the need arises fibroblasts can give rise, by division, to more fibroblasts. They are, however, regarded to be specialized cells and cannot convert themselves to other cell types.

The mechanism of the production of collagen fibres by fibroblasts has been extensively studied. Amino acids necessary for synthesis of fibres are taken into the cell. Under the influence of ribosomes located on rough endoplasmic reticulum the amino acids are bonded together to form polypeptide chains (α-chains) (Fig. 4.6). A procollagen molecule is formed by joining together of three such chains. Molecules of procollagen are transported to the exterior of the cell where they are acted upon by enzymes (released by the fibroblast) to form tropocollagen. Collagen fibres are formed by aggregation of tropocollagen molecules. Vitamin C and oxygen are necessary for collagen formation, and wound repair may be interfered with if either of these is deficient. In this connection it may be noted that fibroblast are themselves highly resistant to damaging influences and are not easily destroyed.

There are observations that indicate that the orientation of collagen fibres depends on the stresses imposed on the tissue. If fibroblasts growing in tissue culture are subjected to tension in a particular direction, the cells exposed to the tension multiply faster than others; they orientate themselves along the line of stress; and lay down fibres in that direction. It follows that in the embryo collagen fibres would tend to be laid down wherever they are required to resist a tensile force. In this way tendons, ligaments etc., will tend to develop wherever they are called for. (This cannot, of course, be a complete explanation. Genetic factors must play a prominent role in development of these structures).

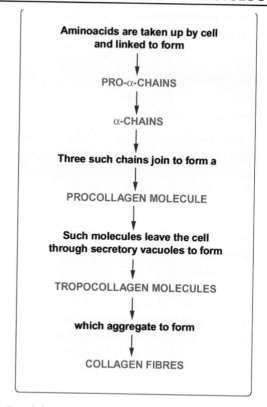

Fig. 4.6. Scheme to show how collagen fibres are synthesized.

Myofibroblasts

Under EM some cells resembling fibroblasts have been shown to contain actin and myosin arranged as in smooth muscle, and are contractile. They have been designated as *myofibroblasts*. In tissue repair such cells probably help in retraction and shrinkage of scar tissue

Undifferentiated Mesenchymal Cells

Embryonic connective tissue is called *mesenchyme*. It is made up of small cells with slender branching processes that join to form a fine network (Fig. 4.7).

It is from such a tissue that the various elements of mature connective tissue are derived. As more specialized types of cells (e.g., fibroblasts) are formed they lose the ability to transform

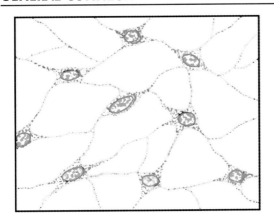

Fig. 4.7. Mesenchymal cells.

themselves into other types. At one time it was believed that fibroblasts were relatively undifferentiated cells, and that when the need arose they could transform themselves into other types. However, it is now believed that mature fibroblasts are not able to do so. It is also believed that some undifferentiated mesenchymal cells persist as such and these are the cells from which other types can be formed when required.

Pigment cells

Pigment cells are easily distinguished as they contain brown pigment (melanin) in their cytoplasm (Fig. 4.8). They are most abundant in connective tissue of the skin, and in the choroid and iris of the eyeball. Along with pigment containing epithelial cells they give the skin, the iris, and the choroid their dark colour. Variations in the number of pigment cells, and in the amount of pigment in them accounts for differences in skin colour of different races, and in different individuals.

Of the many cells that contain pigment in their

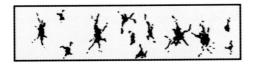

Fig. 4.8. Pigment cells.

cytoplasm only a few are actually capable of synthesizing melanin. Such cells, called *melanocytes*, are of neural crest origin. The remaining cells are those that have engulfed pigment released by other cells. Typically, such cells are star shaped (stellate) with long branching processes. In contrast to melanocytes such cells are called *chromatophores* or *melanophores*. They are probably modified fibroblasts.

Pigment cells prevent light from reaching other cells. The importance of this function in relation to the eyeball is obvious. Pigment cells in the skin protect deeper tissues from the effects of light (specially ultraviolet light). The darker skin of races living in tropical climates is an obvious adaptation for this purpose.

Fat Cells (Adipocytes)

Although some amount of fat (lipids) may be present in the cytoplasm of many cells, including fibroblasts, some cells store fat in large amounts and become distended with it (Fig. 4.12). These are called *fat cells*, *adipocytes*, or *lipocytes*. Aggregations of fat cells constitute *adipose tissue* which is described on page 66.

Macrophage cells

Macrophage cells of connective tissue are part of a large series of cells present in the body that have similar functions. These collectively form the *mononuclear phagocyte system* (Chapter 5).

Macrophage cells of connective tissue are also called *histiocytes* or *clasmatocytes* (Fig. 4.9).

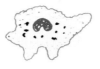

Fig. 4.9.
Macrophage cell
(histiocyte)

They have the ability to phagocytose (eat up) unwanted material. Such material is usually organic: it includes bacteria invading the tissue, and damaged tissues. Macrophages also phagocytose inorganic particles injected into the body (e.g., India ink).

In ordinary preparations of tissue it is difficult to distinguish macrophages from other cells. However, if an animal is injected with India ink (or trypan blue, or lithium carmine) particles of it are taken up into the cytoplasm of macrophages, thus making them easy to recognize.

Macrophages are usually described as 'fixed' when they are attached to fibres; or as motile (or 'free'). Fixed macrophages resemble fibroblasts in appearance, but free macrophages are rounded. However, all macrophages are capable of becoming mobile when suitably stimulated. The nuclei of macrophages are smaller, and stain more intensely than those of fibroblasts. They are often kidney shaped. With the EM the cytoplasm is seen to contain numerous lysosomes (page 19) which help in 'digesting' material phagocytosed by the macrophage. Sometimes macrophages may fuse together to form multinucleated **giant cells**.

Apart from direct phagocytic activity, macrophages play an important role in immunological mechanisms. These are considered in Chapter 5.

Mast Cells

These are small round or oval cells (also called **mastocytes**, or **histaminocytes**)(Fig. 4.10). The

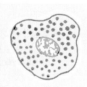

Fig. 4.10.
Mast cell.

nucleus is small and centrally placed. Irregular microvilli (filopodia) are present on the cell surface. The distinguishing feature of these cells is the presence of numerous granules in the cytoplasm. The granules can be demonstrated with the PAS stain. They also stain with dyes like toluidine blue or alcian blue: with them the nuclei stain blue, but the granules stain purple to red. (When components of a cell or tissue stain in a colour different from that of the dye used, the staining is said to be **metachromatic**). On the basis of the staining reactions the granules are known to contain acid mucopolysaccharides. With the EM the 'granules' are seen to be vesicles, each of which is surrounded by a membrane. (In other words they are membrane bound vesicles).

Mast cells are believed to release various substances when appropriately stimulated. The most important of these is histamine. Release of histamine is associated with the production of allergic reactions when a tissue is exposed to an antigen to which it is sensitive (because of previous exposure). In this context it is believed that the cell membranes of mast cells contain antibodies which react with the antigen. This leads to rupture of the cells with discharge of histamine. The discharge in turn leads to local reactions like urticaria, or to severe general reactions like anaphylactic shock.

Apart from histamine mast cells may contain various enzymes, and factors that attract eosinophils or neutrophils.

Mast cells differ considerably in size and in number from species to species, and at different sites in the same animal. They are most frequently seen around blood vessels and nerves. Mast cells are probably related in their origin to basophils of blood. They may represent modified basophil cells.

Lymphocytes

Lymphocytes represent one variety of leucocytes (white blood cells) present in blood. Large aggregations of lymphocytes are present in lymphoid tissues. They reach connective tissue from these sources, and are specially numerous when the tissue undergoes inflammation. Lymphocytes play an important role in defence of the body against invasion by bacteria and other organisms. They have the ability to recognize substances that are foreign to the host body; and to destroy these invaders by producing antibodies against them. Lymphocytes will be considered in detail in Chapter 5. Here it will suffice to note that lymphocytes are derived from stem cells present in bone marrow. They are of two types. *B-lymphocytes* pass through blood to reach other tissues directly. Some B-lymphocytes mature into *plasma cells* described below. The second type of lymphocytes, called *T-lymphocytes*, travel (through blood) from bone marrow to the thymus. After undergoing a process of maturation in this organ they again enter the blood stream to reach other tissues. Both B-lymphocytes and T-lymphocytes can be seen in connective tissue.

Other Leucocytes

Apart from lymphocytes two other types of leucocytes may be seen in connective tissue. *Monocytes* are closely related in function to macrophages. *Eosinophils* (so called because of the presence of eosinophilic granules in the cytoplasm) are found in the connective tissue of many organs. They increase in number in allergic disorders.

Plasma Cells or Plasmatocytes

Very few plasma cells can be seen in normal connective tissue. Their number increases in the

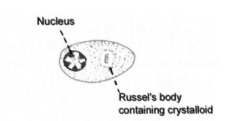

Fig. 4.11. Plasma cell.

presence of certain types of inflammation. It is believed that plasma cells represent B-lymphocytes that have matured and have lost their power of further division.

With the light microscope a plasma cell is seen to be small and rounded (Fig. 4.11). It can be recognized by the fact that the chromatin in its nucleus forms four or five clumps near the periphery (of the nucleus) thus giving the nucleus a resemblance to a cart-wheel. The cytoplasm is basophilic. With the EM the basophilia is seen to be due to the fact that the cytoplasm is filled with rough endoplasmic reticulum, except for a small region near the nucleus where a well developed Golgi complex is located.

Both these features are indicative of the fact that plasma cells are engaged in considerable synthetic activity. They produce antibodies which may be discharged locally; may enter the circulation; or may be stored within the cell itself in the form of inclusions called *Russell's bodies*.

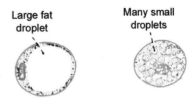

Fig. 4.12. Comparison of a normal fat cell with one in brown fat.

ADIPOSE TISSUE

Structure of Adipose Tissue

Adipose tissue is basically an aggregation of fat cells, also called adipocytes (page 63). Each fat cell contains a large droplet of fat that almost fills it (Fig. 4.12). As a result the cell becomes rounded. (When several fat cells are closely packed, they become polygonal because of mutual pressure: See Fig. 4.13). The cytoplasm of the cell forms a thin layer just deep to the plasma membrane. The nucleus is pushed against the plasma membrane and is flattened.

Fat cells can be seen easily by spreading out a small piece of fresh omentum taken from an animal, on a slide. They are best seen in regions where the layer of fat is thin. The fat content can be brightly stained by using certain dyes (Sudan III, Sudan IV) (Fig. 4.14). During the preparation of usual class room slides, the tissues have to be treated with fat solvents (like xylene or benzene) which dissolve out the fat, so that in such preparations fat cells look like rounded empty spaces (Fig. 4.13). The fat content of the cells can be preserved by cutting sections after freezing the tissue (frozen sections): in this process the tissue is not exposed to fat solvents.

Fat cells may be scattered singly in some situations, but they are usually aggregated into groups that form lobules of adipose tissue. The cells are supported by reticular fibres, and the lobules are held together by areolar tissue. Adipose tissue is richly supplied with blood, and is rich in enzyme systems.

Distribution of Adipose Tissue

Adipose tissue is distributed as follows.

1. It is present in the superficial fascia over most

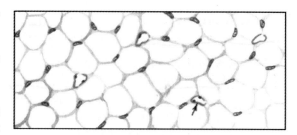

Fig. 4.13. Adipose tissue as seen in a routine paraffin section. The cells look empty as the fat dissolves during processing of tissue.

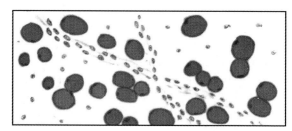

Fig. 4.14. Fat cells in a stretch preparation of omentum stained with a specific stain for fat (Sudan IV).

of the body. This subcutaneous layer of fat is called the ***panniculus adiposus***. It is responsible for giving a smooth contour to the skin. However, fat is not present in the superficial fascia of the eyelids, the scrotum and the penis. The distribution of subcutaneous fat in different parts of the body is also different in the male and female and is responsible (to a great extent) for the differences in body contours in the two sexes. In women it forms a thicker and more even layer: this is responsible for the soft contours of the female body. Subcutaneous fat is not present in animals who have a thick coat of fur.

2. Adipose tissue fills several hollow spaces in the body. These include the orbits, the axillae and the ischiorectal fossae. In the adult much of the space in marrow cavities of long bones is filled by fat in the form of yellow bone marrow. Much fat is also present in synovial folds of many joints filling spaces that would otherwise have been empty during certain phases of movement.

3. Fat is present around many abdominal organs, specially the kidneys (***perinephric fat***).

4. Considerable amounts of fat may be stored in the greater omentum, and in other peritoneal folds.

Functions of Adipose Tissue

Various functions have been attributed to adipose tissue.

(a) It acts as a store house of nutrition, fat being deposited when available in excess; and being removed when deficient in the diet.

(b) In many situations fat performs a mechanical function. The fat around the kidneys keeps them in position. If there is a sudden depletion of this fat the kidneys may become mobile (***floating kidney***). The fat around the eyeball performs an important supporting function and allows the eyeball to move smoothly. In the palms and soles, and over the buttocks fat has a cushioning effect protecting underlying tissues from pressure. In such areas adipose tissue may contain many elastic fibres.

It has been observed that in situations in which the presence of fat serves an important mechanical function, this fat is the last to be depleted in prolonged starvation.

(c) The subcutaneous fat has been regarded as an insulation against heat loss, and would certainly perform this function if the layer of adipose tissue is thick. This may be one reason why girls (who have a thicker layer of subcutaneous fat) feel less cold than boys at the same temperature. The whale (a warm blooded mammal) can survive in very cold water because it has a very thick layer of subcutaneous fat.

(d) Some workers feel that adipose tissue contributes to warmth, not so much by acting as an insulator, but by serving as a heat generator. The heat generated can be rapidly passed on to neighbouring tissues because of the rich blood supply of adipose tissue.

Some further details about Adipose Tissue

Some earlier workers regarded fat cells to be merely fibroblasts that had accumulated fat in their cytoplasm. They believed that after the fat was discharged the fat cell reverted to a fibroblast. However, most authorities now believe that fat cells are derived from specific cells (***lipoblasts***) arising during development from undifferentiated mesenchymal cells: they regard adipose tissue to be a specialized tissue. Some observations that point in this direction are as follows.

(a) When an animal puts on fat it is because of an increase in the size of fat cells rather than an increase in their number.

(b) Mature adipose tissue does not appear to have any capacity for regeneration. If a pad of fat is partially excised compensatory hypertrophy cannot be observed in the remaining part.

(c) In man the fat in fats cells is in the form of triglyceride: it consists mainly of oleic acid, and of smaller amounts of lineolic and palmitic acids. The composition of fat differs from species to species and is influenced by diet. The esterification of triglyceride results in the liberation of large amounts of heat.

Removal of fat from adipose tissue (for use by the body) is under nervous and hormonal control. Sympathetic nerve endings are present in adipose tissue. Fat cells bear receptors for various hormones that regulate release of fat (insulin, glucocorticoids, thyroid hormone, norepinephrine).

Brown Adipose Tissue

In some parts of the body adipose tissue has a brownish colour (in distinction to the yellowish colour of ordinary fat). The cells in this type of tissue differ from those in ordinary adipose tissue as follows.

(**a**) They are smaller than in typical adipose tissue.

(**b**) The fat in the cytoplasm occurs in the form of several small droplets. Hence brown fat is also called *multilocular adipose tissue* (while the typical variety is described as *unilocular adipose tisue*).

(**c**) The cytoplasm and nucleus of the cell are not pushed to the periphery. The cytoplasm contains numerous mitochondria (which are few in typical fat cells).

Brown adipose tissue is abundant in the new born, but most of it is lost during childhood. Brown fat is also abundant in hibernating animals in whom it serves mainly as a heat generator when the animal comes out of hibernation.

Mucoid Tissue

In contrast to all the connective tissues described so far the most conspicuous component of mucoid tissue is a jelly like ground substance rich in hyaluronic acid. Scattered through this ground substance there are star-shaped fibroblasts, some delicate collagen fibres and some rounded cells (Fig. 4.15). This kind of tissue is found in the umbilical cord. The vitreous of the eyeball is a similar tissue.

SUMMARY OF THE FUNCTIONS OF CONNECTIVE TISSUES

Mechanical Functions

1. In the form of loose connective tissue, it holds together structures like skin, muscles,

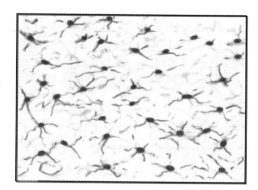

Fig. 4.15. Mucoid tissue.

blood vessels etc. It binds together various layers of hollow viscera. In the form of areolar tissue and reticular tissue it forms a framework that supports the cellular elements of various organs like the spleen, lymph nodes, and glands, and provides capsules for them.

2. The looseness of areolar tissue facilitates movement between structures connected by it. The looseness of superficial fascia enables the movement of skin over deep fascia. In hollow organs this allows for mobility and stretching.

3. In the form of deep fascia connective tissue provides a tight covering for deeper structures (specially in the limbs and neck) and helps to maintain the shape of these regions.

4. In the form of ligaments it holds bone ends together at joints.

5. In the form of deep fascia, intermuscular septa and aponeuroses, connective tissue provides attachment for the origins and insertions of many muscles.

6. In the form of tendons it transmits the pull of muscles to their insertion.

7. Thickened areas of deep fascia form retinacula which hold tendons in place at the wrist and ankle.

8. Both areolar tissue and fascial membranes provide planes along which blood vessels, lymphatics, and nerves travel. The superficial fascia provides passage to vessels and nerves going to the skin, and supports them.

9. In the form of dura mater it provides support to the brain and spinal cord.

Other functions

(**a**) In the form of adipose tissue it provides a store of nutrition. In cold weather the fat provides insulation and helps to generate heat.

(**b**) Because of the presence of cells of the immune system (macrophages and plasma cells), connective tissue helps the body to fight against invading foreign substances (including bacteria) by destroying them, or by producing antibodies against them.

(**c**) Because of the presence of fibroblasts connective tissue helps in laying down collagen fibres necessary for wound repair.

(**d**) By virtue of the presence of undifferentiated mesenchymal cells connective tissue can help in regeneration of tissues (e.g., cartilage and bone) by providing cells from which specialized cells can be formed.

(**e**) Deep fascia plays a very important role in facilitating venous return from the limbs (specially the lower limbs). When muscles of the limb contract, their outward expansion is limited by the deep fascia. As a result, veins deep to the fascia are pressed upon. Because of the presence of valves in the veins, this pressure causes blood to flow towards the heart. In this way deep fascia enables muscles to act as pumps that push venous blood towards the heart.

Some diseases of Connective Tissue

Mutations in genes that are responsible for production of collagen can lead to a number of diseases. The main feature of these diseases is that there is reduced strength in the tissues concerned. Collagen plays an important role in giving strength to bone (Chapter 7). When collagen is not properly formed bones are weak and break easily. This condition is called *osteogenesis imperfecta*.

In other collagen diseases the skin may become abnormally extensible, and joints may be lax (because of improperly formed ligaments (*Ehlers Danlos syndrome*).

Mutations in genes coding for fibrillin can result in abnormalites in organs where elastic fibres play an important role. For example, there may be subluxations of the lens (due to weakness of the suspensory ligament). The tunica media of the aorta may be weak and this can lead to rupture of the vessel. It appears that fibrillin has something to do with the control of bone growth, and when fibrillin is deficient the person becomes abnormally tall. The features mentioned above constitute *Marfan's syndrome*.

The Blood and the Mononuclear Phagocyte System

5

Blood is regarded as a modified connective tissue because the cellular elements in it are separated by a considerable amount of 'intercellular substance' (see below); and because some of the cells in it have close affinities to cells in general connective tissue.

The Plasma

In contrast to all other connective tissues, the 'intercellular substance' of blood is a liquid called

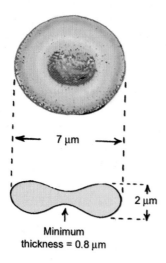

Fig. 5.1. Average dimensions of an erythrocyte. The erythrocyte is seen in surface view (A), and in profile (B)

plasma. The cellular elements float freely in the plasma. Plasma consists of water in which are dissolved *colloids* and *crystalloids*. The colloids are proteins including prothrombin (associated with the clotting of blood), immunoglobulins (involved in immunological defence mechanisms), hormones etc. The crystalloids are ions of sodium, chloride, potassium, calcium, magnesium, phosphate, bicarbonate etc. Several other substances like glucose and amino acids are also present.

About 55% of the total volume of blood is plasma, the rest being constituted by the cellular elements described below.

Cellular Elements of Blood

The cellular or formed elements of blood are of three main types. These are *red blood corpuscles* or *erythrocytes*, *white blood corpuscles* or *leucocytes*, and *blood platelets*. We refer to them as 'cellular' or 'formed' elements rather than as cells because of the fact that red blood corpuscles are not strictly cells (see below). However, in practice, the terms red blood cells and white blood cells are commonly used.

We have seen that about 55% of the total volume

of blood is accounted for by plasma. Most of the remaining 45% is made up of red blood corpuscles, the leucocytes and platelets constituting less than 1% of the volume. If we take one cubic millimetre (mm³ = microlitre or μl) of blood we find that it contains about five million erythrocytes. In comparison there are only about 7000 leucocytes in the same volume of blood.

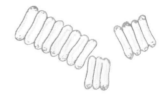

Fig. 5.2. Erythrocytes in rouleaux formation.

ERYTHROCYTES
(Red Blood Corpuscles)

When seen in surface view each erythrocyte is a circular disc having a diameter of about 7 μm (6.5-8.5 μm). When viewed from the side it is seen to be biconcave, the maximum thickness being about 2 μm (Fig. 5.1). Erythrocytes are cells that have lost their nuclei (and other organelles). They are bounded by a plasma membrane. They contain a red coloured protein called *haemoglobin*. It is because of the presence of haemoglobin that erythrocytes (and blood as a whole) are red in colour. Haemoglobin plays an important role in carrying oxygen from the lungs to all tissues of the body. In a healthy person there are about 15 g of haemoglobin in every 100 ml of blood.

When erythrocytes are seen in a film of blood spread out on a slide, they appear yellow (or pale red) in colour. Their rims (being thicker) appear darker than the central parts. When suspended in a suitable medium erythrocytes often appear to be piled over one another: this is described as *rouleaux formation* (Fig. 5.2). If a piece of transparent tissue (e.g., omentum) of a living animal is placed under a microscope, and a capillary focused, erythrocytes can be seen moving through the capillary. When thus examined it is seen that erythrocytes can alter their shape to pass through capillaries that are much narrower than the diameter of the erythrocytes.

Erythrocytes maintain their normal shape only if suspended in an isotonic solution. If the surrounding medium becomes hypotonic the cells absorb water, swell up, and ultimately burst: this is called *haemolysis*. Alternatively, if erythrocytes are placed in a hypertonic solution, they shrink and their surfaces develop irregularities (*crenation*). Such cells are sometimes called *echinocytes*.

Erythrocytes are formed in bone marrow from where they enter the blood stream. Each erythrocyte has a life of about 100 to 120 days at the end of which it is removed from blood by cells of the mononuclear phagocyte system (specially in the spleen and bone marrow). The constituents of erythrocytes are broken down and reused to form new erythrocytes.

Like cell membranes of other cells, the plasma membranes of erythrocytes are composed of lipids and proteins. Several types of proteins are present, including *ABO antigens* responsible for a person's blood group.

The shape of erythrocytes is maintained by a cytoskeleton made up of the protein *spectrin*. Spectrin filaments are anchored to the cell membrane by another protein *ankyrin*. Actin filaments and some other proteins are also present.

Haemoglobin consists of molecules of *globulin* bound to an iron containing porphyrin called *haem*. Each globulin molecule is made up of a group of four polypeptide chains. The composition of the polypeptide chains is variable, and as a result several types of haemoglobin can exist. Most of normal adult haemoglobin is classified as Haemoglobin A (HbA). Haemoglobin A (HbA$_2$) is also present. Abnormal forms of haemoglobin include haemoglobin S (in sickle cell disease).

Apart from haemoglobin, erythrocytes contain enzyme systems which control pH by adjusting sodium levels within the erythrocytes. They derive energy by anaerobic metabolism of glucose and by ATP generation (via a hexose monophosphate shunt).

Fetal erythrocytes are nucleated and contain a different form of haemoglobin (HbF). However, in the later part of fetal life the erythrocytes are progressively replaced by those of the adult type.

Anaemia

Deficiency of haemoglobin in blood is called *anaemia*. Anaemia is commonly produced by deficiency of iron in diet. In this kind of anaemia red blood cells are small (*microcytic*) and pale staining (*hypochromic*). Another cause of anaemia is recurrent bleeding from any cause (e.g., excessive menstrual bleeding, infestation with hook worms etc.). Anaemia can also result from excessive destruction of red blood cells (*haemolytic anaemia*). This is more likely to occur when red blood cells are abnormal. One such abnormality is caused by absence of ankyrin (see above) so that red blood cells become spherical (*spherocytosis*) rather than biconcave. Excessive cell destruction also occurs in sickle cell disease (see above), and in malaria.

LEUCOCYTES
(White Blood Corpuscles)

Differences between Erythrocytes and Leucocytes

Leucocytes are different from erythrocytes in several ways.

(**a**) They are true cells, each leucocyte having a nucleus, mitochondria, Golgi complex, and other organelles.

(**b**) They do not contain haemoglobin and, therefore, appear colourless in unstained preparations.

(**c**) Unlike erythrocytes which do not have any mobility of their own, leucocytes can move actively.

(**d**) As a corollary of (c) erythrocytes do not normally leave the vascular system, but leucocytes can move out of it to enter surrounding tissues. In fact blood is merely a route by which leucocytes travel from bone marrow to other destinations.

(**e**) Most leucocytes have a relatively short life span (page 74).

Features of different types of leucocytes

Leucocytes are of various types. Some of them have granules in their cytoplasm and are, therefore, called *granulocytes*. Depending on the staining characters of their granules granulocytes are further divided into *neutrophil leucocytes* (or *neutrophils*), *eosinophil leucocytes* (or *eosinophils*), and *basophil leucocytes* (or *basophils*).

Apart from these granulocytes there are two

types of agranular leucocytes. These are *lymphocytes* and *monocytes* (Fig. 5.10).

Apart from the presence or absence of granules, and their nature, the different types of leucocytes show various other differences. In describing the differences it is usual for text books to consider all features of one type of leucocyte together. However, in practice, it is more useful to take the features one by one and to compare each feature in the different types of leucocytes as given below.

Relative number

We have seen that there are about 7000 leucocytes (range 5000-10000) in every cubic millimetre (=mm^3=μl) of blood. Of these about two thirds (60-70%) are neutrophils, and about one fourth (20-30%) are lymphocytes. The remaining types are present in very small numbers. The eosinophils are about 3%, the basophils about 1%, and the monocytes about 5%. The relative and absolute numbers of the different types of leucocytes vary considerably in health; and to a more marked degree in disease. Estimations of their numbers provide valuable information for diagnosis of many diseases. In this connection it is to be stressed that absolute numbers are more significant than percentages. In a healthy individual neutrophils are 3000-6000/μl; lymphocytes 1500-2700/μl; monocytes 100-700/μl; eosinophils 100-400/μl; and basophils 25-200/μl.

Relative size

Leucocytes are generally examined in thin films of blood that are spread out on glass slides. In the process of making such films the cells are flattened and, therefore, appear somewhat larger than they are when suspended in a fluid medium. In a dry film all types of granulocytes, and

monocytes are about 10 μm in diameter. Most lymphocytes are distinctly smaller (6-8 μm) and are called small lymphocytes, but some (called large lymphocytes) measure 12-15 μm.

Nuclei

In lymphocytes the nucleus is spherical, but may show an indentation on one side (Fig. 5.3). It stains densely in small lymphocytes, but tends to be partly euchromatic in large lymphocytes. In monocytes the nucleus is ovoid and may be indented: it is placed eccentrically. In basophils the nucleus is S-shaped. The nucleus of the eosinophil leucocyte is made up of two or three lobes that are joined by delicate strands. In neutrophil leucocytes the nucleus is very variable in shape and consists of several lobes (up to 6): that is why these cells are also called *polymorphonuclear leucocytes*, or simply *polymorphs*. The number of lobes increases with the life of the cell. (Also see sex chromatin, page 42).

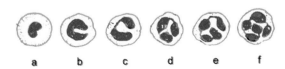

Fig. 5.3. Neutrophile leucosytes (b to f) showing varying numbers of lobes in their nuclei. A metamyelocyte is shown at 'a' for comparison.

Cytoplasm

The cytoplasm of a lymphocyte is scanty and forms a thin rim around the nucleus. It is clear blue in stained preparations. In monocytes the cytoplasm is abundant. It stains blue, but in contrast to the 'transparent' appearance in lymphocytes the cytoplasm of monocytes is like frosted glass. Granules are not present in the cytoplasm of lymphocytes or of monocytes. The cytoplasm of granulocytes is marked by the

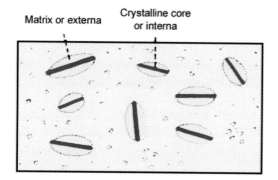

Fig. 5.4. Granules of eosinophil leucocyte
as seen by EM.

presence of numerous granules. In neutrophils
the granules are very fine and stain lightly with
both acidic and basic dyes. The granules of
neutrophils are really lysosomes: they are of
various types depending upon the particular
enzymes present in them. The granules of
eosinophil leucocytes are large and stain brightly
with acid dyes (like eosin). These are also
lysosomes. With the EM the granules are seen to
contain a *crystalloid* (Fig.5.4). The outer part
or *matrix* of each granule contains lysosomal
enzymes. The crystalline core has proteins that
are responsible for red staining. In basophil
leucocytes the cytoplasm contains large spherical
granules that stain with basic dyes; are PAS
positive; and stain metachromatically with some
dyes.

Other cell organelles including mitochondria,
Golgi complex and endoplasmic reticulum are
present in the cytoplasm of leucocytes.
Microtubules are present and probably play a role
in movements of leucocytes. Mitochondria are
particularly abundant in monocytes. Organelles
are sparse in small lymphocytes, but are much
more conspicuous in large lymphocytes.

Motility and Phagocytosis

All leucocytes are capable of amoeboid
movement. Neutrophils and monocytes are the
most active. The eosinophil and basophil
leucocytes move rather slowly. Lymphocytes in
blood show the least power of movement.
However, when they settle on solid surfaces they
become freely motile and can pass through
various tissues.

Because of their motility leucocytes easily pass
through capillaries into surrounding tissues, and
can migrate through the latter. Neutrophils
collect in large numbers at sites of infection. Here
they phagocytose bacteria and use the enzymes
in their lysosomes to destroy the bacteria.
Eosinophils are phagocytic, but their ability to
destroy bacteria is less than that of neutrophils.
Monocytes are also actively phagocytic. Most
monocytes in blood are, in fact, macrophages on
their way to other tissues from bone marrow
(page 87).

Leucocytes in circulating blood are in an inactive
state. To leave the circulation a leucocyte first
adheres to endothelium, and then traverses the
vessel wall. Cytokines (see page 81) which are
present in diseased areas greatly stimulate
adhesion of leucocytes to endothelium and their
migration through the vessel wall.

Life span

We have seen that erythrocytes have a life span
of about 100-120 days. The life of a neutrophil
leucocyte is only about 15 hours. Eosinophils live
for a few days, while basophils can live for 9 to
18 months. The life span of lymphocytes is
variable. Some live only a few days (*short-lived
lymphocytes*) while others may live several years
(*long-lived lymphocytes*).

SOME FURTHER FACTS ABOUT GRANULOCYTES

Some further facts about Neutrophils

1. The granules of neutrophils are of three types. The first formed, or primary, granules are similar to those in lysosomes (page 19). They contain acid hydrolases. They also contain *myeloperoxidase* which is antibacterial. Secondary granules contain substances that are secreted into extracellular spaces and stimulate an inflammatory reaction. Tertiary granules are concerned with adhesion of leucocytes to other cells and their phagocytosis.

2. Neutrophils contain abundant glycogen which provides energy to the cells after they leave the blood stream.

3. Neutrophils die soon after they have phagocytosed materials. Lysosomal enzymes are then released into surrounding tissue causing liquefaction. Pus thus formed consists of dead neutrophils and fluid.

4. Neutrophils bear receptors that can recognize and adhere to foreign particles and bacteria. After adhesion, the neutrophil sends out pseudopodia that surround the foreign matter and phagocytose it (see page 19).

5. Neutrophils are attracted by *chemotaxins* that are produced by dead cells present in areas where there is infection.

6. The motility of neutrophils depends on changing patterns of actin filaments in their cytoplasm.

Some Further Facts About Basophils

1. We have seen, above, that the staining characters of the granules of basophils are very similar to those of mast cells (page 64). Like the granules of mast cells basophils contain histamine. Many authorities, therefore, regard basophils to be precursors of mast cells. (However, differences in reactions to monoclonal antibodies suggest that even though basophils and mast cells are closely related they may be distinct cell types).

2. In addition to histamine, basophils contain heparin, chondroitin sulphate and leukotriene 3 (see below) which are also present in mast cells. Antibodies (produced by lymphocytes in the presence of antigens) get attached to the cell membranes of basophils and mast cells, and this leads to release of histamine into surrounding tissue. This phenomenon is described as the *immediate hypersensitivity reaction*. This reaction can lead to conditions like urticaria, asthma or allergic rhinitis.

For interactions between basophils and eosinophils see below.

Some Further Facts About Eosinophils

1. The number of eosinophils (in blood and tissues) is greatly increased in some allergic conditions, and in parasitic infestations.

2. Eosinophils have a functional correlation with basophils (and mast cells) as follows.

(a) We have seen that when stimulated by antigens mast cells release histamine (and other substances) into tissues, and set up an allergic reaction. Eosinophils are attracted (chemotactically) to the matter released by mast cells. They try to reduce and localize the allergic reaction by neutralizing histamine. They also release factors that prevent further degranulation of mast cells. Leukotriene 3 released by mast cells is also inhibited by eosinophils.

3. In addition to the main granules (which are large), EM studies reveal small granules in mature eosinophils. These granules have been shown to contain the enzymes acid phosphatase and aryl sulphatase. These enzymes are probably secreted into surrounding tissues.

4. The number of eosinophils (in blood and in tissues) shows a circadian rhythm, being greatest in the morning and least in the afternoon.

FURTHER FACTS ABOUT LYMPHOCYTES

We have seen that lymphocytes are numerous and constitute about 20-30% of all leucocytes in blood. Large numbers of lymphocytes are also present in bone marrow, and as aggregations in various lymphatic tissues.

The distinction between small and large lymphocytes has been mentioned. Small lymphocytes with dense nuclei, and sparse cytoplasm and organelles, are regarded as resting cells. Large lymphocytes include two types of cells. Some of them are *lymphoblasts* that are capable of dividing to form small lymphocytes.

Other large lymphocytes are mature cells that have been stimulated because of the presence of antigens.

Formation and Circulation of Lymphocytes

In the embryo lymphocytes are derived from mesenchymal cells present in the wall of the yolk sac, in the liver and in the spleen. These stem cells later migrate to bone marrow. Lymphocytes formed from these stem cells (in bone marrow) enter the blood. Depending on their subsequent behaviour they are classified into two types.

(**1**) Some of them travel in the blood stream to reach the thymus. Here they divide repeatedly and undergo certain changes. They are now

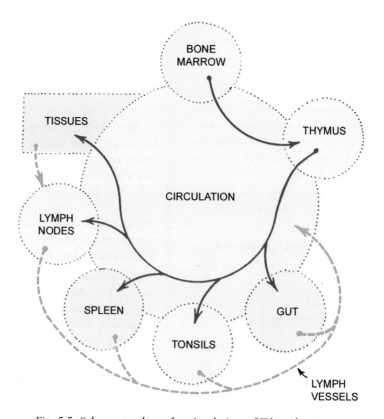

Fig. 5.5. Scheme to show the circulation of T-lymphoctes.

called *T-lymphocytes* ('T' from thymus). These T-lymphocytes, that have been 'processed' in the thymus re-enter the circulation to reach lymphoid tissue in lymph nodes, spleen, tonsils and intestines.

In lymph nodes T-lymphocytes are found in the diffuse tissue around lymphatic nodules. In the spleen they are found in white pulp (Chapter 11). From these masses of lymphoid tissue many lymphocytes pass into lymph vessels, and through them they go back into the circulation. In this way lymphocytes keep passing out of blood into lymphoid tissue (and bone marrow), and back from these into the blood. About 85% of lymphocytes seen in blood are T-lymphocytes (Fig. 5.5).

(2) Lymphocytes of a second group arising from stem cells in bone marrow enter the blood stream, but do not go to the thymus. They go directly to lymphoid tissues (other than the thymus). Such lymphocytes are called *B-lymphocytes* ('B' from *bursa of Fabricus*, a diverticulum of the cloaca in birds: in birds B-lymphocytes are formed here). In contrast to T-lymphocytes which lie in the diffuse lymphoid tissue of the lymph nodes and spleen, B-lymphocytes are seen in lymphatic nodules. The germinal centres are formed by actively dividing B-lymphocytes, while the dark rims of lymphatic nodules are formed by dense aggregations of B-lymphocytes. Like T-lymphocytes, B-lymphocytes also circulate between lymphoid tissues and the blood stream (Fig. 5.6).

It has been suggested that B-lymphocytes also

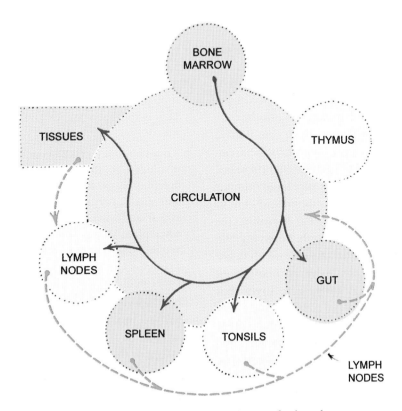

Fig. 5.6. Scheme to show the circulation of B-lymphocytes.

undergo a process of maturation (similar to that of T-lymphocytes in the thymus), but the site at which this happens is not certain. Most workers are of the opinion that maturation of B-lymphocytes takes place in the bone marrow itself. Another site suggested for this is mucosa associated lymphoid tissue of the gut (Chapter 11).

Lymphocytes & The Immune System

Lymphocytes are an essential part of the *immune system* of the body that is responsible for defence against invasion by bacteria and other organisms. In contrast to granulocytes and monocytes which directly attack invading organisms, lymphocytes help to destroy them by producing substances called *antibodies*. These are protein molecules that have the ability to recognize a 'foreign' protein (i.e., a protein not normally present in the individual). The foreign protein is usually referred to as an *antigen*. An antigen may be part of an invading bacterium or other organism. It may be cellular (as when blood is transfused from one person to another, or when a tissue is transplanted from one person to another). It will be appreciated that there can be a very large number of such foreign proteins. The body itself also contains a very large number of proteins of its own. For any defence system to be effective it is necessary that lymphocytes should be able to distinguish between the proteins of the individual and those that are foreign to it. Every antigen can be neutralized only by a specific antibody. It follows that lymphocytes must be capable of producing a very wide range of antibodies; or rather that there must be a very wide variety of lymphocytes each variety programmed to recognize a specific antigen and to produce antibodies against it.

This function of antibody production is done by B-lymphocytes. When stimulated by the presence of antigen the cells enlarge and get converted to plasma cells. The plasma cells produce antibodies.

Antibodies are also called *immunoglobulins*. These are Y-shaped proteins. One end (called the *Fab fraction*) binds to antigen. The other end (Fc) can attach itself to any cell that has suitable receptors on its surface. Immunoglobulins are of five main types viz., IgG, IgM, IgA, IgE and IgD.

Antibodies enter the circulation and act against the antigen in various ways as follows.

(a) They directly bind with the antigen (agglutination) and make it inactive or destroy it.

(b) The antibody may get attached to other cells (e.g., macrophages, neutrophils) conferring on them the ability to detect antigen and ingest it.

(c) The antibody may bind to other B-lymphocytes and stimulate their transformation to plasma cells which produce more antibody.

(d) Some B-lymphocytes to which antibody gets attached have a long life. These cells (and their progeny) are able to 'remember' antigens that have once invaded the body, and react more strongly to them if they invade the body again. This is the basis for long term immunisation against diseases.

B-lymphocytes, plasma cells, and the antibodies produced by them are the basis of what is described as the *humoral immune response* to antigens. Initially, all B-lymphocytes produce similar antibodies, but subsequently specialization takes place to produce antibodies for specific antigens only. Those B-lymphocytes that produce antibodies against normal body proteins are eliminated.

T-lymphocytes are also concerned with immune responses, but their role is somewhat different from that of B-lymphocytes. T-lymphocytes specialize in recognizing cells that are foreign to the host body. These may be fungi, virus infected cells, tumour cells, or cells of another individual. T-lymphocytes have surface receptors which recognize specific antigens (there being many varieties of T-lymphocytes each type recognizing a specific antigen). When exposed to a suitable stimulus the T-lymphocytes multiply and form large cells which can destroy abnormal cells by direct contact, or by producing cytotoxic substances called *cytokines* or *lymphokines* (See below). From the above it will be seen that while B-lymphocytes defend the body through blood borne antibodies, T-lymphocytes are responsible for cell mediated immune responses (*cellular immunity*). T-lymphocytes can also influence the immune responses of B-lymphocytes as well as those of other T-lymphocytes; and also those of non-lymphocytic cells.

Like B-lymphocytes some T-lymphocytes also retain a memory of antigens encountered by them, and they can respond more strongly when the same antigens are encountered again.

The destruction of foreign cells by T-lymphocytes is responsible for the 'rejection' of tissues or organs grafted from one person to another. Such rejection is one of the major problems in organ transplantation.

Investigations using sophisticated techniques have established that T-lymphocytes can be divided into several categories as follows.

(a) *Cytotoxic T-cells (TC cells)* attack and destroy other cells by release of lysosomal proteins. They have the ability to recognize proteins that are foreign to the host body.

(b) *Delayed type hypersensitivity related T-cells* synthesize and release lymphokines when they come in contact with antigens. Lymphokines attract macrophages into the area. They also stimulate macrophages to destroy the antigen. One type of cytokine called interleukin-2 stimulates the proliferation of both B-lymphocytes and T-lymphocytes.

(c) *Helper T-cells* (or *TH cells*) play a rather indirect role in stimulating production of antibodies by B-lymphocytes. When a macrophage ingests an antigen some products of antigen breakdown pass to the cell surface. Here they combine with special molecules (Class II MHC molecules) present in the cell membrane. This complex of antigen remnant and MHC protein, present on the macrophage, can be recognized by helper T-cells. When helper T-cells come in contact with this complex they look for B-lymphocytes capable of producing antibody against the particular antigen. They then stimulate these B-lymphocytes to multiply so that large numbers of B-lymphocytes capable of producing antibody against the particular antigen are produced. This is how immunity against the particular antigen is acquired. Helper T-cells are specifically destroyed by the virus responsible for AIDS resulting in a loss of immunity (See below).

(d) *Suppresser T-cells* (or *TS cells*) have a role opposite to that of helper T-cells. They suppress the activities of B-lymphocytes and of other T-lymphocytes. The possibility of such suppression allows fine control of the activities of lymphocytes.

(e) *Natural killer cells* are similar to cytotoxic T-cells, but their actions are less specific than those of the latter. These cells can destroy virus infected cells and some tumour cells. Their structure is somewhat different from that of typical lymphocytes.

Natural killer cells are regarded by some as a third variety of lymphocytes (in addition to B-lymphocytes and T-lymphocytes) as markers in them are different from those in typical T-lymphocytes (See below).

Markers for cells of immune system

Many proteins that are specific to cells of the immune system are now recognized. These may be cytosolic or cell membrane proteins. Using antibodies specific to these proteins it is possible to identify many varieties of lymphocytes and macrophages. The proteins are called *cluster designation (CD) molecules*, and are designated by number (CD-1, CD-2 etc.).

The virus (HIV) which causes the disease called

5.7. CYTOKINES PRODUCED BY DIFFERENT CELLS

CELL TYPE	CYTOKINES PRODUCED										
	IL-1	IL-2	IL-3	IL-5	IL-6	IL-8	IL-9	G-CSF	M-CSF	GM-CSF	Stem cell factor
T-LYMPHOCYTES		+	+	+	+					+	
MONOCYTES	+				+	+	+	+	+		
ENDOTHELIUM								+	+		+
FIBROBLASTS	+				+	+		+	+		+

5.8. CYTOKINES THAT STIMULATE PRODUCTION OF BLOOD CELLS OR ACTIVATE THEM

CELL TYPE	CYTOKINES STIMULATING THEM										
	IL-2	IL-3	IL-5	IL-6	IL-8	IL-9	IL-11	G-CSF	M-CSF	GM-CSF	Erythro-poietin
GRANULOCYTE PRECURSORS								+		+	
EOSINOPHIL & BASOPHIL PRECURSORS			+								
NEUTROPHIL ACTIVATION					+						
MONOCYTE ACTIVATION	+										
MONOCYTE PRECURSORS							+		+	+	
ERYTHROCYTE PRECURSORS						+					+
MEGAKARYOCYTE PRECURSORS		+		+		+					+
T-CELL PRODUCTION	+										

AIDS (acquired immune deficiency syndrome) attaches itself to the protein CD-4 present on the cell membrane, and destroys cells bearing this protein. Reduction in the number of CD-4 bearing lymphocytes is an important indicator of the progress of AIDS.

Cytokines (Lymphokines)

We have seen that T-lymphocytes produce cytokines that affect other cells. The main function of these cytokines is to stimulate production of blood cells and their precursors. Apart from T-cells, cytokines are also produced by monocytes, macrophages, some fibroblasts, and some endothelial cells. Some cytokines that have been identified are as follows.

1. Interleukins are of eleven known types (IL-1 to IL-11).

2. Granulocyte macrophage colony stimulating factor (GM-CSF).

3. Granulocyte colony stimulating factor (G-CSF).

4. Macrophage colony stimulating factor (M-CSF).

5. Stem cell factor.

6. Erythropoietin.

The cytokines produced by different types of cells are summarized in Table 5.7. The cytokines stimulating production of different blood cells are given in Table 5.8.

Lukaemias

Lukaemia is a condition in which there is uncontrolled production of leucocytes by bone marrow. It is a malignant, life threatening, condition. Leucocyte precursors, normally confined to bone marrow, are seen in large numbers in peripheral blood.

Lukaemias are of different types depending on the type of leucocytes, or leucocyte precursors,

that are proliferating. When progress of the disease is slow (chronic lukaemia) the proliferating cells get time to differentiate, and they can be recognized. However, in acute lukaemias the peripheral blood is flooded with undifferentiated precursors of leucocytes.

BLOOD PLATELETS

Blood platelets are round, oval, or irregular discs about 3 μm in diameter. They are also known as **thrombocytes**. The discs are biconvex. Each disc is bounded by a plasma membrane within which there are mitochondria and membrane bound vesicles. There is no nucleus. In ordinary blood films the platelets appear to have a clear outer zone (**hyalomere**) and a granular central part (**granulomere**).

Platelets are concerned with the clotting of blood. As soon as blood is shed from a vessel, platelets stick to each other and to any available surfaces (specially to collagen fibres). Platelets break down into small granules and threads of fibrin appear around them.

There are about 250,000 to 500,000 platelets per μl of blood. The life of a platelet is about 10 days.

Electronmicroscopy shows that the cell membrane of a platelet is covered by a thick coat of glycoprotein. The presence of this coat facilitates adhesion of the platelet to other surfaces. Apart from the usual organelles the cytoplasm contains microtubules, actin filaments, and myosin filaments which are of importance in clot retraction (See below).

The cytoplasm also contains three main types of membrane bound vesicles (or granules) as follows. **Alpha granules** contain **fibrin** and various other proteins. They also contain a *platelet derived growth factor*. *Delta granules* (or dense granules) contain 5-hydroxytryptamine, calcium ions, ADP and ATP. *Lambda granules* contain lysosomal enzymes (acid hydrolases). A few peroxisomes are also present. During clotting of blood, platelets adhere to one another forming a *platelet plug* that assists in stopping the bleeding. Fibrin is released from alpha granules. Under the influence of various factors fibrin is converted into filaments which form a clot. The actin and myosin filaments (present in platelets) cause the fibrin clot to contract (*clot retraction*). At later stages clot removal is aided by lysosomal enzymes present in platelets.

Deficiency of blood platelets is called *thrombocytopaenia*. It is associated with prolonged bleeding after minor injury. Spontaneous bleeding may occur into skin or other tissues.

FORMATION OF BLOOD (HAEMOPOIESIS)

In embryonic life blood cells are first formed in relation to mesenchymal cells surrounding the yolk sac. After the second month of intrauterine life blood formation starts in the liver; later in the spleen; and still later in the bone marrow. At first lymphocytes are formed along with other cells of blood in bone marrow, but later they are formed mainly in lymphoid tissues. In postnatal life blood formation is confined to bone marrow and lymphoid tissue. However, under conditions in which the bone marrow is unable to meet normal requirements, blood cell formation may start in the liver and spleen. This is referred to as *extramedullary haemopoiesis*.

There has been considerable controversy regarding the origin of various types of blood cells. The *monophyletic theory* holds that all types of blood cells are derived from a common *stem cell*; while according to the *polyphyletic theory* there are several independent types of stem cells. There is no doubt that in the embryo all blood forming cells are derived from mesenchyme, and that the earliest stem cells are capable of forming all types of blood cells. Subsequently the potency of stem cells becomes restricted.

Details of the structure of developing blood cells are beyond the scope of this book. The purpose of the account that follows is mainly to make the student familiar with numerous terms that are used in this connection. We will first study the terms traditionally used for developing blood cells. Some terms based on recent researches will be introduced later.

We have already seen that there are embryonic stem cells that are pleuripotent. Arising from them there are the following.

(a) *Haemopoietic stem cells* or *haemocytoblasts*, that are present (in postnatal life) only in bone marrow and give rise to all blood cells other than lymphocytes.

(b) *Lymphopoietic stem cells* that are present in bone marrow and in lymphoid tissues and give rise to lymphocytes. (Stages in the development of blood cells are illustrated in Fig. 5.10).

Formation of Erythrocytes

Precursor cells of the erythrocyte series are called *erythroblasts* or *normoblasts*. The earliest identifiable precursors of erythrocytes are large cells called *proerythrocytes*. These are succeeded by slightly smaller cells called *early erythroblasts*: these cells do not contain haemoglobin and their cytoplasm is basophil. As haemoglobin begins to be formed some areas of

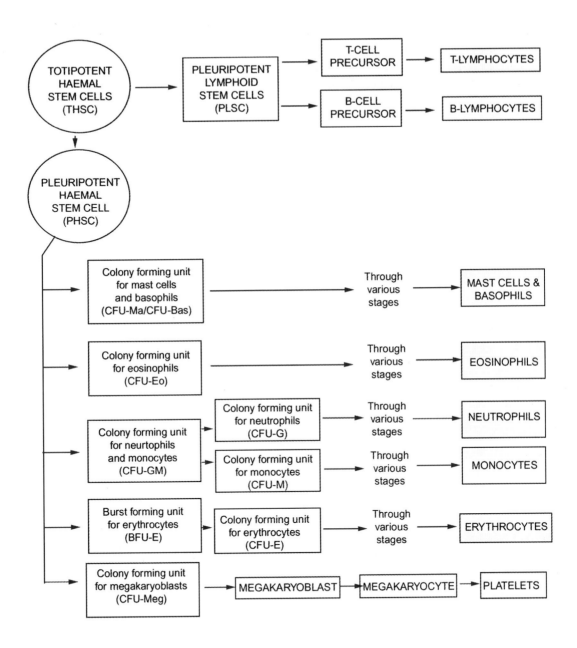

Fig. 5.9. Scheme to show terms currently being used for designating precursors of blood cells.

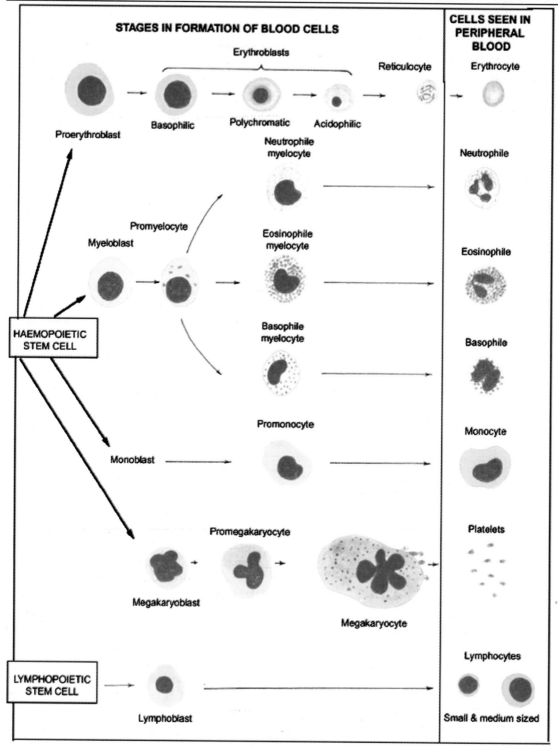

Fig. 5.10. Stages in formation of blood cells (Traditional terms used).

cytoplasm become eosinophil while others remain basophil: such cells are called *intermediate erythroblasts*. As more and more haemoglobin is formed the entire cytoplasm becomes acidophil: these cells are the *final erythroblasts*. Note that during these changes the erythroblasts become progressively smaller. At this stage their nuclei shrink and are thrown out of the cells. The cytoplasm now has a reticular appearance (produced by RNA remaining within it): these cells are, therefore, called *reticulocytes*. Reticulocytes leave the bone marrow and enter the blood stream. Here they lose their reticulum within a day or two and become mature erythrocytes.

Formation of granulocytes

It is believed that neutrophil, eosinophil and basophil leucocytes arise from a common early derivative of the haemopoietic stem cell which is called a *myeloblast*. (It is, however, possible that there may be separate types of myeloblasts for each type of granulocyte). The myeloblast matures into a larger cell called a *promyelocyte* which is marked by the presence of large granules (lysosomes) in its cytoplasm. The promyelocyte now gives rise to *myelocytes* in which the granules are smaller and *specific* so that at this stage neutrophil, eosinophil and basophil myelocytes can be recognized. The nucleus now undergoes transformation dividing into two or three lobes in eosinophil cells; and forming up to six lobes in neutrophils. With the nuclei assuming their distinctive appearance the myelocytes become mature granulocytes.

Formation of Monocytes

Monocytes are also formed in bone marrow from haemopoietic stem cells. Recent evidence (see below) suggests a common origin of monocytes and granulocytes. Early stages in the formation of monocytes are referred to as *monoblasts*. These change into *promonocytes* and finally into mature *monocytes*. We have already noted that the stem cells that give rise to monocytes also give rise to other cells of the mononuclear phagocyte system.

Formation of Platelets

The precursor cells of blood platelets are called *megakaryoblasts*. The megakaryoblast enlarges to form a *promegakaryocyte*. Still further enlargement converts it into a *megakaryocyte*: this cell may be 50 to 100 μm in diameter, and has a multi-lobed nucleus. The nucleus is polyploid because of repeated divisions that are not accompanied by divisions of cytoplasm. Platelets are formed by separation of small masses of cytoplasm from this large cell. Each mass of cytoplasm is covered by cell membrane and contains some endoplasmic reticulum. In this way the cytoplasm of a megakaryocyte becomes subdivided into many small portions each forming one platelet.

Some Recent Insights Into Haemopoiesis

Blood cell formation is currently a subject of great interest to research workers. The methods being used to investigate the subject include cell or organ culture, and experiments based on replacement of bone marrow. Some facts that have emerged as a result of these studies are as follows.

1. Adult bone marrow contains a small number of cells that are totipotent i.e., they can give origin to all types of blood cells. *Totipotent stem cells* can also divide to form new cells of their own type. Totipotent stem cells give rise to *lymphocytic stem cells* and to *pleuripotent haemal stem cells*.

2. Lymphocytic stem cells given origin to all lymphocytes (T and B).

3. Pleuripotent haemal stem cells give origin to three types of cells as follows.

(**a**) Cells that are precursors of erythrocytes.

(**b**) Cells that are precursors of granulocytes *as well as* those of monocytes.

(**c**) Cells that are precursors of megakaryoblasts, and hence of platelets.

A complex terminology has developed for various precursors of blood cells. Unfortunately, there is lack of uniformity in its use, and much of it is based on experiments on rodents. Applicability to humans requires confirmation. In spite of these reservations, it is necessary for medical students to be aware of these developments. Some of the terms used are shown in Fig. 5.9. We will not go into details of these terms here. However, two terms need explanation.

(**1**) *Colony forming units* (CFU) are those cells that multiply to form colonies of a particular type of blood cell.

(**2**) The earliest precursors of erythrocytes multiply very rapidly. This 'explosive' growth gives these cells the name *burst forming units* (BFU).

An important question engaging the attention of reseach workers is the stage up to which blood cell precursors are *self renewing* (i.e., they can divide to forms more cells of their own type). Some authorities hold that only totipotent stem cells have this power, while others believe that some cell types lower down the line may also be self renewing. In leukaemias, one line of treatment is to destroy all cells in the bone marrow of the patient by radiation, and to then tranfuse marrow cells from a normal donor. The procedure has so far had only limited success because most of the transplanted cells survive only for a limited period (as they are not self renewing).

MONONUCLEAR PHAGOCYTE SYSTEM

Distributed widely through the body there are a series of cells that share the property of being able to phagocytose unwanted matter including bacteria and dead cells. These cells also play an important role in defence mechanisms, and in carrying out this function they act in close collaboration with lymphocytes. In the past some of the cells of this system have been included under the term *reticulo-endothelial system*, but this term has now been discarded as it is established that most endothelial cells do not act as macrophages. The term *macrophage system* has also been used for cells of the system, but with the discovery of a close relationship between these cells and mononuclear leucocytes of blood the term *mononuclear phagocyte system* (or *monocyte phagocyte system*) has come into common usage. It is now known that all macrophages are derived from stem cells in bone marrow that also give origin to mononuclear cells of blood.

Cells of mononuclear phagocyte system

The various cells that are usually included in the mononuclear phagocyte system are as follows.

1. Monocytes of blood, and their precursors in bone marrow (monoblasts, promonocytes).

2. Macrophage cells (histiocytes) of connective tissue.

3. Littoral cells (von Kupffer cells) interspersed among cells lining the sinusoids of the liver; and cells in walls of sinusoids in the spleen and lymph nodes.

4. Microglial cells of the central nervous system.

5. Macrophages in pleura, peritoneum, alveoli of lungs, spleen, and in synovial joints.

6. Free macrophages present in pleural, peritoneal and synovial fluids.

7. Dendritic cells of the epidermis, and similar highly branched cells in lymph nodes, spleen and thymus. These are now grouped as *antigen presenting cells* (see below).

Structure of Cells

All cells of the mononuclear phagocyte system have some features in common. They are large cells (15-25 μm) in diameter. The nucleus is euchromatic. Granular and agranular endoplasmic reticulum, Golgi complex and mitochondria are present, as are endocytic vesicles and lysosomes. The cells have irregular surfaces which bear filopodia (irregular microvilli). Most of the cells are more or less oval in shape, but the dendritic cells are highly branched.

Macrophages often form aggregations. In relation to the peritoneum and pleura such aggregations are seen as *milky spots*; and in the spleen they form ellipsoids around small arteries. When they come in contact with large particles, macrophages may fuse to form multinuclear giant cells (*foreign body giant cells*). In the presence of organisms like tubercle bacilli the cells may transform to *epitheloid cells.* (These are involved in T-cell mediated immune responses).

As already mentioned monocytes can be classified into various types depending on the markers present in them, and their relationship to cytokines (Tables 5.7, 5.8).

Origin of cells

All cells of the system are believed to arise from stem cells in bone marrow (classified as CFU-G/M stem cells). From bone marrow they pass into blood where they are seen as monocytes. From blood they pass into the tissues concerned.

Functions of the mononuclear phagocyte system

(a) Participation in defence mechanisms

As already stated the cells have the ability to phagocytose particulate matter, dead cells, and organisms. In the lungs, alveolar macrophages engulf inhaled particles and are seen as *dust cells*. In the spleen and liver, macrophages destroy aged and damaged erythrocytes.

(b) Role in immune responses

(1) All mononuclear phagocytes bear antigens on their surface (class II MHC antigens). Antigens phagocytosed by macrophages are partially digested by lysosomes. Some remnants of these pass to the cell surface where they form complexes with the MHC antigens. This complex has the ability to stimulate T-lymphocytes.

(2) Certain T-lymphocytes produce macrophage activating factors (including interleukin-2) that influence the activity of macrophages. Macrophages when thus stimulated synthesize and secrete cytokines which stimulate the proliferation and maturation of further lymphocytes.

(3) When foreign substances (including organisms) enter the body, antibodies are produced against them (by lymphocytes). These antibodies adhere to the organisms. Macrophages bear receptors (on their surface) that are able to recognize these antibodies. In this way macrophages are able to selectively

destroy such matter by phagocytosis, or by release of lysosomal enzymes.

From the above it will be seen that lymphocytes and macrophages constitute an integrated immune system for defence of the body.

(4) When suitably stimulated mononuclear phagocytes secrete a tumour necrosing factor (TNF) which is able to kill some neoplastic cells.

(5) Macrophages influence the growth and differentiation of tissues by producing several growth factors and differentiation factors.

Functional Classification

From a functional point of view mononuclear phagocytes are divided into two main types.

(a) With the exception of dendritic cells all the cell types listed on page 86 are classified as *highly phagocytic cells*.

(b) The dendritic mononuclear phagocytes (now called dendritic antigen presenting cells) are capable of phagocytosis, but their main role is to initiate immune reactions in lymphocytes present in lymph nodes, spleen and thymus (in the manner discussed above). It has been postulated that *all* dendritic cells are primarily located in the skin. From here they pick up antigens and migrate to lymphoid tissues where they stimulate lymphocytes against these antigens. They are therefore referred to as antigen presenting cells (APCs). Most APCs are derived from monocytes, but some are derived from other sources.

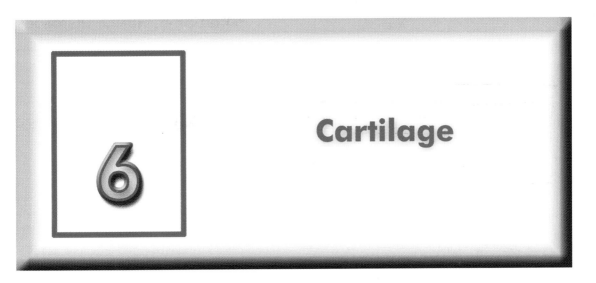

Cartilage

Cartilage is a tissue that forms the 'skeletal' basis of some parts of the body e.g., the auricle of the ear, or the lower part of the nose. Feeling these parts readily demonstrates that while cartilage is sufficiently firm to maintain its form, it is not rigid like bone. It can be bent, returning to its original form when the bending force is removed.

Cartilage is considered to be a modified connective tissue. It resembles ordinary connective tissue in that the cells in it are widely separated by a considerable amount of intercellular material or *matrix*. The latter consists of a homogeneous *ground substance* within which fibres are embedded. (Some authorities use the term matrix as an equivalent of ground substance, while others include embedded fibres under the term). Cartilage differs from typical connective tissue mainly in the nature of the ground substance: this is firm and gives cartilage its characteristic consistency. Three main types of cartilage can be recognized depending on the number and variety of fibres in the matrix. These are, *hyaline cartilage*, *fibrocartilage*, and *elastic cartilage*.

As a rule the free surfaces of hyaline cartilage are covered by a fibrous membrane called the *perichondrium*, but fibrocartilage is not.

Before we consider the features of individual varieties of cartilage we shall examine some features of cartilage cells and of the matrix.

Cartilage Cells

The cells of cartilage are called *chondrocytes*. They lie in spaces (or *lacunae*) present in the matrix. At first the cells are small and show the features of metabolically active cells. The nucleus is euchromatic. Mitochondria, endoplasmic reticulum and Golgi complex are prominent. Some authorities use the term *chondroblasts* for these cells. (This term is used mainly for embryonic cartilage producing cells). As the cartilage cells mature they enlarge often reaching a diameter of 40 μm or more. The nuclei become heterochromatic and organelles become less prominent. The cytoplasm of chondrocytes may also contain glycogen, and lipids.

Ground Substance

The ground substance of cartilage is made up of complex molecules containing proteins and carbohydrates (proteoglycans, page 58). These molecules form a meshwork which is filled by water and dissolved salts.

* protein carbohydrate complexes

The carbohydrates are chemically *glycosaminoglycans* (GAG). They include chondroitin sulphate, keratan sulphate and hyaluronic acid. The core protein is *aggrecan*. The proteoglycan molecules are tightly bound. Along with the water content, these molecules form a firm gel that gives cartilage its firm consistency.

Collagen Fibres of Cartilage

The collagen fibres present in cartilage are (as a rule) chemically distinct from those in most other tissues. They are described as Type II collagen (page 59). However, fibrocartilage, and the perichondrium, contain the normal Type I collagen.

Type II Collagen fibres

HYALINE CARTILAGE Type II collagen fibres

Hyaline cartilage is so called because it is transparent (hyalos = glass). Its intercellular substance appears to be homogeneous, but using special techniques it can be shown that many collagen fibres are present in the matrix. In haematoxylin and eosin stained preparations the matrix is stained blue i.e., it is basophilic. However, the matrix just under the perichondrium is acidophilic (Fig. 6.1). The structure of the matrix has been described above.

Towards the centre of a mass of hyaline cartilage the chondrocytes are large and are usually present in groups (of two or more). The groups are formed by division of a single parent cell. The cells tend to remain together as the dense matrix prevents their separation. Groups of cartilage cells are called *cell-nests* or *isogenous cell groups*. Immediately around lacunae housing individual chondrocytes, and around

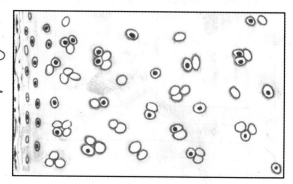

Fig. 6.1. Hyaline cartilage. Note groups of chondroctes surrounded by homogenous matrix. Perichondrium is seen at the left end of the figure.

cell nests the matrix stains deeper than elsewhere giving the appearance of a capsule. This deep staining matrix is newly formed and is called the *territorial matrix* or *lacunar capsule*. In contrast the pale staining matrix separating cell nests is the *interstitial matrix*. Towards the periphery of the cartilage the cells are small, and elongated in a direction parallel to the surface. Just under the perichondrium the cells become indistinguishable from fibroblasts.

Embedded in the ground substance of hyaline cartilage, there are numerous collagen fibres. The fibres are arranged so that they resist tensional forces. Hyaline cartilage has been compared to a tyre. The ground substance (corresponding to the rubber of the tyre) resists compressive forces, while the fibres (corresponding to the treads of the tyre) resist tensional forces.

Distribution of Hyaline Cartilage

Hyaline cartilage is widely distributed in the body as follows.

(1) Costal cartilages

These are bars of hyaline cartilage that connect the ventral ends of the ribs to the sternum, or to adjoining costal cartilages. They show the typical structure of hyaline cartilage described above.

The cellularity of costal cartilage decreases with age.

(2) Articular Cartilage

The articular surfaces of most synovial joints are lined by hyaline cartilage. These articular cartilages provide the bone ends with smooth surfaces between which there is very little friction. They also act as shock absorbers. Articular cartilages are not covered by perichondrium. Their surface is kept moist by synovial fluid which also provides nutrition to them.

Near the free surface of articular cartilage (called the **superficial stratum**, the **tangential stratum**, or **zone 1)** the cell are small and flattened parallel to the surface. Just deep to the superficial stratum there is another layer called the **intermediate stratum**, the **transitional stratum**, or **zone 2**. In this layer the cells are larger and more rounded: they may lie singly or in groups. On proceeding towards the deep surface of the cartilage (which is attached to bone) the cells become still larger and may be arranged in vertical columns (**radiate stratum**, or **zone 3**). The deepest layer of the cartilage (just next to bone) has a calcified matrix. (Compare with epiphyseal cartilage, Chapter 7).

The matrix of articular cartilage is pervaded by numerous collagen fibres. Those near the surface of the cartilage run tangentially and are believed to be orientated along lines of stress.

(3) Other sites where Hyaline Cartilage is found

(a) The skeletal framework of the larynx is formed by a number of cartilages. Of these the thyroid cartilage, the cricoid cartilage and the arytenoid cartilage are composed of hyaline cartilage.

(b) The walls of the trachea and large bronchi contain incomplete rings of cartilage. Smaller bronchi have pieces of cartilage of irregular shape in their walls (Fig. A25).

(c) Parts of the nasal septum, and of the lateral wall of the nose are made up of pieces of hyaline cartilage.

(d) In growing children long bones consist of a bony **diaphysis** (corresponding to the shaft) and of one or more bony **epiphyses** (corresponding to bone ends or projections). Each epiphysis is connected to the diaphysis by a plate of hyaline cartilage called the epiphyseal plate. This plate is essential for bone growth. Its structure and significance are considered in detail in Chapter 7.

FIBROCARTILAGE Type I

On superficial examination this type of cartilage (also called **white fibrocartilage**) looks very much like dense fibrous tissue (Fig. 6.2). However, in sections it is seen to be cartilage because it contains typical cartilage cells surrounded by capsules. The matrix is pervaded by numerous collagen bundles amongst which there are some fibroblasts. The fibres merge with those of surrounding connective tissue, there being no perichondrium over the cartilage. This *the most numerous cells of Connective tissue*

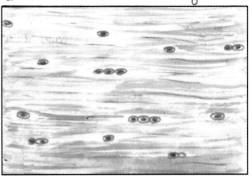

Fig. 6.2. Fibrocartilage. Cartilage cells are embedded amongst thick bundles of collagen fibres.

kind of cartilage has great tensile strength combined with considerable elasticity. The collagen in fibrocartilage is different from that in hyaline cartilage in that it is Type I collagen (identical to that in connective tissue), and not Type II.

White fibrocartilage is found at the following sites.

(1) Fibrocartilage is most conspicuous in secondary cartilaginous joints or symphyses. These include the joints between bodies of vertebrae (where the cartilage forms intervertebral discs); the pubic symphysis; and the manubriosternal joint.

(2) In some synovial joints the joint cavity is partially or completely subdivided by an articular disc. These discs are made up of fibrocartilage. (Examples are discs of the temporo-mandibular and sternoclavicular joints, and menisci of the knee joint). *something of crescent shape*

(3) The glenoidal labrum of the shoulder joint and the acetabular labrum of the hip joint are made of fibrocartilage.

(4) In some situations where tendons run in deep grooves on bone, the grooves are lined by fibrocartilage. Fibrocartilage is often present where tendons are inserted into bone.

ELASTIC CARTILAGE *type II*

Elastic cartilage (or yellow fibrocartilage) is similar in many ways to hyaline cartilage. The main difference is that instead of collagen fibres, the matrix contains numerous elastic fibres (page 60) which form a network (Fig. 6.3). The fibres are difficult to see in haematoxylin and eosin stained sections, but they can be clearly visualized

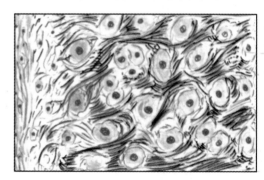

Fig. 6.3. Elastic cartilage. Note chondrocytes surrounded by bundles of elastic fibres, The section has been stained by Verheoff's method in which elastic fibres are stained bluish black.

if special methods for staining elastic fibres are used. The surface of elastic cartilage is covered by perichondrium. *Collagen fibre Type I*

Elastic cartilage possesses greater flexibility than hyaline cartilage, and readily recovers its shape after being deformed.

The sites where elastic cartilage is found are as follows.

(1) It forms the 'skeletal' basis of the auricle (or pinna) (Fig. A49), and of the lateral part of the external acoustic meatus.

(2) The wall of the medial part of the auditory tube is made of elastic cartilage.

Imp (3) The epiglottis (Fig. A47) and two small laryngeal cartilages (corniculate and cuneiform) consist of elastic cartilage. The apical part of the arytenoid cartilage contains elastic fibres but the major portion of it is hyaline.

Note that all the sites mentioned above are concerned either with the production or reception of sound.

SOME ADDITIONAL FACTS ABOUT CARTILAGE

1. Cartilage is derived (embryologically) from mesenchyme. Some mesenchymal cells differentiate into cartilage forming cells or **chondroblasts**. Chondroblasts produce the intercellular matrix as well as the collagen fibres that form the intercellular substance of cartilage. Chondroblasts that become imprisoned within this matrix become chondrocytes. Some mesenchymal cells that surround the developing cartilage form the **perichondrium**. Apart from collagen fibres and fibroblasts the perichondrium contains cells that are capable of transforming themselves into cartilage cells when required.

2. Newly formed cartilage grows by multiplication of cells throughout its substance: this kind of growth is called **interstitial growth**. Interstitial growth is possible only as long as the matrix is sufficiently pliable to allow movement of cells through it. As cartilage matures the matrix hardens and the cartilage cells can no longer move widely apart: in other words interstitial growth is no longer possible. At this stage, when a cartilage cell divides the daughter cells remain close together forming cell nests. Further growth of cartilage now takes place only by addition of new cartilage over the surface of existing cartilage: this kind of growth is called **appositional growth**. It is possible because of the presence of cartilage forming cells in the deeper layers of the perichondrium. (We shall see later that bone grows entirely by apposition).

3. Cartilage has very limited ability for regeneration (after destruction by injury or disease). Defects in cartilage are usually filled in by fibrous tissue.

4. During fetal life cartilage is much more widely distributed than in the adult. The greater part of the skeleton is cartilaginous in early fetal life. The ends of most long bones are cartilaginous at the time of birth, and are gradually replaced by bone. The replacement is completed only after full growth of the individual (i.e., by about 18 years of age).

Replacement of cartilage by bone is called **ossification**; details of this process are considered in Chapter 7. Ossification of cartilage has to be carefully distinguished from **calcification** in which the matrix hardens because of the deposition in it of calcium salts, but true bone is not formed.

Calcification of hyaline cartilage is often seen in old people. The costal cartilages or the large cartilages of the larynx are commonly affected. In contrast to hyaline cartilage, elastic cartilage and fibrocartilage do not undergo calcification. Although articular cartilage is a variety of hyaline cartilage it does not undergo calcification or ossification.

5. With advancing age the collagen fibres of hyaline cartilage (which are normally difficult to see) become much more prominent, so that in some places hyaline cartilage is converted to fibrocartilage. It has been said that the transformation of hyaline cartilage to fibrocartilage is one of the earliest signs of ageing in the body.

6. Cartilage is usually described as an avascular tissue. However, the presence of **cartilage canals**, through which blood vessels may enter cartilage, is well documented. Each canal contains a small artery surrounded by numerous venules and capillaries. Cartilage cells receive their nutrition by diffusion from vessels in the perichondrium or in cartilage canals. Cartilage canals may also play a role in the ossification of cartilage by carrying bone forming cells into it.

7

Bone

Some Features of Gross Structure

If we examine a longitudinal section across a bone (such as the humerus) we see that the wall of the shaft is tubular and encloses a large *marrow cavity*. The wall of the tube is made up of a hard dense material which appears, on naked eye examination, to have a uniform smooth texture with no obvious spaces in it. This kind of bone is called *compact bone*. It is seen further, that compact bone is thickest midway between the two ends of the bone and gradually tapers towards the ends.

When we examine the bone ends we find that the marrow cavity does not extend into them. They are filled by a meshwork of tiny rods or plates of bone and contain numerous spaces, the whole appearance resembling that of a sponge. This kind of bone is called *spongy* or *cancellous bone* (cancel= cavity). The spongy bone at the bone ends is covered by a thin layer of compact bone, thus providing the bone ends with smooth surfaces. Small bits of spongy bone are also present over the wall of the marrow cavity.

Where the bone ends take part in forming joints they are covered by a layer of articular cartilage (already described on page 91). With the exception of the areas covered by articular cartilage, the entire outer surface of bone is covered by a membrane called the *periosteum*. The wall of the marrow cavity is lined by a membrane called the *endosteum*.

The marrow cavity and the spaces of spongy bone (present at the bone ends) are filled by a highly vascular tissue called *bone marrow* At the bone ends the marrow is red in colour. Apart from blood vessels this *red marrow* contains

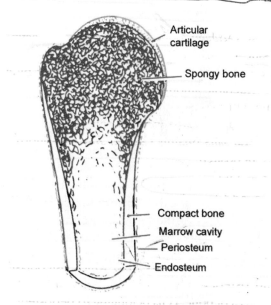

Fig. 7.1. Some features of bone structure as seen in a longitudinal section through one end of a long bone.

numerous masses of blood forming cells (haemopoietic tissue). In the shaft of the bone of an adult, the marrow is yellow. This *yellow marrow* is made up predominantly of fat cells. Some islands of haemopoietic tissue may be seen here also. In bones of a fetus, or of a young child, the entire bone marrow is red. The marrow in the shaft is gradually replaced by yellow marrow with increasing age.

BASIC FACTS ABOUT BONE STRUCTURE

In this section we will consider elementary features of the histology of bone. Details of some aspects of structure are discussed in later sections.

Elements Comprising Bone Tissue

Like cartilage, bone is a modified connective tissue. It consists of bone cells or *osteocytes* that are widely separated from one another by a considerable amount of intercellular substance. The latter consists of a homogeneous ground substance or matrix in which collagen fibres and mineral salts (mainly calcium and phosphorus) are deposited.

In addition to mature bone cells (osteocytes) two additional types of cells are seen in developing bone. These are bone producing cells or *osteoblasts*, and bone removing cells or *osteoclasts*. Other cells present include *osteoprogenitor cells* from which osteoblasts and osteocytes are derived; cells lining the surfaces of bone; cells belonging to periosteum; and cells of blood vessels and nerves which invade bone from outside. Details of the various

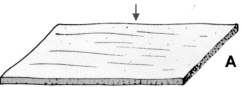

The unit of bone structure is called a lamellus

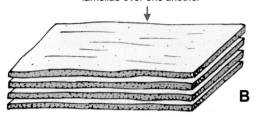

Bone acquires thickness by stacking of lamellae over one another

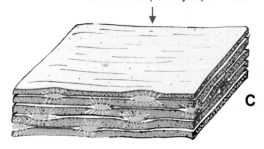

Between adjoining lamellae there are spaces called lacunae. These spaces are occupied by cells of bone (osteocytes)

Fig. 7.2. Scheme to show how lamellae constitute bone.

elements comprising bone are considered in subsequent sections.

Lamellar Bone

When we examine the structure of any bone of an adult, we find that it is made up of layers or *lamellae*. This kind of bone is called *lamellar bone*. Each lamellus is a thin plate of bone consisting of collagen fibres and mineral salts that are deposited in a gelatinous ground substance. Even the smallest piece of bone is made up of several lamellae placed over one another.

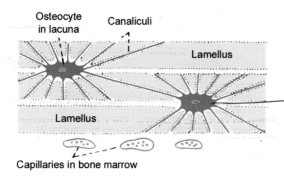

Fig. 7.3. Diagram to show the relationship of osteocytes to bone lamellae.

Between adjoining lamellae we see small flattened spaces of *lacunae*.

Each lacuna contains one osteocyte. Spreading out from each lacuna there are fine canals or *canaliculi* that communicate with those from other lacunae. The canaliculi are occupied by delicate cytoplasmic processes of osteocytes.

The lamellar appearance of bone depends mainly on the arrangement of collagen fibres. The fibres of one lamellus run parallel to each other;

but those of adjoining lamellae run at varying angles to each other. The ground substance of a lamellus is continuous with that of adjoining lamellae.

Lacunae.

Woven Bone

In contrast to mature bone, newly formed bone does not have a lamellar structure. The collagen fibres are present in bundles that appear to run randomly in different directions, interlacing with each other. Because of the interlacing of fibre bundles this kind of bone is called *woven bone*. All newly formed bone is woven bone. It is later replaced by lamellar bone.

> Abnormal persistence of woven bone is a feature of Paget's disease. Bones are weak and there may be deformities.

We have seen that bone may be classified as compact or cancellous, and as lamellar or woven. On the basis of the manner of its development, bone can also be classified as *cartilage bone* or

endo chondrial Ossification

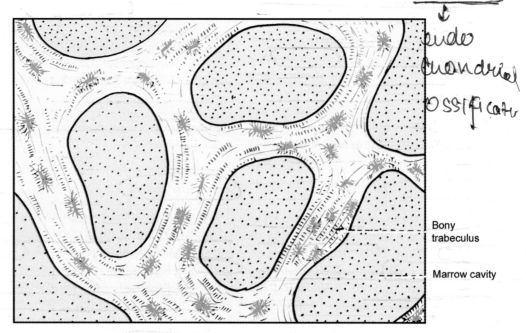

Fig. 7.4A. Structure of cancellous bone (diagrammatic). Also see Fig. 7.4B.

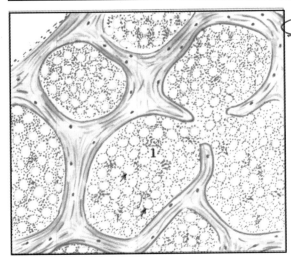

Fig. 7.4B. Structure of cancellous bone as seen in a section. 1-Bone maarrow.

as ***membrane bone*** as described on page 105.

Structure of Cancellous Bone

The bony plates or rods that form the meshwork of cancellous bone are called ***trabeculae.*** Each trabeculus is made up of a number of lamellae (described above) between which there are lacunae containing osteocytes. Canaliculi, containing the processes of osteocytes, radiate from the lacunae.

The trabeculae enclose wide spaces which are filled in by bone marrow. They receive nutrition from blood vessels in the bone marrow (Fig. 7.4 A,B)

Structure of Compact Bone

When we examine a section of compact bone we find that this type of bone is also made up of lamellae, and is pervaded by lacunae (containing osteocytes), and by canaliculi (Fig. 7.5A). Most of the lamellae are arranged in the form of concentric rings that surround a narrow ***Haversian canal*** present at the centre of each ring. The Haversian canal is occupied by blood vessels, nerve fibres, and some cells. One Haversian canal and the lamellae around it

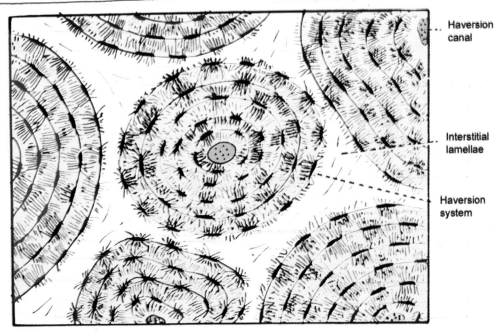

Haversion canal

Interstitial lamellae

Haversion system

Fig. 7.5A. Structure of compact bone (diagrammatic).

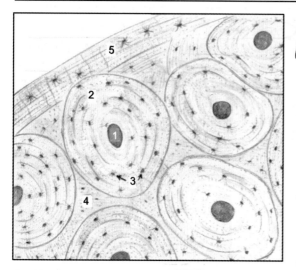

Fig. 7.5B. Structure of compact bone as seen in a ground section. 1= Haversian canal. 2=Concentric lamellae forming Haversian system. 3= Lacunae. 4. Interstitial lamellae. 5. Circumferential lamellae.

constitute a **Haversian system** or **osteon**.

Compact bone consists of several such osteons. Between adjoining osteons there are angular intervals that are occupied by **interstitial lamellae**. These lamellae are remnants of osteons the greater parts of which have been destroyed (as explained later). Near the surface of compact bone the lamellae are arranged parallel to the surface: these are called **circumferential lamellae**.

When we examine longitudinal sections through compact bone (Fig. 7.6) we find that the Haversian canals (and, therefore, the osteons) run predominantly along the length of the bone. The canals branch and anastomose with each other. They also communicate with the marrow cavity, and with the external surface of the bone through channels that are called the **canals of Volkmann**. Blood vessels and nerves pass through all these channels so that compact bone is permeated by a network of blood vessels that provide nutrition to it.

From what has been said above it will be appreciated that there is an essential similarity in the structure of cancellous and compact bone. Both are made up of lamellae. The difference lies in the relative volume occupied by bony lamellae and by the spaces. In compact bone the spaces are small and the solid bone is abundant; whereas in cancellous bone the spaces are large and actual bone tissue is sparse.

FURTHER DETAILS OF BONE STRUCTURE

Cells of Bone

Osteoprogenitor cells

These are stem cells of mesenchymal origin that can proliferate and convert themselves into osteoblasts whenever there is need for bone formation. They resemble fibroblasts in appearance. In the fetus such cells are numerous at sites where bone formation is to take place. In the adult, osteoprogenitor cells are present over bone surfaces (on both the periosteal and endosteal aspects).

Osteoblasts

These are bone forming cells derived from osteoprogenitor cells. They are found lining growing surfaces of bone, sometimes giving an epithelium-like appearance. However, on closer examination it is seen that the cells are of varied shapes (oval, triangular, cuboidal etc.) and that there are numerous gaps between adjacent cells.

The nucleus of an osteoblast is ovoid and euchromatic. The cytoplasm is basophilic because of the presence of abundant rough endoplasmic reticulum. This, and the presence of a well developed Golgi complex, signifies that

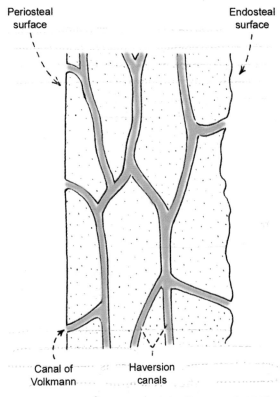

Fig. 7.6. Schematic longitudinal section through compact bone to show Haversian canals and the canals of Volkmann.

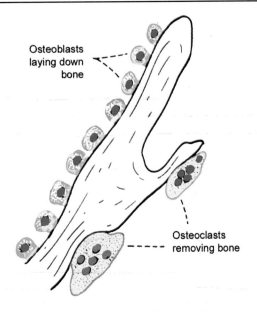

Fig. 7.7. Relationship of osteoblasts and osteoclasts to developing bone.

A benign tumour arising from osteoblasts is called an *osteoma*. A malignant tumour arising from the same cells is called an *osteosarcoma*. Osteosarcomas are most commonly seen in bones adjoining the knee joint. They can spread to distant sites in the body through the blood stream.

the cell is engaged in considerable synthetic activity. Numerous slender cytoplasmic processes radiate from each cell and come into contact with similar processes of neighbouring cells.

Osteoblasts are responsible for laying down the organic matrix of bone including the collagen fibres. They are also responsible for calcification of the matrix. Alkaline phosphatase present in the cell membranes of osteoblasts plays an important role in this function. Osteoblasts are believed to shed off *matrix vesicles* which possibly serve as points around which formation of hydroxyapatite crystals (see below) takes place. Osteoblasts may indirectly influence the resorption of bone by inhibiting or stimulating the activity of osteoclasts (see below).

Osteocytes

These are the cells of mature bone. They lie in the lacunae of bone and represent osteoblasts that have become imprisoned in the matrix during bone formation (page 108). Delicate cytoplasmic processes arising from osteocytes establish contacts with other osteocytes and with bone lining cells present on the surface of bone.

In contrast to osteoblasts, osteocytes have eosinophilic or lightly basophilic cytoplasm. This is to be correlated with (a) the fact that these cells have negligible secretory activity; and (b) the presence of only a small amount of endoplasmic reticulum in the cytoplasm.

Osteocytes are present in greatest numbers in

*[handwritten top margin: * Receptors for para thyroid harmone → Osteocytic]*

young bone, the number gradually decreasing with age.

The functions attributed to osteocytes are that (a) they probably maintain the integrity of the lacunae and canaliculi, and thus keep open the channels for diffusion of nutrition through bone (See page 102); and (b) that they play a role in removal or deposition of matrix and of calcium when required.

[handwritten: Blood Ca Level.]

Osteoclasts *[handwritten: Greek origin → Clast. come from Macrophage Monocyte System]*

These are bone removing cells. They are found in relation to surfaces where bone removal is taking place. (Bone removal is essential for maintaining the proper shape of growing bone). At such locations the cells occupy pits called *resorption bays* or *lacunae of Howship*. Osteoclasts are very large cells (20 to 100 μm or even more in diameter). They have numerous nuclei: up to 20 or more. The cytoplasm shows numerous mitochondria and lysosomes containing acid phosphatase. At sites of bone resorption the surface of an osteoclast shows many folds which are described as *ruffled membrane*. Removal of bone by osteoclasts involves demineralization and removal of matrix. Bone removal can be stimulated by factors secreted by osteoblasts, by macrophages, or by lymphocytes. It is also stimulated by the parathyroid hormone.

Recent studies have shown that osteoclasts are derived from monocytes of blood. It is not certain whether osteoclasts are formed by fusion of several monocytes, or by repeated division of the nucleus, without division of cytoplasm.

[handwritten: Crack the crystaline Ca + Locks from the moisture]

Bone Lining Cells

These cells form a continuous epithelium-like layer on bony surfaces where active bone deposition or removal is not taking place. The cells are flattened. They are present on the periosteal surface as well as the endosteal surface. They also line spaces and canals within bone. It is possible that these cells can change to osteoblasts when bone formation is called for. (In other words many of them are osteoprogenitor cells).

Organic & Inorganic Constituents of Bone Matrix

The ground substance (or matrix) of bone consists of an organic matrix in which are deposited mineral salts.

The Organic Matrix *[handwritten: mineral Salts r deposited fibres is cartilage]*

This consists of a ground substance in which collagen fibres are embedded. The *ground substance* consists of glycosamino-glycans, proteoglycans and water. Two special glycoproteins osteonectin and osteocalcin are present in large quantity. They bind readily to calcium ions and, therefore, play a role in mineralization of bone. Various other substances including chondroitin sulphates, phospholipids and phosphoproteins are also present.

The *collagen fibres* are similar to those in connective tissue (Type I collagen). (They are sometimes referred to as osteoid collagen). The fibres are usually arranged in layers, the fibres within a layer running parallel to one another. Collagen fibres of bone are synthesized by osteoblasts.

The matrix of bone is more dense than elsewhere immediately around the lacunae, forming capsules around them, similar to those around chondrocytes in cartilage. The term osteoid is applied to the mixture of organic ground substance and collagen fibres (before it is mineralized).

The Inorganic Ions

The ions present are predominantly calcium and phosphorus (or phosphate). Magnesium, carbonate, hydroxyl, chloride, fluoride, citrate, sodium and potassium are also present in significant amounts. Most of the calcium, phosphate and hydroxyl ions are in the form of needle shaped crystals that are given the name hydroxyapatite $(Ca_{10} [PO_4]_6 [OH]_2)$. Hydroxyapatite crystals lie parallel to collagen fibres and contribute to the lamellar appearance of bone. Some amorphous calcium phosphate is also present.

About 65% of the dry weight of bone is accounted for by inorganic salts, and 35% by organic ground substance and collagen fibres. (Note that these percentages are for dry weight of bone. In living bone about 20% of its weight is made up by water). About 85% of the total salts present in bone are in the form of calcium phosphate; and about 10% in the form of calcium carbonate. Ninety seven percent of total calcium in the body is located in bone. .

The calcium salts present in bone are not 'fixed'. There is considerable interchange between calcium stored in bone and that in circulation. When calcium level in blood rises calcium is deposited in bone; and when the level of calcium in blood falls calcium is withdrawn from bone to bring blood levels back to normal. These exchanges take place under the influence of hormones (parathormone produced by the parathyroid glands) and calcitonin produced by the thyroid gland: See Chapter 20).

The nature of mineral salts of bone can be altered under certain conditions. If the content of fluoride ions in drinking water is high, the fluoride content of bone increases considerably. This can lead to drastic alterations in bone, including the outgrowth of numerous abnormal projections (exostoses); narrowing of foramina leading to compression of nerves, or even of the spinal cord;

and abnormalities in histological structure. This condition called fluorosis is seen in many parts of India.

Normal calcium and phosphorus are easily substituted by radioactive calcium (Ca^{45}) or radioactive phosphorus (P^{32}) if the latter are ingested. Calcium can also be replaced by radioactive strontium, radium or lead. Presence of radioactive substances in bone can lead to the formation of tumours and to leukaemia. All these changes occur in individuals who are exposed to radioactivity from any source: in particular from a nuclear explosion.

Radioisotopes of calcium and phosphorus can also serve a useful purpose when used with care. If these substances are administered to an animal they get deposited wherever new bone is being formed. Areas of such deposits can be localized, in sections, by a process called *autoradiography*. In this way radioactive isotopes can be used for study of the patterns of bone growth.

Some Further Details about Osteons

During bone formation the first formed osteons do not have a clear lamellar structure, but consist of woven bone. Such osteons are described as *primary osteons* (or *atypical Haversian systems*). Subsequently, the primary osteons are replaced by *secondary osteons* (or *typical Haversian systems*) having the structure already described.

We have seen that osteons run in a predominantly longitudinal direction (i.e., along the long axis of the shaft). However, this does not imply that osteons lie parallel to each other. They may follow a spiral course, may branch, or may join other osteons. In transverse sections osteons may appear circular, oval or ellipsoid.

The number of lamellae in each osteon is highly variable. The average number is six.

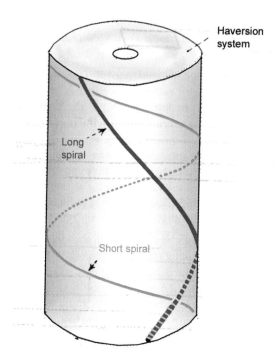

Fig. 7.8. Scheme to show orientation of fibres in adjacent lamellae of a Haversion system.

In an osteon collagen fibres in one lamellus usually run either longitudinally or circumferentially (relative to the long axis of the osteon). Typically, the direction of fibres in adjoining lamellae is alternately longitudinal and circumferential. It is because of this difference in direction of fibres that the lamellar arrangement is obvious in sections. It has been claimed that in fact fibres in all lamellae follow a spiral course, the 'longitudinal' fibres belonging to a spiral of a long 'pitch'; and the 'circumferential' fibres to spirals of a short 'pitch' (Fig. 7.8).

The place where the periphery of one osteon comes in contact with another osteon (or with interstitial lamellae) is marked by the presence of a ***cement line***. Along this line there are no collagen fibres, the line consisting mainly of inorganic matrix. For significance of cement lines see page 110.

The various lacunae within an osteon are

connected with one another through canaliculi which also communicate with the Haversian canal. The peripheral canaliculi of the osteon do not (as a rule) communicate with those of neighbouring osteons: they form loops and turn back into their own osteon. A few canaliculi that pass though the cement line provide communications leading to interstitial lamellae.

The lacunae and canaliculi are only partially filled in by osteocytes and their processes. The remaining space is filled by a fluid which surrounds the osteocytes. This space is in communication with the Haversian canal and provides a pathway along which substances can pass from blood vessels in the Haversian canal to osteocytes.

The phenomenon of birefringence has been referred to on page 58. When a transverse section of compact bone is examined with polarized light each osteon shows two bright bands that cross each other (Fig. 7.9). This birefringence is an indication of the very regular arrangement of collagen fibres (and the crystals related to them) within the lamellus.

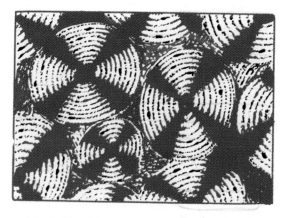

Fig. 7.9. Compact bone seen with polarized light.

THE PERIOSTEUM

We have seen that the external surface of any bone is, as a rule, covered by a membrane called periosteum. (The only parts of the bone surface devoid of periosteum are those that are covered with articular cartilage). The periosteum consists of two layers, outer and inner. The outer layer is a fibrous membrane. The inner layer is cellular. In young bones the inner layer contains numerous osteoblasts, and is called the *osteogenetic layer*. (This layer is sometimes described as being distinct from periosteum). In the periosteum covering the bones of an adult osteoblasts are not conspicuous, but osteoprogenitor cells present here can form osteoblasts when need arises e.g., in the event of a fracture. Periosteum is richly supplied with blood. Many vessels from the periosteum enter the bone and help to supply it (But see page 117).

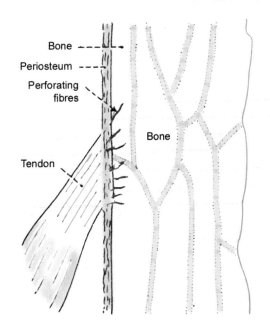

Bone

Periosteum

Perforating
fibres

Bone

Tendon

Fig. 7.10. Diagram to show the perforating fibres
(of Sharpey)

Functions of Periosteum

1. The periosteum provides a medium through which muscles, tendons and ligaments are attached to bone. In situations where very firm attachment of a tendon to bone is necessary, the fibres of the tendon continue into the outer layers of bone as the *perforating fibres of Sharpey*. The parts of the fibres that lie within the bone are ossified: they have been compared to 'nails' that keep the lamellae in place.

2. Because of the blood vessels passing from periosteum into bone, the periosteum performs a nutritive function. (However, see page 117).

3. Because of the presence of osteo-progenitor cells in its deeper layer the periosteum can form bone when required. This role is very important during development (page 107). It is also important in later life for repair of bone after fracture.

4. The fibrous layer of periosteum is sometimes described as a *limiting membrane* that prevents bone tissue from 'spilling out' into neighbouring tissues. This is based on the observation that if periosteum is torn osteogenic cells may extend into surrounding tissue forming bony projections (*exostoses*). Such projections are frequently seen on the bones of old persons. The concept of the periosteum as a limiting membrane helps to explain how ridges and tubercles are formed on the surface of a bone. At sites where a tendon pulls upon periosteum the latter tends to be lifted off from bone. The 'gap' is filled by proliferation of bone leading to the formation of a tubercle. (Such views are, however, hypothetical).

CORRELATION OF BONE STRUCTURE & SOME OF ITS MECHANICAL PROPERTIES

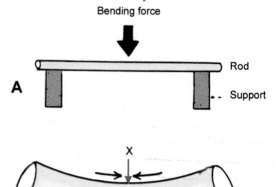

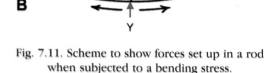

Fig. 7.11. Scheme to show forces set up in a rod when subjected to a bending stress.

Living bone is a very strong material that can withstand severe stresses. These stresses include compression, tension, bending and twisting. It has been estimated that bone is about three times as strong as wood, and about half as strong as steel.

When any force is applied to a rod-shaped structure so that it tends to bend the rod (Fig.7.11A) different kinds of forces are set up in different parts of the rod (Fig. 7.11B). At point 'X' (in the figure) the material of the rod tends to be compressed, while at 'Y' the material tends to be pulled apart. Midway between 'X' and 'Y' the two forces neutralize each other so that there is very little stress on material in the centre of the rod. This means that the resistance of the rod to bending would not be affected if material in the centre of the rod was removed; or if, in other words, the rod were to be replaced by a tube. It is for this reason that shafts of long bones can be tubular without any loss of strength. At the same time a tubular design confers the advantage of much lesser weight than for a solid bone of the same dimensions.

The stresses on any particular bone (or part of it) can be very complex. The structure of each part of a bone is adapted to these stresses bone being thickest along lines of maximum stress, and absent in areas where there is no stress. This applies not only to the gross structure of a bone, but also to its microscopic structure. The fact that the trabeculae of cancellous bone are arranged along the lines of stress has been recognized since long: this fact is known as **Wolff 's law**. In some situations (e.g., at the upper end of the femur) the trabeculae appear to be arranged predominantly in two planes at right angles to each other. It has been suggested that trabeculae in one plane resist compressive forces, and those

in the other direction resist tensile forces. In this context it is interesting to note that a clear pattern of trabeculae is seen in the femur of a child only after it begins to walk.

Within compact bone, osteons (and the collagen fibres within them) are also arranged so as to most efficiently counteract the stresses imposed on them. The spiral arrangement of fibres in osteons (page 102) is probably a device to allow bones to withstand severe twisting strains.

The stresses on different parts of a bone can be greatly altered in abnormal conditions. Following a fracture, if the two segments of a bone unite at an abnormal angle, it is seen that (over a period of time) the entire internal architecture of the bone becomes modified to adjust to the changed directions of stresses imposed.

Role of Inorganic Salts in Providing Strength to Bone

Mineral salts can be removed from bone by treating it with weak acids. Chelating agents (e.g., ethylene diamine tetraacetic acid or EDTA) are also used. The process, called *decalcification*, is necessary for preparing sections of bone. When mineral salts are removed by decalcification the tissue becomes soft and pliable: a long bone like the fibula, or a rib, can even be tied into a knot. This shows that the rigidity of bone is due mainly to the presence in it of mineral salts.

Conversely, the organic substances present in bone can be destroyed by heat (as in burning). The form of the bone remains intact, burning). The form of the bone remains intact, but the bone becomes very brittle and breaks easily. It follows that the organic matter contributes substantially to the strength of bone. Resistance to tensile forces is due mainly to the presence of collagen fibres.

FORMATION OF BONE

All bone is of mesodermal origin. The process of bone formation is called **ossification**. We have seen (page 93) that formation of most bones is preceded by the formation of a cartilaginous model, which is subsequently replaced by bone. This kind of ossification is called **endochondral ossification**; and bones formed in this way are called **cartilage bones**. In some situations (e.g., the vault of the skull) formation of bone is not preceded by formation of a cartilaginous model. Instead bone is laid down directly in a fibrous membrane. This process is called **intramembranous ossification**; and bones formed in this way are called **membrane bones**. The bones of the vault of the skull, the mandible, and the clavicle are membrane bones.

Intramembranous ossification

The various stages in intramembranous ossification are as follows.

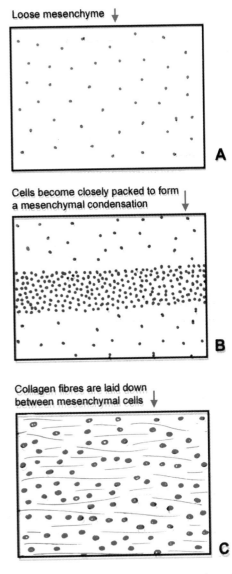

Loose mesenchyme

A

Cells become closely packed to form a mesenchymal condensation

B

Collagen fibres are laid down between mesenchymal cells

C

Fig. 7.12. Scheme to show how the mesenchymal basis of bone is formed.

(1) At the site where a membrane bone is to be formed the mesenchymal cells become densely packed (i.e., a **mesenchymal condensation** is formed) (Fig. 7.12B).

(2) The region becomes highly vascular.

(3) Some of the mesenchymal cells lay down bundles of collagen fibres in the mesenchymal condensation. In this way a membrane is formed

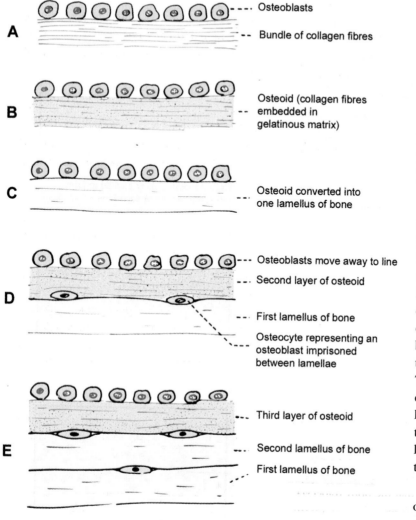

A --- Osteoblasts
--- Bundle of collagen fibres

B --- Osteoid (collagen fibres embedded in gelatinous matrix)

C --- Osteoid converted into one lamellus of bone

D --- Osteoblasts move away to line
--- Second layer of osteoid
--- First lamellus of bone
--- Osteocyte representing an osteoblast imprisoned between lamellae

E --- Third layer of osteoid
--- Second lamellus of bone
--- First lamellus of bone

Fig. 7.13. Scheme to show how bony lamellae are laid down over one another.

(Fig.7.12C).

4. Some mesenchymal cells (possibly those that had earlier laid down the collagen fibres) enlarge and acquire a basophilic cytoplasm, and may now be called osteoblasts. They come to lie along the bundles of collagen fibres. These cells secrete a gelatinous matrix in which the fibres get embedded. The fibres also swell up. Hence the fibres can no longer be seen distinctly. This mass of swollen fibres and matrix is called *osteoid*

(Fig.7.13B).

5. Under the influence of osteoblasts calcium salts are deposited in osteoid. As soon as this happens the layer of osteoid can be said to have become one lamellus of bone (Fig. 7.13C).

6. Over this lamellus, another layer of osteoid is laid down by osteoblasts. The osteoblasts move away from the lamellus to line the new layer of osteoid. However, some of them get caught between the lamellus and the osteoid (Fig. 7.13D). The osteoid is now ossified to form another lamellus. The cells trapped between the two lamellae become osteocytes (Fig. 7.13D).

7. In this way a number of lamellae are laid down one over another, and these lamellae together form a trabeculus of bone (Fig. 7.13E).

8. If we consider the arrangement of collagen bundles in a membrane we will see that the appearance is somewhat like that in Fig. 7.14A. If we further imagine the process of bone formation, described above, to be occurring along each of these bundles it will be apparent that bone formed will also follow the same pattern. In this way typical cancellous bone will be formed. Cancellous bone is converted into

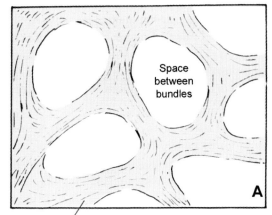

Fig. 7.14. Conversion of a fibrous membrane (A) into spongy bone (B). Note that the bony trabecylae follow the same pattern as the fibre bundles (in A).

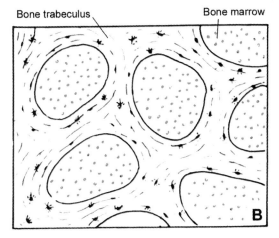

compact bone as described on page 109.

The description of intramembranous ossification given above has been simplified for easy comprehension. In fact the first formed bone may not be in the form of regularly arranged lamellae. The elements are irregularly arranged and form woven bone.

Endochondral Ossification

The essential steps in the formation of bone by endochondral ossification are as follows.

1. At the site where the bone is to be formed, the mesenchymal cells become closely packed to form a mesenchymal condensation (Fig. 7.15A).

2. Some mesenchymal cells become chondroblasts and lay down hyaline cartilage (Fig. 7.15B). Mesenchymal cells on the surface of the cartilage form a membrane called the perichondrium. This membrane is vascular and contains osteoprogenitor cells.

3. The cells of the cartilage are at first small and irregularly arranged. However, in the area where bone formation is to begin, the cells enlarge considerably (Fig.7.16).

4. The intercellular substance between the enlarged cartilage cells becomes calcified, under the influence of alkaline phosphatase, which is secreted by the cartilage cells. The nutrition to the cells is thus cut off and they die, leaving behind empty spaces called *primary areolae* (Fig.7.17).

5. Some blood vessels of the perichondrium (which may be called periosteum as soon as bone is formed) now invade the cartilaginous matrix.

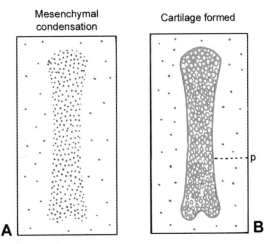

Fig. 7.15. Endochondral ossification. Formation of cartilaginous model. p =perichondrium.

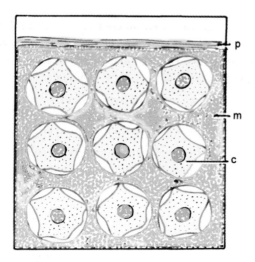

Fig. 7.16. Early stage in endochondral ossification. The cartilage cells (c) are separated by matrix (m). p=perichondrium.

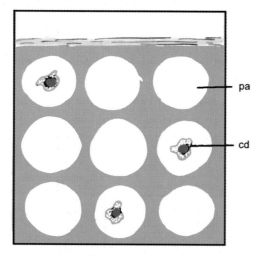

Fig. 7.17. Endochondral ossification. The matrix has calcified. Cartilage cells are dead (cd) leaving empty spaces called primary alveolae (pa).

They are accompanied by osteo-progenitor cells. This mass of vessels and cells is called the **periosteal bud**. It eats away much of the calcified matrix forming the walls of the primary areolae, and thus creates large cavities called **secondary areolae**, also called **medullary spaces** (Fig. 7.18).

6. The walls of secondary areolae are formed

by thin layers of calcified matrix that have not by thin layers of calcified matrix that have not been dissolved. The osteoprogenitor cells become osteoblasts and arrange themselves along the surfaces of these bars, or plates, of calcified matrix (Fig.7.19A).

7. These osteoblasts now lay down a layer of ossein fibrils embedded in a gelatinous ground substance (i.e., osteoid), exactly as in intra-membranous ossification (Fig. 7.19B). This osteoid is calcified and a lamellus of bone is formed (Fig. 7.19C).

8. Osteoblasts now lay down another layer of osteoid over the first lamellus. This is also calcified. Thus two lamellae of bone are formed. Some osteoblasts that get caught between the two lamellae become osteocytes. As more lamellae are laid down bony trabeculae are formed (Fig. 7.19D).

It may be noted that the process of bone formation in endochondral ossification is exactly the same as in intramembranous ossification. The calcified matrix of cartilage only acts as a support

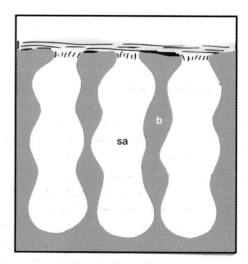

Fig. 7.18. Endochondral ossification. Some primary areolae have fused to form larger spaces called secondary areolae (sa) which are separated by bars of calcified matrix.

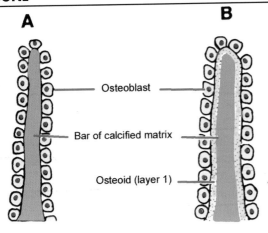

A

Osteoblast

Bar of calcified matrix

Osteoid (layer 1)

B

C

Osteoblast

1st lamellus

2nd lamellus

Osteoid (layer 2)

Osteoid (layer 3)

Osteocyte

D

Fig. 7.19. Endochondral ossification. Four stages in formation of bony lamellae.

for the developing trabeculae and is not itself converted into bone.

9. At this stage the ossifying cartilage shows a central region (1 in Fig. 7.20) where bone has been formed. As we move away from this area we see (a) a region where cartilaginous matrix has been calcified and surrounds dead and dying cartilage cells (2 in Fig. 7.20); (b) a zone of hypertrophied cartilage cells in an uncalcified matrix (3); and (c) normal cartilage (4) in which there is considerable mitotic activity. If we see the same cartilage some time later (Fig.7.20) we find that ossification has now extended into zone 2, and simultaneously the matrix in zone 3 has

become calcified. The deeper cells of zone 4 have meanwhile hypertrophied, while the more superficial ones have multiplied to form zone 5. In this way formation of new cartilage keeps pace with the loss due to replacement by bone. The total effect is that the ossifying cartilage progressively increases in size.

Conversion of Cancellous Bone to Compact Bone

All newly formed bone is cancellous. It is converted into compact bone as follows.

Each space between the trabeculae of cancellous bone comes to be lined by a layer of osteoblasts. The osteoblasts lay down lamellae of bone as already described. The first lamellus

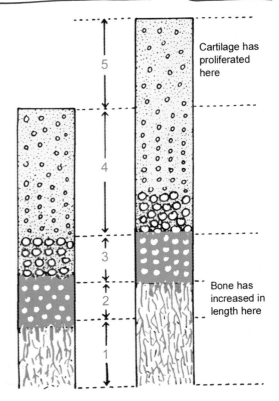

Cartilage has proliferated here

Bone has increased in length here

Fig. 7.20. Scheme to show how bones grow in length.

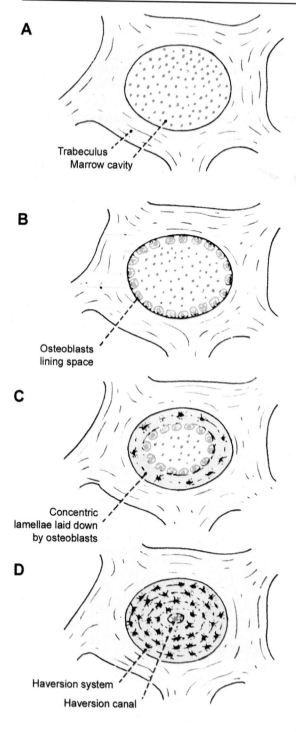

A

Trabeculus
Marrow cavity

B

Osteoblasts
lining space

C

Concentric
lamellae laid down
by osteoblasts

D

Haversion system

Haversion canal

Fig. 7.21. Steps in the conversion of spongy bone to
compact bone.

is formed over the inner wall of the original space and is, therefore, shaped like a ring. Subsequently, concentric lamellae are laid down inside this ring thus forming an osteon. The original space becomes smaller and smaller and persists as a Haversian canal.

The first formed Haversian systems are called *atypical Haversian systems* or *primary osteons*. These osteons do not have a typical lamellar structure, and their chemical composition may also be atypical.

Primary osteons are soon invaded by blood vessels and by osteoclasts which bore a new series of spaces through them. These new spaces are again filled in by bony lamellae, under the influence of osteoblasts, to form *secondary osteons* (or *typical Haversian systems*). The process of formation and destruction of osteons takes place repeatedly as the bone enlarges in size; and continues even after birth. In this way the internal structure of the bone can be repeatedly remodelled to suit the stresses imposed on the bone.

From the above it will be obvious that interposed in between osteons of the newest series there will be remnants of previous generations of osteons. The interstitial lamellae of compact bone (page 98) represent such remnants.

When a newly created cavity begins to be filled in by lamellae of a new osteon, the first formed layer is atypical in that it has a very high density of mineral deposit. This layer can subsequently be identified as a *cement line* that separates the osteon from previously formed elements. As the cement line represents the line at which the process of bone erosion stops and at which the process of bone formation begins, it is also called a *reversal line.* From the above it will be clear why cement lines are never present around primary osteons, but are always present around subsequent generations of osteons.

HOW BONES GROW

While considering the growth of cartilage (page 93) we have seen that a hard tissue like bone can grow only by deposition of new bone over existing bone i.e., by apposition. We will now consider some details of the method of bone growth in some situations.

Growth of Bones of Vault of Skull

In the bones of the vault of the skull (e.g., the parietal bone) ossification begins in one or more small areas called ***centres of ossification***. Bone is formed as described on page 104. At first it is in the form of narrow trabeculae or spicules. These spicules increase in length by deposition of bone at their ends. As the spicules lengthen they radiate from the centre of ossification to the periphery. Gradually the entire mesenchymal condensation is invaded by this spreading process of ossification and the bone assumes its normal shape. However, even at birth the radiating arrangement of trabeculae is obvious.

The mesenchymal cells lying over the developing bone differentiate to form the *memb* periosteum (page 103).

The embryonic parietal bone, formed as described above, has to undergo considerable growth. After ossification has extended into the entire membrane representing the embryonic parietal bone, this bone is separated from neighbouring bones by intervening fibrous tissue (in the region of the sutures). Growth in size of the bone can occur by deposition of bone on the edges adjoining sutures (Fig. 7.22). Growth in thickness and size of the bone also occurs when the overlying periosteum forms bone (by the process of intramembranous ossification described above) over the outer surface of the

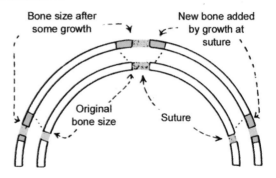

Fig. 7.22. Growth of skull bones at surures.

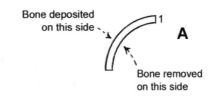

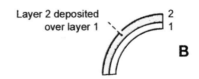

As layer 3 is deposited on layer 2, layer 1 is removed

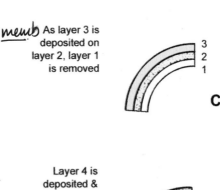

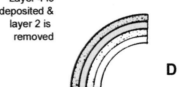

Fig. 7.23. Scheme to show how skull bones grow.

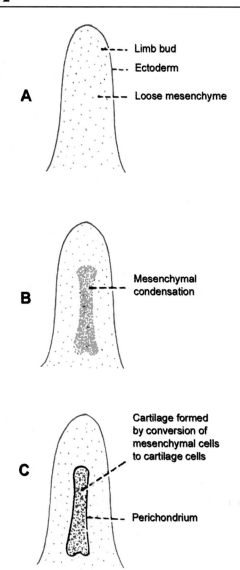

Fig. 7.24. Formation of a typical long bone:
establishment of cartilaginous model.

Development of a Typical Long Bone

In the region where a long bone is to be formed the mesenchyme first lays down a cartilaginous model of the bone. This cartilage is covered by perichondrium. Endochondral ossification starts in the central part of the cartilaginous model (i.e., at the centre of the future shaft).

This area is called the *primary centre of ossification*. Gradually, bone formation extends from the primary centre towards the ends of shaft. This is accompanied by progressive

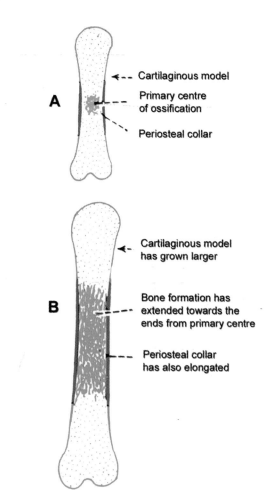

Fig. 7.25. Formation of a tpical long bone:
primary centre of ossification and periosteal collar.

bone.

Simultaneously, there is removal of bone from the inner surface. In this way, as the bone grows in size, there is simultaneous increase in the size of the cranial cavity.

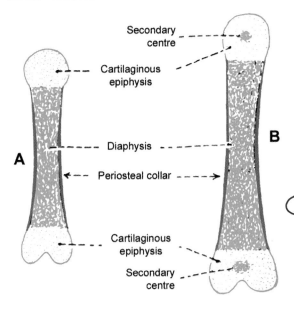

Fig. 7.26. Formation of a typical long bone:
secondary centres of ossification.

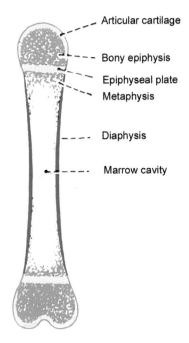

Fig. 7.27. Formation of a typical long bone:
bony epiphyses and epiphyseal plates.

enlargement of the cartilaginous model.

Soon after the appearance of the primary centre, and the onset of endochondral ossification in it, the perichondrium (which may now be called periosteum) becomes active. The osteoprogenitor cells in its deeper layer lay down bone on the surface of the cartilaginous model by *intramembranous ossification*. This periosteal bone completely surrounds the cartilaginous shaft and is, therefore, called the *periosteal collar* (Fig.7.25A).

The periosteal collar is first formed only around the region of the primary centre, but rapidly extends towards the ends of the cartilaginous model (Fig. 7.25B). It acts as a splint, and gives strength to the cartilaginous model at the site where it is weakened by the formation of secondary areolae. We shall see that most of the shaft of the bone is derived from this periosteal collar and is, therefore, membranous in origin.

At about the time of birth the developing bone consists of (a) a part called the *diaphysis* (or shaft), that is bony, and has been formed by extension of the primary centre of ossification, and (b) ends that are cartilaginous (Fig.7.26A). At varying times after birth *secondary centres* of endochondral ossification appear in the cartilages forming the ends of the bone (Fig. 7.26B). These centres enlarge until the ends become bony (Fig. 7.27). More than one secondary centre of ossification may appear at either end. The portion of bone formed from one secondary centre is called an *epiphysis.*

For a considerable time after birth the bone of the diaphysis and the bone of any epiphysis are separated by a plate of cartilage called the *epiphyseal cartilage*, or *epiphyseal plate*. This is formed by cartilage into which ossification has not extended either from the diaphysis or from the epiphysis. We shall see that this plate plays a vital role in growth of the bone.

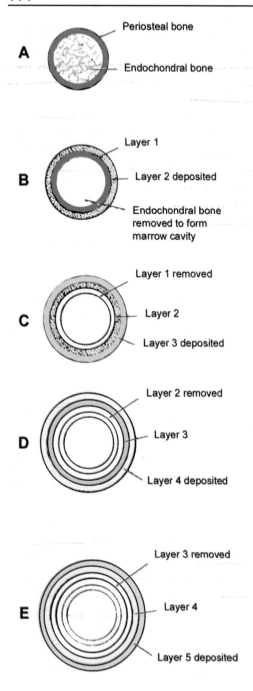

A
— Periosteal bone
— Endochondral bone

B
— Layer 1
— Layer 2 deposited
— Endochondral bone removed to form marrow cavity

C
— Layer 1 removed
— Layer 2
— Layer 3 deposited

D
— Layer 2 removed
— Layer 3
— Layer 4 deposited

E
— Layer 3 removed
— Layer 4
— Layer 5 deposited

Fig. 7.28. Scheme to show a long bone grows in thickness.

Growth of a Long Bone

A growing bone increases both in length and in girth.

We have seen that the periosteum lays down a layer of bone around the shaft of the cartilaginous model. This periosteal collar gradually extends to the whole length of the diaphysis. As more layers of bone are laid down over it, the periosteal bone becomes thicker and thicker. However, it is neither necessary nor desirable for it to become too thick. Hence, osteoclasts come to line the internal surface of the shaft and remove bone from this aspect. As bone is laid down outside the shaft it is removed from the inside. The shaft thus grows in diameter, and at the same time its wall does not become too thick (Figs. 7.28 A-E). The osteoclasts also remove trabeculae lying in the centre of the bone that were formed by endochondral ossification. In this way, a *marrow cavity* is formed. As the shaft increases in diameter there is a corresponding increase in the size of the marrow cavity. This cavity also extends towards the ends of the diaphysis, but does not reach the epiphyseal plate. Gradually most of the bone formed from the primary centre (i.e., of endochondral origin) is removed, except near the bone ends, so that the wall of the shaft is ultimately made up entirely of periosteal bone formed by the process of intramembranous ossification.

To understand how a bone grows in length, we will now take a closer look at the epiphyseal plate. Depending on the arrangement of cells, three zones can be recognized (Fig. 7.29).

(a) *Zone of resting cartilage*: Here the cells are small and irregularly arranged.

(b) *Zone of proliferating cartilage*. This is also called the *zone of cartilage growth*. In this zone the cells are larger, and undergo repeated mitosis. As they multiply, they come to be arranged in parallel columns, separated by

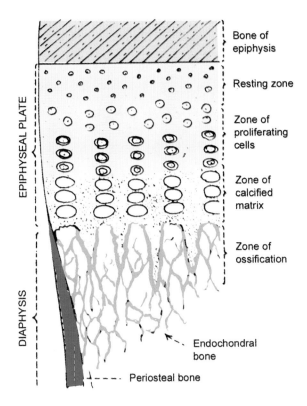

Fig. 7.29. Structure of an epiphyseal plate.

bars of intercellular matrix.

(c) *Zone of calcification*. This is also called the *zone of cartilage transformation*. In this zone the cells become still larger and the matrix becomes calcified.

Next to the zone of calcification, there is a zone where cartilage cells are dead and the calcified matrix is being replaced by bone. Growth in length of the bone takes place by continuous transformation of the epiphyseal cartilage to bone (Figs. 7.20, 7.30) in this zone (i.e., on the diaphyseal surface of the epiphyseal cartilage). At the same time, the thickness of the epiphyseal cartilage is maintained by the active multiplication of cells in the zone of proliferation. When the bone has attained its full length, cells in the cartilage stop proliferating. The process of calcification, however, continues to extend

into it until the whole of the epiphyseal plate is converted into bone. The bone substance of the diaphysis and that of the epiphysis then become continuous. This is called *fusion of the epiphysis*.

Metaphysis

The portion of the diaphysis adjoining the epiphyseal plate is called the metaphysis (Fig. 7.27). It is a region of active bone formation and, for this reason, it is highly vascular. The metaphysis does not have a marrow cavity. Numerous muscles and ligaments are usually attached to the bone in this region. Even after bone growth has ceased, the calcium turnover function of bone is most active in the metaphysis, which acts as a store house of calcium. The metaphysis is frequently the site of infection.

Nutritional and Hormonal Factors Influencing Bone Growth

For normal development and maintenance of bone adequate amounts of calcium,

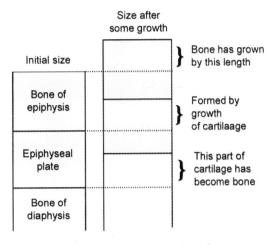

Fig. 7.30. Scheme to show how a long bone grows in length at the epiphyseal plate.

phosphorus and of vitamins A, C and D should be present in the diet of an individual. Deficiency of calcium leads to reduced mineral content of bone (*osteoporosis*). Vitamin D influences calcium levels by its influence on intestinal absorption. Deficiency of this vitamin causes *osteomalacia* in adults and *rickets* in children.

Deficiency of vitamin C interferes with synthesis of collagen and of proteoglycans present in bone matrix. Bone trabeculae and cortical bone are reduced in thickness. Bones become weak and healing of fractures is interfered with. Vitamin A is necessary for a proper balance between bone deposition and removal; both deficiency and excess are harmful.

Various hormones influence bone growth. Parathyroid hormone and thyro-calcitonin which control calcium levels in blood indirectly affect bone. Growth hormone (somatotropin) produced by the adenohypophysis influences bone growth. When excessive it leads to *giantism* (in growing individuals), and to *acromegaly* (in adults). Growth is also influenced by the thyroid hormones and by secretions of the ovaries, the testes, and the adrenal cortex.

> The collagen fibres of bone may be defective as a result of a genetic abnormality. This leads to *osteogenesis imperfecta* (page 69) in which bones are weak and fracture easily.

BLOOD SUPPLY OF BONE

A long bone receives three sets of arteries.

1. A *nutrient artery* (or more accurately a *diaphyseal nutrient artery*) pierces the shaft near its middle and enters the marrow cavity. Sometimes more than one nutrient artery may

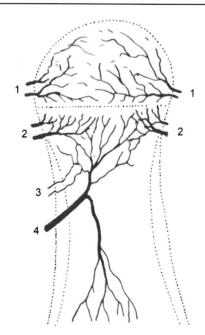

Fig. 7.31.Scheme to show the arteries supplying a long bone. 1-epiphyseal; 2-metaphyseal; 3-periosteal; 4-nutrient. The veins (not shown) accompany the arteries.

be present. The opening for the nutrient artery is called the *nutrient foramen*. The foramen leads into a canal that passes obliquely through the shaft. The canal is directed away from the growing end of the bone (i.e., the end where the epiphysis fuses with the shaft later than at the other end). Within the marrow cavity the artery divides into ascending and descending branches.

2. Several arteries enter the bone near either end. Some of these are *epiphyseal arteries*, while others are *metaphyseal arteries*.

3. Several small arteries arise from periosteal vessels and enter the bone through minute foramina (Fig. 7.31).

Branches of all these arteries form a rich sinusoidal plexus in bone marrow. Many branches from the plexus enter Haversian canals through communications of the latter with the marrow cavity. Periosteal arteries reach the Haversian canals through the canals of Volkmann.

Traditionally the nutrient artery has been regarded as the main artery of supply to bone. However, it is now known that a much greater volume of blood enters the bone through the epiphyseal and metaphyseal arteries, and that the nutrient arteries can be tied without damage to the bone.

It has also been held that periosteal vessels play an important role in the blood supply of bone and that considerable amount of blood flows inwards from the periosteum towards the marrow cavity. Recent investigations throw doubt on this view, and show that most blood vessels passing between bone and periosteum are veins, the flow being mainly outwards. However, from a practical point of view the periosteal vessels are of importance and removal of periosteum can cause necrosis of underlying bone.

The marrow cavity contains a large central venous sinus. This sinus is drained by numerous veins that accompany the arteries.

Apart from bone tissue proper, blood vessels to bone supply bone marrow, the periosteum, the articular cartilages (from their deep surfaces) and the epiphyseal plate. The epiphyseal plate is supplied on the metaphyseal side by metaphyseal arteries, and on the epiphyseal side by epiphyseal arteries. The epiphyseal and metaphyseal arteries remain distinct as long as the epiphyseal plate is intact, but after its disappearance the two sets of arteries anastomose with one another. Lymphatic vessels are present in periosteum, but not in bone substance. Nerve fibres accompany blood vessels into the marrow cavity and into Haversian canals. They are most numerous near joints.

nutrient foramen
present in the diaphysis of the bone in
foetal stage & pierce the periosteum

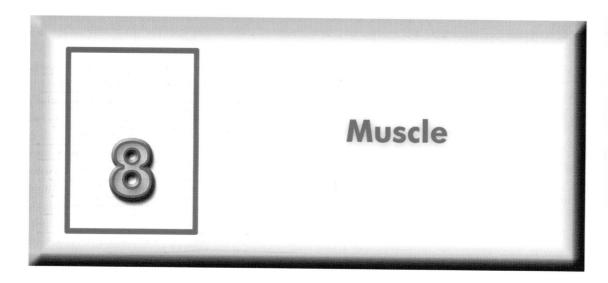

Muscle

Introductory Remarks

Muscle tissue is composed predominantly of cells that are specialized to shorten in length by contraction. This contraction results in movement. It is in this way that virtually all movements within the body, or of the body in relation to the environment, are ultimately produced.

Muscle tissue is made up basically of cells that are called *myocytes*. Myocytes are elongated in one direction and are, therefore, often referred to as *muscle fibres*. We shall see, however, that in some cases muscle fibres are made up of several myocytes joined to each other; or of greatly elongated myocytes containing multiple nuclei.

The force generated by contraction of a muscle fibre is transmitted to other structures through connective tissue. Each muscle fibre is closely invested by connective tissue which is continuous with that around other muscle fibres. Because of this fact the force generated by different muscle fibres gets added together. In some cases a movement may be the result of simultaneous contraction of thousands of muscle fibres.

The connective tissue framework of muscle also provides pathways along which blood vessels and nerves reach muscle fibres.

From the point of view of its histological structure muscle is of three types.

(1) The first variety of muscle tissue is present mainly in the limbs and in relation to the body wall. Because of its close relationship to the bony skeleton, this variety is called *skeletal muscle*. When examined under a microscope fibres of skeletal muscle show prominent transverse striations. Skeletal muscle is, therefore, also called *striated muscle*. Skeletal muscle can normally be made to contract under our will (to perform movements we desire). It is, therefore, also called *voluntary muscle*. Skeletal muscle is supplied by somatic motor nerves.

(2) The second variety of muscle is present mainly in relation to viscera. It is seen most typically in the walls of hollow viscera. As fibres of this variety do not show transverse striations it is called *smooth muscle*, or *non-striated muscle*. As a rule, contraction of smooth muscle is not under our control; and smooth muscle is, therefore, also called *involuntary muscle*. It is supplied by autonomic nerves.

(3) The third variety of muscle is present exclusively in the heart and is called *cardiac muscle*. It resembles smooth muscle in being

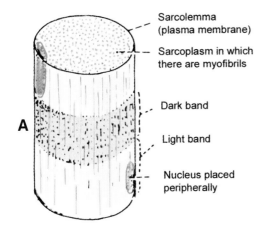

Sarcolemma
(plasma membrane)

Sarcoplasm in which
there are myofibrils

Dark band

Light band

Nucleus placed
peripherally

A

Fig. 8.1A. Scheme to show the structure of a muscle
fibre. Also see Figs. 8.1B and 8.1C.

It will be obvious that the various terms described above are not entirely satisfactory there being numerous contradictions. Some 'skeletal' muscle has no relationship to the skeleton being present in situations such as the wall of the oesophagus, or of the anal canal. The term striated muscle is usually treated as being synonymous with skeletal muscle, but we have seen that cardiac muscle also has striations. In many instances the contraction of skeletal muscle may not be strictly voluntary (e.g., in sneezing or coughing; respiratory movements; maintenance of posture). Conversely, contraction of smooth muscle may be produced by voluntary effort as in passing urine.

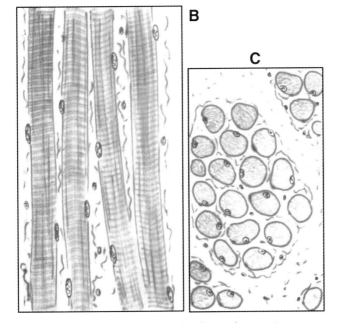

B

C

Figs. 8.1B and 8.1C showing skeletal muscle seen in
longitudinal section and transverse section.

involuntary; but it resembles striated muscle in that the fibres of cardiac muscle also show transverse striations. Cardiac muscle has an inherent rhythmic contractility the rate of which can be modified by autonomic nerves that supply it.

SKELETAL MUSCLE

Elementary Facts about Skeletal Muscle

Skeletal muscle is made up essentially of long, cylindrical 'fibres'. The length of the fibres is highly variable, the longest being as much as 30 cm in length. The diameter of the fibres also varies considerably (10 to 60 μm: usually 50-60 μm). Each 'fibre' is really a syncytium with hundreds of nuclei along its length. (The 'fibre' is formed, during development, by fusion of numerous myoblasts). The nuclei are elongated and lie along the periphery of the fibre, just under the cell membrane (which is called the **sarcolemma**). The cytoplasm (or **sarcoplasm**) is filled with numerous longitudinal fibrils that are called **myofibrils**. In transverse sections through muscle fibres, prepared by

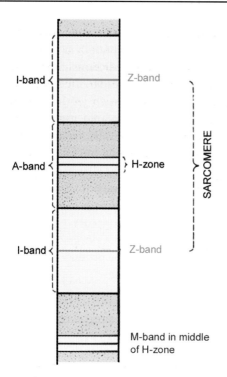

Fig. 8.2. Scheme to show the terminology of transverse bands in a myofibril. Note that the A-band is confined to one sarcomere, but the I-band is made up of parts of two sarcomeres that meet at the Z-band.

stretched) some further details can be made out. Running across the middle of each I-band there is a thin dark line called the **Z-band**. The centre of the A-band is traversed by a lighter band called the **H-band** (or **H-zone**). Running through the centre of the H-band a thin dark line can be made out. This is the **M-band**. (The significance of the letters Z, H, and M is explained on page 124).

The various bands described are really present in myofibrils. They appear to run transversely across the whole muscle fibre because corresponding bands in adjoining myofibrils lie exactly opposite one another.

The part of a myofibril situated between two consecutive Z-bands is called a **sarcomere**. The significance of the striations of myofibrils has to be understood in terms of their ultrastructure which is described on page 124.

In addition to myofibrils the sarcoplasm of a muscle fibre contains the usual cell organelles which tend to aggregate near the nuclei. Mitochondria are numerous. Substantial amounts of glycogen are also present. Glycogen provides energy for contraction of muscle.

routine methods, the myofibrils often appear to be arranged in groups that are called the *fields of Conheim*. The appearance is now known to be an artefact. The myofibrils are in fact distributed uniformly throughout the fibre.

The most striking feature of skeletal muscle fibres is the presence of transverse striations in them. After staining with haematoxylin the striations are seen as alternate dark and light bands that stretch across the muscle fibre. The dark bands are called **A-bands**, while the light bands are called **I-bands**. (As an aid to memory note that 'A' and 'I' correspond to the second letters in the words dark and light. The significance of these letters is explained on page 123).

In good preparations (specially if the fibres are

Organisation of Muscle Fibres in Muscles

Within a muscle, the muscle fibres are arranged in the form of bundles or fasciculi. The number of fasciculi in a muscle, and the number of fibres in each fasciculus, are both highly variable. In small muscles concerned with fine movements (like those of the eyeball, or those of the vocal folds) the fasciculi are delicate and their number small. In large muscles (in which strength of contraction is the main consideration) fasciculi are coarse and numerous.

Muscles differ in the way their fasciculi are arranged. Some muscles (e.g., the sartorius) are strap-like, the fasciculi running the whole length

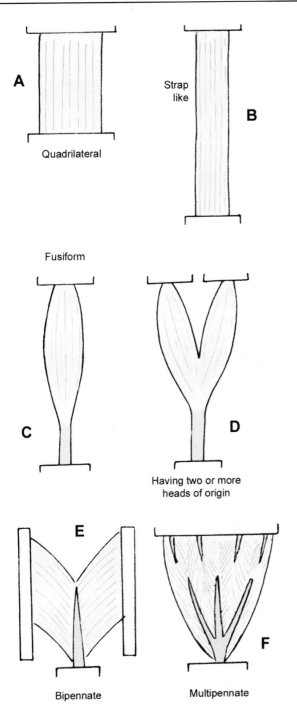

A — Quadrilateral

B — Strap like

Fusiform

C

D — Having two or more heads of origin

E — Bipennate

F — Multipennate

Fig. 8.3. Scheme to show some ways in which the fasciculi of a skeletal muscle may be arranged.

of the muscle. Other muscles are fusiform, the fasciculi being attached at one or both ends to tendons. In still other muscles, the fasciculi are much shorter than the total length of the muscle, and gain attachment to tendinous intersections within the muscle. Some variations in fascicular architecture are illustrated in Figs.8.3 A to F.

Variations in the fascicular architecture are to be correlated with the kind of movements performed by a muscle. A muscle fibre can shorten to about two-thirds of its full length. The total displacement that a muscle can produce is, therefore, proportional to the length of its fibres. In contrast the strength of contraction of a muscle depends on the number of fibres in a muscle (irrespective of their length). In some muscles a large number of short fasciculi are packed into a relatively small total volume (e.g., in a multipennate muscle like the deltoid: Fig.8.3F). Such a muscle can exert much greater force than a long strap muscle having the same total volume.

Connective Tissue Framework of Muscles

Muscles are pervaded by a network of connective tissue fibres that support muscle fibres and unite them to each other. Individual muscle fibres are surrounded by delicate connective tissue that is called the *endomysium*. Individual fasciculi are surrounded by a stronger sheath of connective tissue called the *perimysium*. Connective tissue that surrounds the entire muscle is called the *epimysium*. At the junction of a muscle with a tendon the fibres of the endomysium, the perimysium and the epimysium become continuous with the fibres of the tendon.

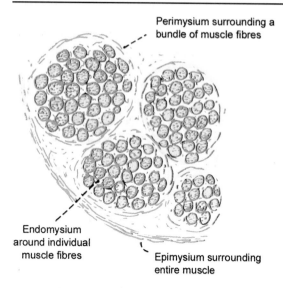

Fig. 8.4. Diagram to show the connective tissue present in relation to skeletal muscle.

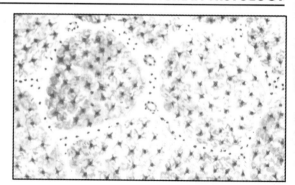

Fig. 8.5A. Transverse section through tendon.

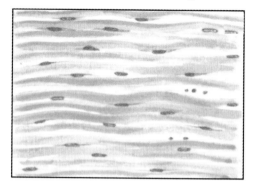

Fig. 8.5B. Longitudinal section through tendon.

Tendons

Tendons are composed of collagen fibres that run parallel to each other. The fibres are arranged in the form of bundles (Figs. 8.5A,B). These bundles are united by areolar tissue, which contains numerous fibroblasts. In longitudinal sections through a tendon the fibroblasts, and their nuclei, are seen to be elongated. In transverse sections, the fibroblasts are stellate. Tendons serve to concentrate the pull of a muscle on a relatively small area of bone. By curving around bony pulleys, or under retinacula, they allow alterations in the direction of pull. Tendons also allow the muscle mass to be placed at a convenient distance away from its site of action. (Imagine what would happen if there were no tendons in the fingers!).

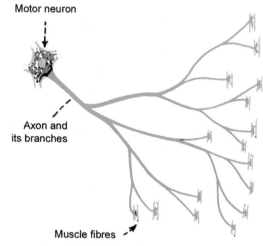

Fig. 8.5C. Scheme to show the concept of a motor unit.

Innervation of Skeletal Muscle

The nerve supplying a muscle enters it (along with the main blood vessels) at an area called the **neurovascular hilus.** This hilus is usually situated nearer the origin of the muscle than the insertion. After entering the muscle the nerve breaks up into many branches that run through the connective tissue of the perimysium and endomysium to reach each muscle fibre. The nerve fibres supplying skeletal muscle are axons arising from large neurons in the anterior (or ventral) grey columns of the spinal cord (or of corresponding nuclei in the brain stem). These *alpha-efferents* have a large diameter and are myelinated. Because of repeated branching of its axon, one anterior grey column neuron may supply many muscle fibres all of which contract when this neuron 'fires'. One anterior grey column neuron and the muscle fibres supplied by it constitute one *motor unit.* The number of muscle fibres in one motor unit is variable. The units are smaller where precise control of muscular action is required (as in ocular muscles), and much larger in limb muscles where force of contraction is more important. The strength with which a muscle contracts at a particular moment depends on the number of motor units that are activated.

The junction between a muscle fibre and the nerve terminal that supplies it is highly specialized and is called a *motor end plate*. The structure of a motor end plate is described in Chapter 9.

Apart from the alpha efferents described above every muscle receives smaller myelinated *gamma-efferents* that arise from gamma neurons in the ventral grey column of the spinal cord. These fibres supply special muscle fibres that are present within sensory receptors called *muscle spindles* (see Chapter 9). These special muscle fibres are called *intrafusal fibres*. Nerves to muscles also carry autonomic fibres that supply smooth muscle present in the walls of blood vessels.

FURTHER DETAILS ABOUT SKELETAL MUSCLE

Origin of terms I-Band and A-Band

We have seen that the light and dark bands of myofibrils (or of muscle fibres) are designated I-bands and A-bands respectively. The letters 'I' and 'A' stand for the terms *isotropic* and *anisotropic* respectively. These terms refer to the way in which any material (e.g., a crystal) behaves with regard to the transmission of light through it. Some materials refract light equally in all directions: they are said to be isotropic. Other materials that do not refract light equally in different planes are anisotropic. These qualities depend on the arrangement of the elements making up the material. In the case of muscle fibres the precise reason for alternate bands being isotropic and anisotropic is not understood. The phenomenon is most probably due to peculiarities in arrangement of molecules within them.

Although striations can be made out in unstained material using ordinary light, they are

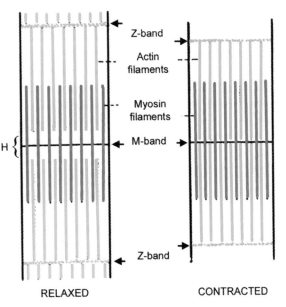

Fig. 8.6. Scheme to show how a myofibril shortens by sliding of actin filaments into the intervals between myosin filaments. Note that the width of the I-band becomes less, and that the H-zone disappears when the myofibril contracts.

much better seen through a microscope using polarized light.

Significance of letters Z, H, M

We have seen that the part of a myofibril between the two Z-bands is called a sarcomere. In other words a Z band is a plate lying between two sarcomeres. The letter 'Z' is from the German word **zwischenschiebe** (zwischen = between; schiebe = disc). The M-band is a plate lying in the middle of the sarcomere. The letter 'M' is from the German word **mittleschiebe** (mittle = middle). The H-band (or zone) is named after Hensen who first described it.

Ultrastructure of Striated Muscle

Each muscle fibre is covered by a plasma membrane that is called the **sarcolemma**. The sarcolemma is covered on the outside by a **basement membrane** (also called the **external lamina**) which establishes an intimate connection between the muscle fibre and the fibres (collagen, reticular) of the endomysium.

The cytoplasm (**sarcoplasm**) is permeated with myofibrils which push the elongated nuclei to a peripheral position. Between the myofibrils there is an elaborate system of membrane lined tubes called the **sarcoplasmic reticulum**. Elongated mitochondria (**sarcosomes**) and clusters of glycogen are also scattered amongst the myofibrils. Perinuclear Golgi bodies, ribosomes, lysosomes, and lipid vacuoles are also present.

Structure of Myofibrils

When examined by EM each myofibril is seen to be made of fine myofilaments. These are of two types: **actin** and **myosin**, made up of molecules of corresponding proteins. (Each myosin filament is about 12 nm in diameter,

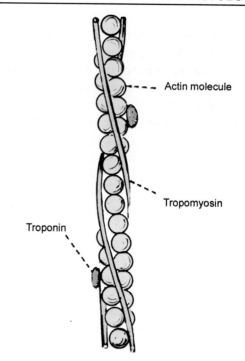

Fig. 8.7. Actin filament (F-actin) made up of globular molecules of G-actin.

while an actin filament is about 8 nm in diameter. They are therefore referred to as thick and thin filaments respectively). The arrangement of actin and myosin filaments within a sarcomere is shown in Fig. 8.6. It will be seen that myosin filaments are confined to the A-band, the width of the band being equal to the length of the myosin filaments. The actin filaments are attached at one end to the Z-band. From here they pass through the I-band and extend into the 'outer' parts of the A-band, where they interdigitate with the myosin filaments. Note that the I-band is made up of actin filaments alone. The H-band represents the part of the A-band into which actin filaments do not extend. The Z-band is really a complicated network at which the actin filaments of adjoining sarcomeres meet. The M-band is produced by fine interconnections between adjacent myosin filaments.

In an uncontracted myofibril, overlap between

actin and myosin filaments is minimal. During contraction the fibril shortens by sliding in of actin filaments more and more into the intervals between the myosin filaments. As a result the width of the I-band decreases, but that of the A-band is unchanged. The H-bands are obliterated in a contracted fibril.

To understand the mechanism by which actin filaments 'slide' into the A-band, it is necessary to examine the structure of actin and myosin filaments in greater detail.

Each **actin filament** is really composed of two subfilaments that are twisted round each other (Fig.8.7). Each subfilament is a chain of globular (rounded) molecules. These globular molecules are G-actin, and the chain formed by them is designated as **f-actin**. Each actin filament has a head end (that extends into the A-band) and a tail end that is anchored to the Z-line (through a protein called α-actinin). The filament also contains two other proteins called **tropomyosin** and **troponin**. Tropomyosin is in the form of a long fibre that winds around actin and stabilizes it. Troponin is a complex made up of several fractions. These complexes are arranged regularly over the actin fibre and represent sites at which myosin binds to actin.

Each **myosin filament** is made up of a large number of myosin molecules. Each molecule is made up of two units, each unit having a head and a tail (Fig.8.8). The tails are coiled over each other. A myosin filament is a 'bundle' of the tails of such molecules. The heads project outwards from the bundle as projections of the myosin filament. The projecting heads are arranged in a regular helical manner.

Because of the manner in which it is formed each myosin fibril can be said to have a head end and a tail end. The tail end is attached to the M-line.

Movement is produced by interaction of actin and myosin filaments as follows. Myosin filaments establish bonds with adjoining actin filaments. After making a bond a head probably 'bends' dragging the actin filament with it. The original

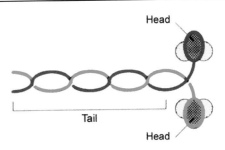

Fig. 8.8. Structure of a myosin molecule. Each molecule has two components (shown in red and green) each consisting of a head and a tail. The tails are coiled over each other. The parts shown in red or green are heavy myosin. Light myosin is shaded yellow.

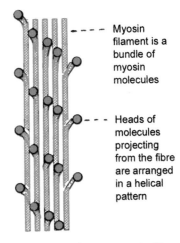

Myosin filament is a bundle of myosin molecules

Heads of molecules projecting from the fibre are arranged in a helical pattern

Fig. 8.9. Diagram to show a myosin filament made up of several molecules of myosin.

bond is now broken, the head unbends, and establishes another bond with the next part of the actin filament. These bonds are made and unmade in rapid succession dragging actin filaments into the intervals between the myosin filaments. This is the probable mechanism for shortening of myofibrils; and hence for the contraction of muscle.

It will be obvious that for successful operation of such a system the actin and myosin filaments must be arranged in a precise geometrical fashion: and this is indeed the case (Fig.8.10). This precision of alignment is achieved through **accessory proteins** which link the diffent components.

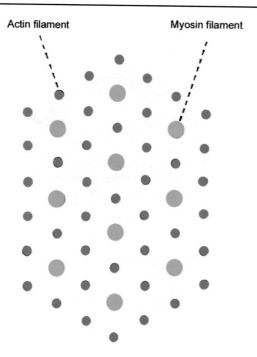

Actin filament   Myosin filament

Fig. 8.10. Schematic T.S. through A-band to show the regular geometric arrangement of actin and myosin filaments. Myosin filaments are arranged in triangular arrays. Each myosin filament is surrounded by six actin filaments.

The energy for repeated binding and release of the heads of myosin molecules to actin is derived from hydrolysis of ATP. ATP binds to the myosin head. When the head comes in contact with actin ATP is hydrolysed to form ADP and phosphate. This leads to firm binding of the head to actin. After a short interval ADP is released by the head, which now separates from actin. Fresh ATP binds to the head and the cycle is repeated.

Other Proteins present in muscle

Several proteins other than actin and myosin are present in muscle. Some of them are as follows.

1. Actinin is present in the region of Z discs. It binds the tail ends of actin-filaments to this disc.

2. Myomesin is present in the region of the M disc. It binds the tail ends of myosin filaments to this disc.

3. Titin links the head ends of myosin filaments to the Z disc. This is a long and elastic protein that can lengthen and shorten as required. It keeps the myosin filament in proper alignment.

4. Desmin is present in intermediate filaments of the cytoskeleton. It links myofibrils to each other, and also to the cell membrane.

Some other proteins are also present.

Each muscle fibre contains a cytoskeleton. The fibres of the cytoskeleton are linked to actin fibres. The cytoskeleton is also linked to the external lamina through glycoproteins present in the cell membrane. Forces generated within the fibre are thus transmitted to the external lamina. The external lamina is in turn attached to connective tissue fibres around the muscle fibre. A number of proteins are responsible for these linkages. Genetic defects is these proteins can result in abnormalities in muscle (muscle dystrophy: page 134).

Sarcoplasmic Reticulum

In the intervals between myofibrils, the sarcoplasm contains an elaborate system of tubules called the sarcoplasmic reticulum (Fig. 8.11). The larger elements of this reticulum run in planes at right angles to the long axes of the myofibrils, and form rings around each myofibril. At the level of every junction between an A and I band the myofibril is encircled by a set of three closely connected tubules which constitute a **muscle triad**. For purposes of description each such triad can be said to be composed of an upper, a middle, and a lower tubule (Fig.8.11). The upper and lower tubules of the triad are connected to the tubules of adjoining triads through a network of smaller tubules. There is one such network opposite each A-band, and another opposite each I-band. These networks, along with the upper and lower tubules of the triad, constitute the sarcoplasmic reticulum. This reticulum is a closed system of tubes.

The middle tube of the triad is an entity independent of the sarcoplasmic reticulum. It is

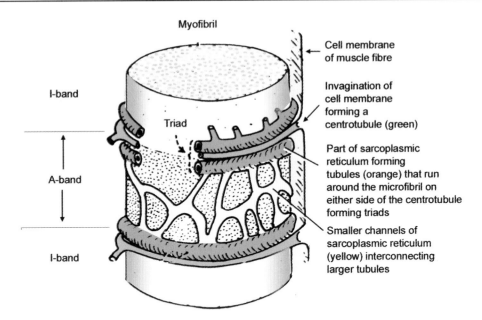

Myofibril

I-band

Triad

A-band

I-band

Cell membrane
of muscle fibre

Invagination of
cell membrane
forming a
centrotubule (green)

Part of sarcoplasmic
reticulum forming
tubules (orange) that run
around the microfibril on
either side of the centrotubule
forming triads

Smaller channels of
sarcoplasmic reticulum
(yellow) interconnecting
larger tubules

Fig. 8.11. Diagram to show the relationship of the sarcoplasmic reticulum, and the T-tubes to a myofibril.

called a **centrotubule** and belongs to what is called the **T-system** of membranes. The centrotubules are really formed by invagination of the sarcolemma into the sarcoplasm. Their lumina are, therefore, in communication with the exterior of the muscle fibre. As already noted the centrotubules permeate the entire muscle fibre as they form networks around myofibrils as part of the muscle triads.

Contraction of muscle is dependent on release of calcium ions into myofibrils. In a relaxed muscle these ions are strongly bound to the membranes of the sarcoplasmic reticulum. When a nerve stimulus reaches a motor end plate the sarcolemma is depolarized. The wave of depolarization is transmitted to the interior of the muscle fibre through the centrotubules. As a result of this wave calcium ions are released from the sarcoplasmic reticulum into the myofibrils causing their contraction.

Red (or Slow Twitch) & White (or Fast Twitch) Muscle

It has been known since long that some skeletal muscle fibres are reddish in colour while others are whitish. As compared to white fibres the contraction of red fibres is relatively slow. Hence red fibres are also called **slow twitch fibres**, or **type I fibres**; while white fibres are also called **fast twitch fibres** or **type II fibres**.

The colour of red fibres is due to the presence (in the sarcoplasm) of a pigment called **myoglobin**. This pigment is similar (but not identical with) haemoglobin. It is present also in white fibres, but in much lesser quantity.

In addition to colour and speed of contraction there are several other differences between red and white fibres. In comparison to white fibres red fibres differ as follows.

Red fibres are narrower than white fibres. Relative to the volume of the myofibrils the sarcoplasm is more abundant. Probably because of this fact the myofibrils, and striations, are less well defined; and the nuclei are not always at the periphery, but may extend deeper into the fibre. Mitochondria are more numerous in red fibres, but the sarcoplasmic reticulum is less extensive. The sarcoplasm contains more glycogen. The capillary bed around red fibres is richer than around white fibres. Differences have also been described in enzyme systems and the respiratory mechanisms in the two types of fibres. Fibres intermediate between red and white fibres have also been described.

In some animals complete muscles may consist exclusively of red or white fibres, but in most mammals, including man, 0muscles contain an admixture of both types. Although red fibres contract slowly their contraction is more sustained, and they fatigue less easily. They predominate in the so called postural muscles (which have to remain contracted over long periods), while white fibres predominate in muscles responsible for sharp active movements.

Type II (white) fibres may be divided into type IIA and type IIB, the two types differing in their enzyme content, and in the chemical nature of their myosin molecules.

Blood Vessels and Lymphatics of Skeletal Muscle

Skeletal muscle is richly supplied with blood vessels. The main artery to the muscle enters it at the neurovascular hilus (page 122). Several other arteries may enter the muscle at its ends or at other places along its length. The arteries form a plexus in the epimysium and in the perimysium, and end in a network of capillaries that surrounds each muscle fibre. This network is richer in red muscle than in white muscle.

Veins leaving the muscle accompany the arteries. A lymphatic plexus extends into the epimysium and the perimysium, but not into the endomysium. The innervation of skeletal muscle has been described on page 122.

CARDIAC MUSCLE

The structure of cardiac muscle has many similarities to that of skeletal muscle; but there are important differences as well.

Similarities between Cardiac & Skeletal Muscle

These are as follows. Like skeletal muscle, cardiac muscle is made up of elongated 'fibres' within which there are numerous myofibrils. The myofibrils (and, therefore, the fibres) show transverse striations similar to those of skeletal muscle. A, I, Z and H bands can be made out in the striations. The connective tissue framework, and the capillary network around cardiac muscle fibres are similar to those in skeletal muscle.

With the EM it is seen that myofibrils of cardiac muscle have the same structure as those of skeletal muscle and are made up of actin and myosin filaments. A sarcoplasmic reticulum, T-system of centrotubules, numerous mitochondria and other organelles are present.

Differences between Cardiac & Skeletal Muscle

These are as follows.

1. The fibres of cardiac muscle do not run in strict parallel formation, but branch and anastomose with other fibres to form a network.

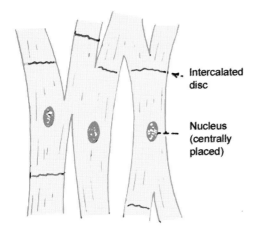

Fig. 8.12A. Cardiac muscle (diagrammatic).
Also see Fig. 8.12B.

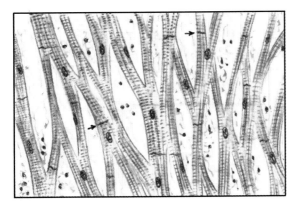

Fig. 8.12B. Cardiac muscle as seen in a section.

2. Each fibre of cardiac muscle is not a multinucleated syncytium as in skeletal muscle, but is a chain of cardiac muscle cells (or *cardiac myocytes*) each having its own nucleus. Each myocyte is about 80 μm long and about 15 μm broad.

3. The nucleus of each myocyte is located centrally (and not peripherally as in skeletal muscle).

4. The sarcoplasm of cardiac myocytes is abundant and contains numerous large mitochondria. The myofibrils are relatively few. At places, the myofibrils merge with each other. As a result of these factors, the myofibrils and

striations of cardiac muscle are not as distinct as those of skeletal muscle. In this respect cardiac muscle is closer to the red variety of skeletal muscle than to the white variety. Other similarities with red muscle are the presence of significant amounts of glycogen and of myoglobin, and the rich density of the capillary network around the fibres.

With the EM it is seen that the sarcoplasmic reticulum is much less prominent than in skeletal muscle. The centrotubules of the T-system lie opposite the Z-bands (and not at the junctions of A and I-bands as in skeletal muscle). The tubules are much wider than in skeletal muscle. Typical triads (page 127) are not present. They are often replaced by *dyads* having one T-tube and one tube of the sarcoplasmic reticulum.

5. With the light microscope the junctions between adjoining cardiac myocytes are seen as dark staining transverse lines running across the muscle fibre. These lines are called *intercalated discs*. Sometimes these discs do not run straight across the fibres, but are broken into a number of 'steps' (Fig. 8.12). The discs always lie opposite the I-bands.

With the EM it is seen that the intercalated discs are formed by cell membranes of adjacent

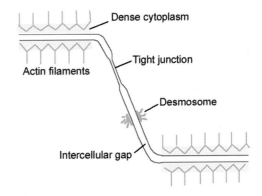

Fig. 8.13. Diagram to show the EM structure of part of an intercalated disc.

myocytes, and by a layer of particularly dense cytoplasm present next to the cell membrane. The ends of actin filaments are embedded in this dense cytoplasm. The cell membranes of adjoining myocytes are connected by numerous desmosomes, gap junctions, and tight junctions. Desmosomes link intermediate filaments present in the cytoskeleton of adjacent cells. Actin filaments of the cells end in relation to tight junctions. Gap junctions allow electrical continuity between adjacent myocytes, and thus convert the cardiac muscle into a *physiological syncytium*.

6. Cardiac muscle is involuntary and is innervated by autonomic fibres (in contrast to skeletal muscle that is innervated by cerebrospinal nerves). Nerve endings terminate near the cardiac myocytes, but motor end plates are not seen.

Isolated cardiac myocytes contract spontaneously in a rhythmic manner. In the intact heart the rhythm of contraction is determined by a pace maker located in the sinuatrial node. From here the impulse spreads to the entire heart through a conducting system made up of a special kind of cardiac muscle. From the above it will be appreciated that a nerve supply is not necessary for contraction of cardiac muscle. Nervous influences do, however, influence the strength and rate of contraction of the heart.

SMOOTH MUSCLE

Basic Facts About Smooth Muscle

Smooth muscle (also called *non-striated, involuntary* or *plain muscle*) is made up of long spindle shaped cells (myocytes) having a broad central part and tapering ends. The nucleus, which is oval or elongated, lies in the

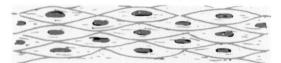
Fig. 8.14a.Smooth muscle cells (diagrammaatic).

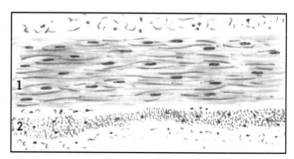
Fig. 8.14b. Smooth musscle as seen in a section. 1-L.S. 2-T.S.

central part of the cell. The length of smooth muscle cells (often called fibres) is highly variable (15 μm to 500 μm).

With the light microscope the sarcoplasm appears to have indistinct longitudinal striations, but there are no transverse striations.

Smooth muscle cells are usually aggregated to form bundles, or fasciculi, that are further aggregated to form layers of variable thickness. In such a layer the cells are so arranged that the thick central part of one cell is opposite the thin tapering ends of adjoining cells. Aggregations of smooth muscle cells into fasciculi and layers is facilitated by the fact that each myocyte is surrounded by a network of delicate fibres (collagen, reticular, elastic) that holds the myocytes together. The fibres between individual myocytes become continuous with the more abundant connective tissue that separates fasciculi or layers of smooth muscle.

Distribution of Smooth Muscle

(a) Smooth muscle is seen most typically in the walls of hollow viscera including the stomach, the intestines, the urinary bladder and the uterus.

(b) It is present in the walls of several structures that are in the form of narrow tubes e.g., arteries, veins, bronchi, ureters, deferent ducts, uterine tubes, and the ducts of several glands.

(c) The muscles that constrict and dilate the pupil are made up of smooth muscle.

(d) Some smooth muscle is present in the orbit (orbitalis); in the upper eyelid (Muller's muscle); in the prostate; in the skin of the scrotum (Dartos muscle). In the skin delicate bundles of smooth muscle are present in relation to hair follicles. These bundles are called the *arrector pili* muscles (Chapter 12).

Variations in Arrangement of Smooth Muscle

Smooth muscle fibres may be arranged in a variety of ways depending on functional requirements.

(a) In some organs (e.g., the gut) smooth muscle is arranged in the form of two distinct layers: an inner circular and an outer longitudinal. Within each layer the fasciculi lie parallel to each other. Such an arrangement allows peristaltic movements to take place for propulsion of contents along the tube.

In some organs (e.g., the ureter) the arrangement of layers may be reversed, the longitudinal layer being internal to the circular one. In yet other situations there may be three layers: inner and outer longitudinal with a circular layer in between.

(b) In some regions (e.g., urinary bladder, uterus) the smooth muscle is arranged in layers, but the layers are not distinctly demarcated from each other. Even within layers the fasciculi tend to run in various directions and may form a network. In these organs contraction of muscle reduces the size of the lumen of the organ and pushes out its contents.

(c) In some tubes (e.g., the bile duct) a thick layer of circular muscle may surround a segment of the tube forming a *sphincter*. Contraction of the sphincter occludes the tube.

(d) In the skin, and in some other situations, smooth muscle occurs in the form of narrow bands.

Innervation of Smooth Muscle

Smooth muscle is innervated by autonomic nerves, both sympathetic and parasympathetic. The two have opposite effects. For example, in the iris, parasympathetic stimulation causes constriction of the pupil, and sympathetic stimulation causes dilatation. It may be noted that sympathetic or parasympathetic nerves may cause contraction of muscle at some sites, and relaxation at other sites.

For further details see below.

Blood vessels & Lymphatics of Smooth Muscle

Blood vessels and lymphatics are present in smooth muscle, but the density of blood vessels is much less than in skeletal muscle (in keeping with much less activity).

Some Further Facts About Smooth Muscle

Ultrastructure

Each smooth muscle cell is bounded by a plasma membrane. Outside the plasma membrane there is an external lamina to which the plasma membrane is adherent. Connective tissue fibres are attached to the lamina (through special proteins). Adjacent smooth muscle cells communicate through gap junctions. The longitudinal striations (see with the light

A

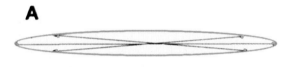

B

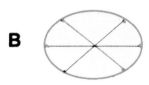

Fig. 8.15. Diagram to show contractile fibres in smooth muscle stretching between anchoring points on the cell membrane. The cell is shown in the relaxed state in A, and in the contracted state in B.

microscope) are due to the presence of delicate myofilaments. These myofilaments are composed mainly of the proteins actin and myosin, but these do not have the highly ordered arrangement seen in striated muscle. Apart from myofibrils the sarcoplasm also contains mitochondria (which provide energy), a Golgi complex, some granular endoplasmic reticulum, free ribosomes, and intermediate filaments (page 21). A sarcoplasmic reticulum, similar to that in skeletal muscle, is present, but is not as developed. Numerous invaginations (caveolae) resembling endocytic vesicles are seen near the surface of each myocyte, but no endocytosis occurs here.

The mechanism of contraction of smooth muscle is different from that of skeletal muscle as follows.

1. The myosin is chemically different from that in skeletal muscle. It binds to actin only if its light chain is phosphorylated. This phosphorylation of myosin is necessary for contraction of smooth muscle.

2. The actin filaments are also different from those in skeletal muscle. Troponin is not present.

3. As compared to skeletal muscle, smooth muscle needs very little ATP for contraction.

4. The mechanisms regulating the flow of calcium ions into smooth muscle are different from those for skeletal muscle. Caveolae present on the surface of smooth muscle cells play a role in this process.

5. Actin and myosin form bundles that are attached at both ends to the points on the cell membrane called anchoring points (or focal densities). When the muscle contracts these points are drawn closer to each other. This converts an elongated smooth muscle cell in one that is oval (Fig. 8.15).

Further Details of Innervation

The relationship of nerve terminals to smooth muscle cells is much less intimate than that in skeletal muscle. Nerve terminals end in direct relation to only some myocytes. It is believed that impulses travel from one myocyte to another through areas where the plasma membranes of adjacent myocytes actually fuse forming a nexus. Gap junctions connect adjacent myocytes and facilitate excitation of one myocyte by another. This arrangement is to correlated with the fact that, as compared to skeletal muscle, smooth muscle contracts rather slowly. The contraction is, however, more sustained. Afferent nerve fibres are also to be seen in smooth muscle.

Multi-unit and Unitary Smooth Muscle

From the point of view of its nerve supply smooth muscle is divided into two main types: multi-unit and unitary.

In multi-unit muscle nerve fibres establish direct contact with several myocytes (but not with all of them). This kind of muscle contracts when an appropriate nerve stimulus reaches it i.e., contraction is neurogenic. Smooth muscle of this kind is present in the iris, in large arteries, and in the ductus deferens.

In contrast to multi-unit muscle, unitary smooth muscle has its own rhythmic contractility that is independent of a nerve supply. The rate of contraction may be determined by pace maker regions present within the muscle. Contraction of this kind of muscle is also stimulated by stretching. In unitary smooth muscle the nerve endings are less numerous than in multi-unit muscle. The role of the nerves is to increase or decrease the rate of rhythmic contraction. Smooth muscle of this kind is present in the stomach, the intestines, the uterus and the ureter.

Intermediate forms of smooth muscle between the two types described above are also present.

Some other functions of Smooth Muscle

It has been shown that in some ways smooth muscle cells resemble fibroblasts. Myocytes can produce collagen, elastic fibres, and other components of connective tissue matrix. The connective tissue matrix seen in smooth muscle is believed to be produced by smooth muscle cells themselves, fibroblasts being usually missing.

OTHER CONTRACTILE CELLS

Apart from muscle some other cells show the presence of contractile proteins (actin and myosin). These are as follows.

Myoepithelial Cells

In relation to some glands contractile cells are present in close relation to secretory elements. Such cells are called *myoepitheliocytes* (or *myoepithelial cells*). They help to squeeze secretions out of secreting elements. Myoepithelial cells may be *stellate*, forming baskets around acini, or may be *fusiform*.

Myoepitheliocytes are seen in salivary glands, the mammary glands, and sweat glands. These cells are of ectodermal origin. With the EM they

are seen to contain actin and myosin filaments. They can be localized histochemically, because they contain the protein *desmin* which is specific to muscle. Myoepithelial cells are innervated by autonomic nerves.

Myofibroblasts

These are described on page 62.

Pericytes

These are spindle shaped cells present around capillaries and venules. Immunochemical methods reveal the presence of actin and myosin in them. Pericytes can give rise to myofibroblasts, and to mesenchymal tissue which can differentiate into fibroblasts, and can form new blood vessels.

SOME CLINICAL CORRELATIONS OF MUSCLE

1. All varieties of muscle can hypertrophy when exposed to greater stress. Hypertrophy takes place by enlargement of existing fibres, and not by formation of new fibres. Skeletal muscle hypertrophies with exercise. Cardiac muscle hypertrophies if the load on a chamber of the heart is increased for any reason. An example is the hypertrophy of muscle in the wall of the left ventricle in hypertension. Hypertrophy of smooth muscle is seen most typically in the uterus where myocytes may increase from a length of about 15 to 20 μm at the beginning of pregnancy to as much as 500 μm towards the end of pregnancy.

2. Smooth muscle and cardiac muscle have very little capacity for regeneration. Any defects produced by injury or disease are usually repaired by formation of fibrous tissue.

Skeletal muscle fibres can undergo some degree

of regeneration. They cannot divide to form new fibres. However, **satellite cells** present in relation to them (just deep to the external lamina) can give rise to new muscle fibres. Satellite cells are regarded as persisting myoblasts. When large segments of a muscle are destroyed the gap is filled in by fibrous tissue.

3. Overactivity of smooth muscle is responsible for many symptoms. Constriction of bronchi leads to asthma. Spasm of smooth muscle can give rise to severe pain (colic) which may originate in the intestines (intestinal colic), ureter (renal colic), or bile duct (biliary colic). These symptoms can be relieved by drugs swhich cause relaxation of smooth muscle.

4. Proliferation of myofibroblasts is seen in tissue repair, and is associated with some diseases including cirrhosis of the liver, fibrosis of the lung, and atheroma of arteries.

5. Some diseases of muscle (referred to as muscular dystrophy) are caused by genetic defects in proteins that link fibres of the cytoskeleton to the external lamina. One such protein is dystrophin, and its absence is associated with a disease called Duchenne muscular dystrophy.

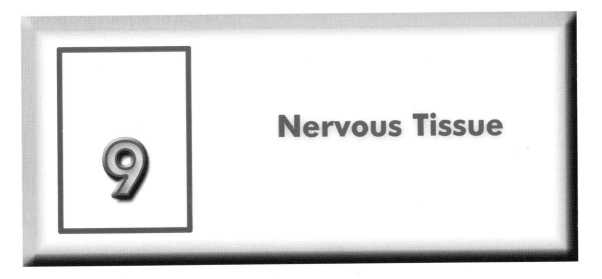

Nervous Tissue

9

TISSUES CONSTITUTING THE NERVOUS SYSTEM

The nervous system is made up, predominantly, of tissue that has the special property of being able to conduct impulses rapidly from one part of the body to another. The specialized cells that constitute the functional units of the nervous system are called *neurons*. Within the brain and spinal cord neurons are supported by a special kind of connective tissue that is called *neuroglia*. Nervous tissue, composed of neurons and neuroglia, is richly supplied with blood. It has been taught that lymph vessels are not present, but the view has recently been challenged.

The nervous system of man is made up of innumerable neurons. The total number of neurons in the human brain is estimated at more than 10^{12}. The neurons are linked together in a highly intricate manner. It is through these connections that the body is made aware of changes in the environment, or of those within itself; and appropriate responses to such changes are produced e.g., in the form of movement or in the modified working of some organ of the body. The mechanisms for some of these relatively simple functions have come to be known as a result of a vast amount of work done by numerous workers for over a century. There is no doubt that higher functions of the brain, like those of memory and intelligence, are also to be explained on the basis of connections

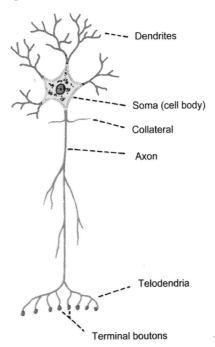

Fig. 9.1. Scheme to show some parts of a neuron.

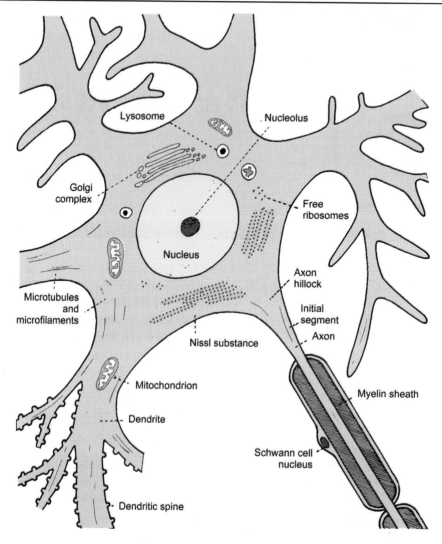

Fig. 9.2. Schematic presentation of some features of the structure of a neuron as seen by EM.

between neurons, but as yet little is known about the mechanisms involved. Neurons are, therefore, to be regarded not merely as simple conductors, but as cells that are specialized for the reception, integration, interpretation and transmission of information.

Nerve cells can convert information obtained from the environment into codes that can be transmitted along their axons. By such coding the same neuron can transmit different kinds of information.

NEURON STRUCTURE

Elementary Structure of a Typical Neuron

Neurons vary considerably in size, shape and other features. However, most of them have some major features in common and these are described below (Figs. 9.1 to 9.4).

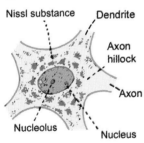

Fig. 9.3A. Neuron stained to show Nissl substance. Note that the Nissl substance extends into the dendrites but not into the axon.

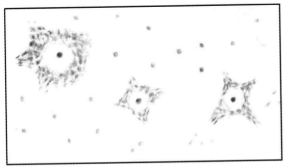

Fig. 9.3B. Section of spinal cord showing large neurons in the ventral grey column.

A neuron consists of a **cell body** which gives off a variable number of **processes** (Fig. 9.1). The cell body is also called the **soma** or **perikaryon**. Like a typical cell it consists of a mass of cytoplasm surrounded by a cell membrane. The cytoplasm contains a large central nucleus (usually with a prominent nucleolus), numerous mitochondria, lysosomes and a Golgi complex (Fig. 9.2). In the past it has

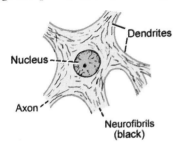

Fig. 9.4. Neuron stained to show neurofibrils. Note that the fibrils extend into both axons and dendrites.

often been stated that centrioles are not present in neurons, but studies with the electron microscope (usually abbreviated to EM) have shown that centrioles are present. In addition to these features, the cytoplasm of a neuron has some distinctive characteristics not seen in other cells. The cytoplasm shows the presence of a granular material that stains intensely with basic dyes; this material is the **Nissl substance** (also called Nissl bodies or granules) (Fig. 9.3). When examined by EM, these bodies are seen to be composed of rough surfaced endoplasmic reticulum (Fig 9.2). The presence of abundant granular endoplasmic reticulum is an indication of the high level of protein synthesis in neurons. The proteins are needed for maintenance and repair, and for production of neurotransmitters and enzymes.

Another distinctive feature of neurons is the presence of a network of fibrils permeating the cytoplasm (Fig. 9.4). These **neurofibrils** are seen, with the EM, to consist of microfilaments and microtubules. (The centrioles present in neurons may be concerned with the production and maintenance of microtubules).

Some neurons contain pigment granules (e.g., neuromelanin in neurons of the substantia nigra). Ageing neurons contain a pigment lipofuscin (made up of residual bodies derived from lysosomes).

The processes arising from the cell body of a neuron are called **neurites.** These are of two kinds. Most neurons give off a number of short branching processes called **dendrites** and one longer process called an **axon.**

The dendrites are characterized by the fact that they terminate near the cell body. They are irregular in thickness, and Nissl granules extend into them. They bear numerous small spines which are of variable shape.

The axon may extend for a considerable distance away from the cell body. The longest axons may be as much as a metre long. Each axon has a uniform diameter, and is devoid of Nissl substance.

In addition to these differences in structure, there is a fundamental functional difference between dendrites and axons. In a dendrite, the nerve impulse travels **towards the cell body** whereas in an axon the impulse travels **away from the cell body.**

The proteins present in dendrites and axons are not identical. This fact is used for

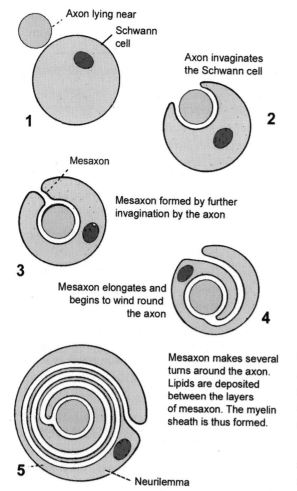

Axon lying near Schwann cell

Axon invaginates the Schwann cell

Mesaxon

Mesaxon formed by further invagination by the axon

Mesaxon elongates and begins to wind round the axon

Mesaxon makes several turns around the axon. Lipids are deposited between the layers of mesaxon. The myelin sheath is thus formed.

Neurilemma

Fig. 9.5. Stages in the formation of the myelin sheath by a Schwann cell.

immunocytochemical identification of dendrites in tissue sections. A protein MAP-2 is present exclusively in dendrites and helps in their identification.

We have seen above that the axon is free of Nissl granules. The Nissl-free zone extends for a short distance into the cell body: this part of the cell body is called the **axon hillock.** The part of the axon just beyond the axon hillock is called the **initial segment** (Fig. 9.2).

During its formation each axon comes to be associated with certain cells that provide a sheath for it. The cells providing this sheath for axons lying outside the central nervous system are called **Schwann cells.** Axons lying within the central nervous system are provided a similar covering by a kind of neuroglial cell called an **oligodendrocyte.** The nature of this sheath is best understood by considering the mode of its formation (Fig. 9.5). An axon lying near a Schwann cell (1) invaginates into the cytoplasm of the Schwann cell (2,3). In this process the axon comes to be suspended by a fold of the cell membrane of the Schwann cell: this fold is called the **mesaxon** (3). In some situations the mesaxon becomes greatly elongated and comes to be spirally wound around the axon, which is thus surrounded by several layers of cell membrane (4,5). Lipids are deposited between adjacent layers of the membrane. These layers of the mesaxon, along with the lipids, form the **myelin sheath.** Outside the myelin sheath a thin layer of Schwann cell cytoplasm persists to form an additional sheath which is called the **neurilemma** (also called the neurilemmal sheath or Schwann cell sheath).

Axons having a myelin sheath are called **myelinated axons.** The presence of a myelin sheath increases the velocity of conduction (for a nerve fibre of the same diameter). It also reduces the energy expended in the process of conduction.

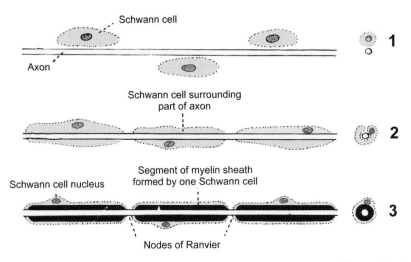

Fig. 9.6. Scheme to show that one Schwann cell forms a short segment of the myelin sheath.

An axon is related to a large number of Schwann cells over its length (Fig. 9.6). Each Schwann cell provides the myelin sheath for a short segment of the axon. At the junction of any two such segments there is a short gap in the myelin sheath. These gaps are called the *nodes of Ranvier.*

There are some axons that are devoid of myelin sheaths. These *unmyelinated axons* invaginate into the cytoplasm of Schwann cells, but the mesaxon does not spiral around them (Fig. 9.7). Another difference is that several such axons may invaginate into the cytoplasm of a single Schwann cell.

An axon may give off a variable number of branches (Fig. 9.1). Some branches, that arise near the cell body and lie at right angles to the axon are called *collaterals.* At its termination the axon breaks up into a number of fine branches called *telodendria* which may end in small swellings (*terminal boutons* or *bouton terminaux*). An axon (or its branches) can terminate in two ways. Within the central nervous system, it always terminates by coming in intimate relationship with another neuron, the junction between the two neurons being called

a *synapse* (page 141). Outside the central nervous system, the axon may end in relation to an effector organ (e.g., muscle or gland), or may end by synapsing with neurons in a peripheral ganglion.

Axons (and some dendrites that resemble axons in structure: see below) constitute what are commonly called *nerve fibres.*

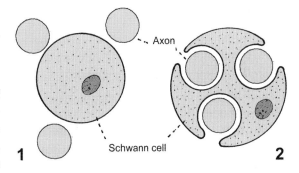

Fig. 9.7. Relationship of unmyelinated axons to a Schwann cell.

Variability in Neuron Structure

Variation in the shape of neuronal cell bodies

Neurons vary considerably in the size and shape of their cell bodies (somata) and in the length and manner of branching of their processes. The cell body varies in diameter from about 5 μm, in the smallest neurons, to as much as 120 μm in the largest ones. The shape of the cell body is dependent on the number of processes arising from it. The most common type of neuron gives off several processes and the cell body is, therefore, ***multipolar*** (Fig. 9.8). Some neurons have only one axon and one dendrite and are ***bipolar.***

Another type of neuron has a single process (which is highly convoluted). After a very short course this process divides into two. One of the divisions represents the axon; the other is functionally a dendrite, but its structure is indistinguishable from that of an axon. This neuron is described as ***unipolar***, but from a functional point of view it is to be regarded as bipolar. (To avoid confusion on this account this kind of neuron has been referred to, in the past, as a ***pseudounipolar*** neuron but this term has now been discarded). Depending on the shapes of their cell bodies some neurons are referred to as ***stellate*** (star shaped) or ***pyramidal.***

In addition to the variations in size and shape, the cell bodies of neurons may show striking variations in the appearance of the Nissl substance. In some neurons, the Nissl substance is very prominent and is in the form of large clumps. In some others, the granules are fine and uniformly distributed in the cytoplasm, while yet other neurons show gradations between these extremes. These differences are correlated with function.

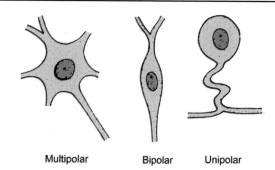

Multipolar   Bipolar   Unipolar

Fig. 9.8. Diagram showing three types of neurons.

Variations in axons

The length of the axon arising from the cell body of a neuron is also subject to considerable variability. Some neurons have long axons, and connect remote regions. These are called ***Golgi type I*** neurons. In other neurons axons are short and end near the cell body. They are called ***Golgi type II*** neurons or ***microneurons***: these are often inhibitory in function. Very rarely, a neuron may not have a true axon.

As stated earlier, axons also differ in the nature of the sheaths covering them, some of them being myelinated and others unmyelinated. Axons also show considerable variation in the diameter of their cross sections (See page 148).

Variations in dendrites

Dendrites arising from a neuronal cell body vary considerably in number, and in the extent and manner of branching. They also differ in the distribution of spines on them. These characteristics are of functional importance. The ***area*** occupied by the dendrites of a neuron is referred to as its ***dendritic field***. Different kinds of neurons have differing dendritic fields (See page 141).

Neurons also show considerable variation in the number and nature of synapses established by them.

FURTHER DETAILS ABOUT NEURONS

Axon hillock and initial segment:

The axon hillock and the initial segment of the axon are of special functional significance. This is the region where action potentials are generated (spike generation) resulting in conduction along the axon. The initial segment is unmyelinated. It often receives axo-axonal synapses that are inhibitory. The plasma membrane here is rich in voltage sensitive channels.

Axoplasmic flow:

The cytoplasm of neurons is in constant motion. Movements of various materials occurs through axons. This *axoplasmic flow* takes place both away from and towards the cell body. The flow away from the cell body is greater. Some materials travel slowly (0.1 to 2 mm a day) constituting a *slow transport.* In contrast other materials (mainly in the form of vesicles) travel 100 to 400 mm a day constituting a *rapid transport.*

Slow transport is unidirectional, away from the cell body. It is responsible for flow of axoplasm (containing various proteins) down the axon. Rapid transport is bi-directional and carries vesicular material and mitochondria. Microtubules play an important role in this form of transport. Retrograde axoplasmic flow may carry neurotropic viruses (e.g., polio) along the axon into the neuronal cell body.

Axoplasmic transport of tracer substances introduced experimentally can help to trace neuronal connections.

Some features of dendrites

(a) As stated earlier dendrites can distinguished immunocytochemically from axons because of the presence in them of microtubule associated protein MAP-2 not present in axons.

(b) Dendritic spines vary in size and shape. Some spines contain aggregations of smooth endoplasmic reticulum (in the form of flattened cisternae with associated dense material). The complex is referred to as the *spine apparatus*.

(c) Actin filaments are present in dendritic spines.

(d) Some variations in the dendritic field are as follows. The field may be *spherical* (as in stellate cells), *hemispherical, disc-like, conical* or *flat*. In some neurons (e.g., pyramidal), the neuron may have two separate dendritic fields. Apart from shape there is considerable variability in *extent* of the dendritic field. Some neurons (e.g., Golgi neurons of the cerebellum) have dendritic fields covering a very wide area. More than eighty per cent of the neuronal surface area (excluding the axon) may be situated on the dendritic tree. The frequency of branching of dendrites is correlated with the number of synapses on them. In some neurons the dendritic spines may number several thousand. Finally, it may be emphasized that the dendritic tree is not a 'fixed' entity, but may undergo continuous remodelling. This affords a basis for modification of neuronal behaviour.

The Synapse

We have seen that synapses are sites of junction between neurons. Synapses may be of various types depending upon the parts of the neurons that come in contact. In the most common type of synapse, an axon terminal establishes contact with the dendrite of a receiving neuron to form an *axodendritic synapse.* Synapses on dendrites may be located on spines or on the smooth areas between spines. The axon terminal may synapse with the cell body (*axosomatic synapse*) or, less commonly, with the axon of the receiving neuron (*axoaxonal synapse*). An axoaxonal synapse may be located either on the initial segment (of the receiving axon) or just proximal to an axon terminal.

In some parts of the brain (e.g., the thalamus) we see some synapses in which the presynaptic

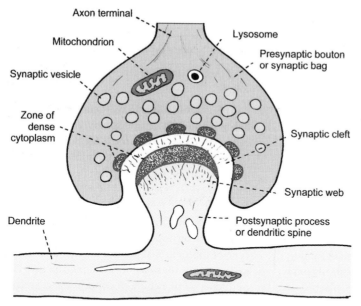

Fig. 9.9. Scheme showing the structure of a typical synapse as seen by EM.

in some other situations. At some sites several synapses may be present around a short length of a dendrite and may be enclosed within a glial capsule. Such a complex is called a *synaptic cartridge*.

A synapse transmits an impulse only in one direction. The two elements taking part in a synapse can, therefore, be spoken of as *presynaptic* and *postsynaptic* (Fig. 9.9). In an axo-dendritic synapse, the terminal enlargement of the axon may be referred to as the *presynaptic bouton* or *synaptic bag*. The region of the dendrite receiving the axon terminal is the *postsynaptic process*. The two are separated by a space called the *synaptic cleft*.

element is a dendrite instead of an axon. Such synapses may be *dendro-axonic* or *dendro-dendritic*. In yet others the soma of a neuron may synapse with the soma of another neuron (*somato-somatic* synapse), or with a dendrite (*somato-dendritic* synapse).

The axon may terminate in a single bulb-like end called a bouton (or *synaptic bag*). Alternatively, the terminal part of the axon may bear a number of such enlargements each of which synapses with the receiving neuron. We have seen that dendrites bear numerous spines. Axon terminals may synapse either with the spines or with smooth portions of the dendrite between the spines. Occasionally, an axon terminal may end by synapsing with the terminal bouton of another axon forming what is called a *serial synapse.* In certain situations several neurons may take part in forming complex synapses. Such areas may be encapsulated by neuroglial cells to form *synaptic glomeruli*. Such glomeruli are found in the cerebellum, the olfactory bulb, the lateral geniculate body and

Delicate fibres or granular material may be seen within the cleft. On either side of the cleft there is a region of dense cytoplasm. On the presynaptic side this dense cytoplasm is broken up into several

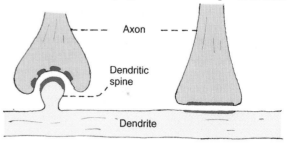

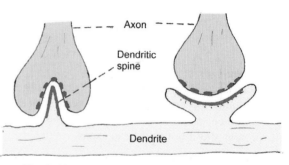

Fig. 9.10. Some variations in the orientation of axodendritic synapses.

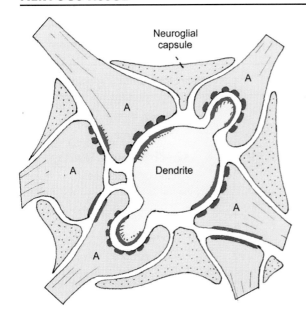

Fig. 9.11. Diagram to show a synaptic glomerulus.

bits. On the postsynaptic side the dense cytoplasm is continuous and is associated with a meshwork of filaments called the *synaptic web.*

The thickened areas of membrane on the presynaptic and postsynaptic sides constitute the *active zone* of a synapse. Neurotransmission takes place through this region. Some variations in the structure of the active zone are described below.

Within the presynaptic bouton numerous synaptic vesicles can be seen. Mitochondria and lysosomes may also be present. The presynaptic bouton contains numerous microtubules (that extend into it from the axon). The tubules end near the presynaptic membrane. Synaptic vesicles are attached to the microtubules by short stalks. The postsynaptic process may also show membranous structures of various shapes, microtubules, filaments and endoplasmic reticulum.

Various proteins and enzymes are present in relation to presynaptic and postsynaptic regions. Some of them (F-actin, spectrin) form a filamentous network that immobilizes vesicles until they are to be released.

Neurotransmitters

The transmission of impulses through synapses involves the release of chemical substances called *neurotransmitters* that are present within synaptic vesicles. When a nerve impulse reaches a terminal bouton neurotransmitter is released into the synaptic cleft. Under the influence of the neurotransmitter the postsynaptic surface becomes depolarized resulting in a nerve impulse in the postsynaptic neuron. In the case of inhibitory synapses, the presence of the neurotransmitter causes hyperpolarisation of the postsynaptic membrane. The neurotransmitter released into the synaptic cleft acts only for a very short duration. It is either destroyed (by enzymes) or is withdrawn into the terminal bouton.

When an action potential reaches the presynaptic terminal, voltage sensitive calcium channels are opened up so that there is an influx of calcium ions leading to a series of chemical changes. As a result of these changes synaptic vesicles pour the neurotransmitter stored in them into the synaptic cleft. The neurotransmitter reaches and binds onto receptor molecules present in the postsynaptic membrane. This alters permeability of the postsynaptic membrane to ions of calcium, sodium, potassium or chloride leading to depolarisation (or hyperpolarisation at inhibitory synapses). The best known (or classical) neurotransmitters responsible for fast but short-lived action of the kind described above are acetylcholine, noradrenaline and adrenaline. For long, all nerve terminals were regarded as either *cholinergic* or *adrenergic*, until it was recognized that these were not the only neurotransmitters present. Other fast neurotransmitters whose presence is now well established are dopamine and histamine.

It is also recognized that apart from the neuro-transmitters mentioned above numerous other chemical substances are associated with synapses. Some of these, which probably act as neuro-transmitters, are serotonin, gama-aminobutyric

Asymmetric / symmetric	Shape of vesicles	Neurotransmitter associated
Asymmetric	Small spherical	Acetyl choline Glutamine Serotonin Some other amines
	Dense cored	Noradrenaline Adrenaline Dopamine
Symmetric	Pleomorphic	GABA Glycine

Fig. 9.12. Classification of synapses on the basis of ultrastructure and neurotransmitters present

acid (GABA), glutamate, aspartate and glycine.

It is now known that at some synapses the effect of a neurotransmitter may last for seconds or even minutes. Repeated synaptic activity can have long lasting effects on the receptor neuron including structural changes such as the formation of new synapses, alterations in the dendritic tree, or growth of axons. Such effects produced under the influence of chemical substances are described as *neuromediation*, the chemical substances concerned being called *neuromediators.* This term includes *neurohormones*, synthesized in neurons and poured into the blood stream through terminals resembling synapses in structure. Similar chemical substances are also poured into the cerebrospinal fluid or into intercellular spaces to influence other neurons in a diffuse manner.

Lastly, some chemical substances associated with synapses do not influence synaptic transmission directly, but influence the effects of transmitters or of neuromediators. Such chemical substances are referred to as *neuromodulators*. Several peptides found in the nervous system probably act as neuromodulators. These include substance P, vasoactive intestinal polypeptide (VIP), somatostatin, cholecystokinin and many others.

Classification of Synapses

We have seen that synapses may be of various types depending on the neuronal elements taking part. They may also be classified on the basis of their ultrastructure, and on the basis of the neurotransmitters released by them. From a physiological standpoint a synapse may be excitatory or inhibitory.

Synapses in different situations can vary considerably in overall shape (Fig. 9.10); in the size, shape and nature of synaptic vesicles and in the configuration of the presynaptic and postsynaptic areas of dense cytoplasm.

Two main types of synapses are recognized on the basis of their ultrastructure.

Asymmetric or Type I synapses: In these synapses the subsynaptic zone of dense cytoplasm is thicker on the presynaptic side. The synaptic cleft is about 30 nm. Such synapses are excitatory.

Symmetric or Type II synapses: In these synapses the subsynaptic zones of dense cytoplasm are thin and of similar thickness on both sides. The synaptic cleft measures about 20 nm.

Various synapses intermediate in structure between these two main types are also encountered.

The vesicles to be seen within synapses can also be of various types. Some vesicles are clear while others have dense cores. They may be pleomorphic (i.e., a mixture of various shapes). The appearance of vesicles can often be correlated with the neurotransmitter present. On the basis of these characters some sub-varieties of Type 1 and Type II synapses that have been recognized are given in Fig. 9.12.

Through its ramifications an axon usually establishes synapses with several different neurons; but in some situations it synapses with one neuron only. Some axons bear boutons that do not come into direct contact with other neurons. Such boutons may represent areas where neurotransmitters are released into surrounding areas, and can have widespread rather than localized effect.

At some sites specialized regions may be seen in relation to synapses. They are mentioned here as they are given specific names.

In some synapses in the retina and internal ear vesicles are arranged around a rod-like element placed at right angles to the cell membrane. This configuration is called a ***synaptic ribbon***. Within some dendritic spines collections of flattened cisternae (endoplasmic reticulum) with associated dense material are seen. These are given the name ***spine apparatus***.

Electrical Synapses

Synapses involving the release of neurotransmitters are referred to as ***chemical synapses***. At some sites one cell may excite another without the release of a transmitter. At such sites adjacent cells have direct channels of communication through which ions can pass from one cell to another altering their electrical status. Such synapses are called ***electrical synapses***.

At the site of an electrical synapse plasma membranes (of the two elements taking part) are closely applied, the gap between them being about 4 nm. Proteins called ***connexins*** project into this gap from the membrane on either side of the synapse. The proteins are so arranged that small open channels are created between the two synaptic elements.

Electrical synapses are common in lower vertebrates and invertebrates. They have been demonstrated at some sites in the brains of mammals (e.g., in the inferior olive and cerebellum).

Junctions between receptors and neurons, or between neurons and effectors, share some of the features of typical synapses and may also be regarded as synapses. Junctions between cardiac myocytes, and between smooth muscle cells, are regarded as electrical synapses.

Influence of neural activity on synapses:

It has been shown that neural activity provides a stimulus for development of new synapses and for increase in their size, specially in early postnatal life. Some experiments show that even in later life (in some situations) brief synaptic activity can have an influence on the subsequent activity of the synapse. This is specially true in areas like the hippocampus and may be associated with memory.

Grey and White Matter

Sections through the spinal cord or through any part of the brain show certain regions that appear whitish, and others that have a darker greyish colour. These constitute the ***white*** and ***grey matter*** respectively. Microscopic examination shows that the cell bodies of neurons are located only in grey matter which also contains

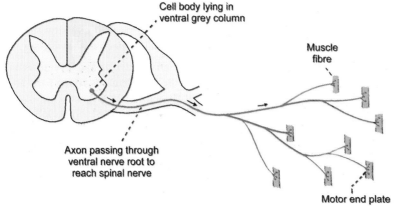

Fig. 9.13. Scheme to show the origin and course of a typical efferent nerve fibre.

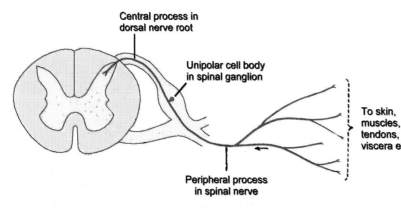

Fig. 9.14. Scheme to show the origin and course of a typical afferent nerve fibre.

of grey matter on the surface. This layer is called the ***cortex.*** Deep to the cortex there is white matter, but within the latter several isolated masses of grey matter are present. Such isolated masses of grey matter present anywhere in the central nervous system are referred to as ***nuclei.*** As grey matter is made of cell bodies of neurons (and the processes arising from or terminating on them) nuclei can be defined as groups of cell bodies of neurons. Aggregations of the cell bodies of neurons may also be found outside the central nervous system. Such aggregations are referred to as ***ganglia.*** Some neurons are located in ***nerve plexuses*** present in close relationship to some viscera. These are, therefore, referred to as ganglionated plexuses.

dendrites and axons starting from or ending on the cell bodies. Most of the fibres within the grey matter are unmyelinated. On the other hand the white matter consists predominantly of myelinated fibres. It is the reflection of light by myelin that gives this region its whitish appearance. Neuroglia and blood vessels are present in both grey and white matter.

The arrangement of the grey and white matter differs at different situations in the brain and spinal cord. In the spinal cord and brainstem the white matter is on the outside whereas the grey matter forms one or more masses embedded within the white matter. In the cerebrum and cerebellum there is an extensive, but thin, layer

The axons arising in one mass of grey matter very frequently terminate by synapsing with neurons in other masses of grey matter. The axons connecting two (or more) masses of grey matter are frequently numerous enough to form recognisable bundles. Such aggregations of fibres are called ***tracts***. Larger collections of fibres are also referred to as ***funiculi, fasciculi*** or ***lemnisci***. (A lemniscus is a ribbon like band). Large bundles of fibres connecting the cerebral or cerebellar hemispheres to the brainstem are called ***peduncles.***

Aggregations of processes of neurons outside

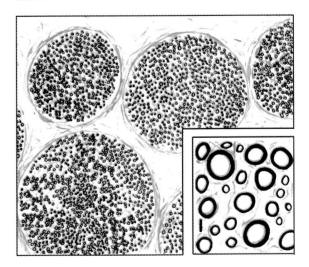

Fig. 9.15A. Section through peripheral nerve stained by a method in which the myelin sheaths become black. The inset shows fibres at high magnification.

the central nervous system constitute *peripheral nerves.*

Neuropil

Many regions of the brain and spinal cord are occupied by a complex meshwork of axon terminals, dendrites and processes of neuroglial cells. This meshwork is called the *neuropil.*

PERIPHERAL NERVES

Peripheral nerves are collections of nerve fibres. These are of two types.

(a) Some nerve fibres carry impulses from the spinal cord or brain to peripheral structures like muscle or gland: they are called *efferent* or *motor* fibres. Efferent fibres are axons of neurons (the cell bodies of which are) located in the grey matter of the spinal cord or of the brainstem.

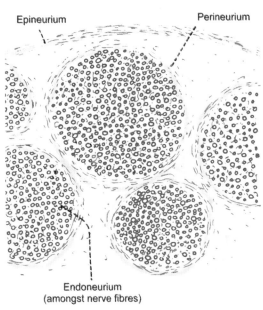

Fig. 9.15B. Diagram to show the connective tissue supporting nerve fibres in a peripheral nerve.

(b) Other nerve fibres carry impulses from peripheral organs to the brain or spinal cord: these are called *afferent* fibres. Many (but not all) afferent fibres are concerned in the transmission of sensations like touch, pain etc.: they are, therefore, also called *sensory* fibres.

Afferent nerve fibres are processes of neurons that are located (as a rule) in sensory ganglia. In the case of spinal nerves these ganglia are located on the dorsal nerve roots. In the case of cranial nerves they are located on ganglia situated on the nerve concerned (usually near its attachment to the brain). The neurons in these ganglia are usually of the unipolar type (page 140). Each unipolar neuron gives off a peripheral process which passes into the peripheral nerve forming an afferent nerve fibre. It also gives off a central process that enters the brain or spinal cord.

From what has been said above it will be clear that the afferent nerve fibres in peripheral nerves are functionally dendrites. However, their histological structure is the same as that of axons.

Basic Structure of Peripheral Nerve Fibres

Each nerve fibre has a central core formed by the axon. This core is called the ***axis cylinder***. The plasma membrane surrounding the axis cylinder is the ***axolemma***. The axis cylinder is surrounded by a myelin sheath (page 138). This sheath is in the form of short segments that are separated at short intervals called the ***nodes of Ranvier*** (Fig. 9.6). The part of the nerve fibre between two consecutive nodes is the ***internode.*** Each segment of the myelin sheath is formed by one Schwann cell. Outside the myelin sheath there is a thin layer of Schwann cell cytoplasm. This layer of cytoplasm is called the ***neurilemma.*** The method of formation of these sheaths has been described on page 138.

Each nerve fibre is surrounded by a layer of connective tissue called the ***endoneurium*** (Fig. 9.15). The endoneurium holds adjoining nerve fibres together and facilitates their aggregation to form bundles or ***fasciculi***. Apart from collagen fibres the endoneurium contains fibroblasts, Schwann cells, endothelial cells and macrophages.

Each fasciculus is surrounded by a thicker layer of connective tissue called the ***perineurium***. The perineurium is made up of layers of flattened cells separated by layers of collagen fibres. The perineurium probably controls diffusion of substances in and out of axons.

A very thin nerve may consist of a single fasciculus, but usually a nerve is made up of several fasciculi. The fasciculi are held together by a fairly dense layer of connective tissue that surrounds the entire nerve and is called the ***epineurium.*** The epineurium contains fat which cushions nerve fibres. Loss of this fat in bedridden patients can lead to pressure on nerve fibres and paralysis.

Classification of Fibres in Peripheral Nerves according to Diameter and Velocity of Conduction

In a transverse section across a peripheral nerve it is seen that the nerve fibres vary considerably in diameter. Fibres of larger diameter are myelinated while those of smallest diameters are unmyelinated. It is well established that by and large fibres of larger diameter conduct impulses more rapidly than those of smaller diameter. Various schemes for classification of nerve fibres on the basis of their diameter and their conduction velocity have been proposed. The best known classification is as follows.

Type A

The fastest conducting fibres are called ***Type A*** fibres. Their conduction velocity is 30 to 120 m/sec; and their diameter varies from 1 to 2 μm. They are myelinated.

Type A fibres are further divided (in descending order of diameter and conduction velocity) into three subtypes: alpha (Aα), delta (Aδ) and gamma (Aγ). Type A fibres subserve both motor and sensory functions as follows:

Motor Type A fibres

1. Aα fibres supply extrafusal fibres in skeletal muscle.

2. Aγ fibres supply intrafusal fibres in muscle spindles.

3. Aδ fibres are collaterals of Aα fibres (to extrafusal fibres) that innervate some intrafusal fibres.

Sensory Type A fibres

1. Aα sensory fibres carry impulses from encapsulated receptors in skin, joints and muscle. They include primary sensory afferents from muscle spindles (also called Group I fibres); and secondary afferents from spindles (also called Group II fibres). Some of them carry impulses from the gut.

Type	Subtype	EFFERENT	AFFERENT
A	Alpha (α)	To extrafusal muscle fibres	From encapsulated receptors in skin, joints, gut Primary sensory fibres from muscle spindles (Group I) Secondary sensory fibres from muscle spindles (Group II)
	Delta (δ)	Some collaterals of Aα fibres to intrafusal muscle fibres	From thermoreceptors and nociceptors
	Gamma (γ)	To intrafusal muscle fibres	
B		Preganglionic autonomic	From skin, viscera From free n. endings in connective tissue of muscle (Group III)
C		Postganglionic autonomic	Interoceptive fibres From thermoreceptors and nociceptors (Group IV)

Fig. 9.16 . Classification of fibres in peripheral nerves.

2. Aδ sensory fibres are afferents from thermo-receptors and nociceptors (pain receptors).

Type B

Type B fibres have a conduction velocity of 4 to 30 m/sec; and their diameter is less than 3 μm. They are myelinated. They are either preganglionic autonomic efferent fibres (motor), or afferent fibres from skin and viscera, and from free nerve endings in connective tissue of muscle (also called Group III fibres).

Type C

In contrast to type A and type B fibres, type C fibres are unmyelinated. They have a conduction velocity of 0.5 to 4 m/sec; and their diameter is 0.5 to 4 μm. These are postganglionic autonomic fibres, and some sensory fibres conveying pain. (These include nociceptive fibres from connective tissue of muscle: Group IV fibres. Note that the terms Group I to IV all refer to afferents from muscle tissue). Some fibres from thermoreceptors and from viscera also fall in this category.

Unmyelinated axons are numerous in dorsal nerve roots and in cutaneous nerves. Many unmyelinated axons are also present in nerves to muscles and in ventral nerve roots. Most autonomic nerve fibres are unmyelinated although myelinated fibres are also present in preganglionic nerves.

The classification of nerve fibres is summarized in Fig. 9.16.

FURTHER DETAILS REGARDING STRUCTURE OF PERIPHERAL NERVES

Further Consideration of the Structure of the Myelin Sheath.

From Fig. 9.17 it will be seen that each layer of plasma membrane helping to form the myelin sheath has an internal or cytoplasmic surface which comes in contact with the internal surface of the next layer; and an external surface that meets the external surface of the next layer. When the myelin sheath is examined with the higher magnifications of the electron microscope it shows alternate thick and thin lines. The thick lines *(called period lines* or *major dense lines)* represent the fused cytoplasmic surfaces of two adjacent layers of the plasma membrane, whereas the thin lines (called *intra-period lines* or *minor dense lines*) represent the fused external surfaces of two adjacent membranes. Some other terms of interest are shown in Fig. 9.17.

Incisures of Schmidt Lanterman

With the light microscope oblique clefts can often be seen in the myelin sheath (Fig. 9.18). These clefts are called the ***Schmidt Lanterman clefts***. Many workers have considered these clefts to be artefacts. However, EM studies show the clefts to be areas where adjoining layers of Schwann cell plasma membrane (forming the myelin sheath) have failed to fuse (Fig. 9.19) leaving (i) a layer of Schwann cell cytoplasm that passes spirally around the axon in the position of the period line; and (ii) a spiral space through which the perineural space communicates with the periaxonal space in the position of the intraperiod line. This space provides a path for passage of substances into the myelin sheath and axon, from the space around the nerve fibre. The clefts enlarge greatly when a nerve fibre undergoes Wallerian degeneration.

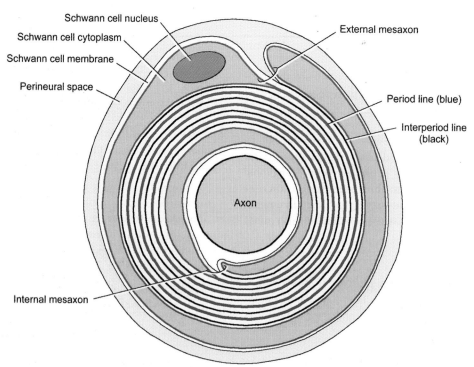

Fig. 9.17. Diagram to explain the significance of period and interperiod lines seen in the myelin sheath at high magnifications of EM.

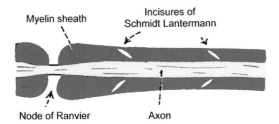

Fig. 9.18. Diagram showing the incisures of Schmidt Lantermann. Also see Fig. 9.19.

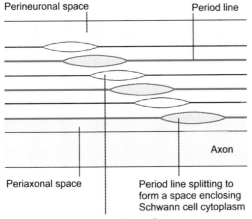

Fig. 9.19. Simplified scheme to show how the incisures of Schmidt Lantermann are formed.

Nodes of Ranvier

We have seen that the myelin sheath is in the form of segments, each segment being formed by one Schwann cell. At the junction of any two such segments there is a gap in the myelin sheath which is called a **node of Ranvier**. The part of the nerve fibre between two such nodes is called the **internode**. The length of the internode is greater in thicker fibres and shorter in thinner ones. It varies from 150 to 1500 μm.

The nerve fibres within a nerve frequently branch. When they do so the bifurcation always lies at a node.

The nodes of Ranvier have great physiological importance. When an impulse travels down a nerve fibre it does not proceed uniformly along the length of the axis cylinder, but jumps from one node to the next. This is called **saltatory conduction**.

(In unmyelinated neurons the impulse travels along the axolemma. Such conduction is much slower than saltatory conduction and consumes more energy).

EM studies reveal several interesting details about the nodes of Ranvier (Fig. 9.20). Immediately next to a node the myelin sheath shows an expansion called the **paranodal bulb**. There are longitudinal furrows on the surface of the paranodal bulb. These furrows are filled in by Schwann cell cytoplasm containing many mitochondria. Finger-like processes of this cytoplasm extend towards the naked part of the axon and come in contact with it. They interdigitate with processes from the

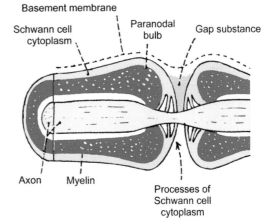

Fig. 9.20. Some details of a node of Ranvier.

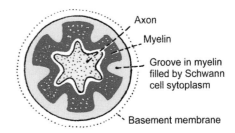

Fig. 9.21. Transverse section across paranodal bulb. Note the fluted appearance of the myelin and of the axon.

neighbouring Schwann cell. In the intervals between these processes the axon is covered by a *gap substance* which plays a role in regulating the flow of the nerve impulse by influencing the passage of ions into, and out of, the axon.

At a node of Ranvier the axon itself is much thinner than in the internode. The part of the axon passing through the paranodal bulb shows infoldings of its axolemma (cell membrane) that correspond to the grooves on the surface of the paranodal bulb (Fig. 9.21).

Chemical composition of myelin

Myelin contains protein, lipids and water. The main lipids present include cholesterol, phospholipids, and glycosphingolipids. Other lipids are present in smaller amounts. Myelination can be seriously impaired, and there can be abnormal collections of lipids, in disorders of lipid metabolism. Various proteins have been identified in myelin sheaths and abnormality in them can be the basis of some neuropathies.

Some facts about myelination

1. It has been observed that myelin sheaths are present only around axons having a diameter more than 1.5 μm in peripheral nerves, and over 1 μm within the central nervous system. However, many axons of these or greater diameter may remain unmyelinated.

2. In general, the larger the axon diameter, the thicker the myelin sheath, and the greater the internodal distance.

3. All Schwann cells associated with a particular axon are believed to be present in relation to it before myelination begins, there being no division of Schwann cells thereafter. Axon diameter and internodal length are also probably determined before myelination begins. However, these dimensions increase with growth.

4. In peripheral nerves Schwann cells accompany nerve fibres as the latter grow towards their destinations. In contrast, in the CNS the axons extend to their destination before oligodendrocytes become associated with them.

5. Myelination does not occur simultaneously in all axons. A myelinated tract becomes fully functional only after its fibres have acquired myelin sheaths.

6. At their exit from the CNS axons in peripheral nerves pass through a central-peripheral transition region where Schwann cells come into relationship with glial cells. This junction normally lies at a node of Ranvier which is called the PNS-CNS compound node (PNS = Peripheral nervous system; CNS = Central nervous system).

Blood Nerve Barrier

Peripheral nerve fibres are separated from circulating blood by a blood-nerve barrier. Capillaries in nerves are non-fenestrated and endothelial cells are united by tight junctions. There is a continuous basal lamina around the capillary. This barrier is reinforced by cell layers present in the perineurium.

Functional relationship between axons and Schwann cells

Schwann cells are not to be regarded merely as a passive covering for axons. A close functional relationship exists between the two as follows.

1. Signals travelling along axons probably influence the differentiation of Schwann cells. Such signals seem to determine proliferation and survival of Schwann cells and also determine whether or not they will form myelin.

2. In contrast, signals arising in Schwann cells can influence the growth of axons and their diameter. Schwann cells are essential for repair of damaged peripheral nerves.

In the preceding sections we have considered some aspects of the normal structure of neurons. We will now consider the changes that take place in neurons when they are injured.

At their peripheral terminations, both afferent and efferent fibres show structural specializations. These are considered on page 155 onwards.

DEGENERATION AND REGENERATION OF NEURONS

When the axon of a neuron is cut across a series of degenerative changes are seen in the axon distal to the injury, in the axon proximal to the injury, and in the cell body.

The changes in the part of the axon distal to the injury are referred to as *anterograde degeneration* or *Wallerian degeneration*. They take place in the entire length of this part of the axon. A few hours after injury the axon becomes swollen and irregular in shape, and in a few days it breaks up into small fragments (Fig. 9.22). The neurofibrils within it break down into granules. The myelin sheath breaks up into small segments. It also undergoes chemical changes that enable degenerating myelin to be stained selectively. The region is invaded by numerous macrophages which remove degenerating axons, myelin and cellular debris. These macrophages probably secrete substances that cause proliferation of Schwann cells. The Schwann cells increase in size and produce a large series of membranes that help to form numerous tubes. We shall see later that these tubes play a vital role in regeneration of nerve fibres.

Degenerative changes in the neuron proximal to the injury are referred to as *retrograde degeneration*. These changes take place in the cell body and in the axon proximal to injury.

The cell body of the injured neuron undergoes a series of changes that constitute the phenomenon of *chromatolysis*. The cell body enlarges tending to become spherical. The nucleus moves from the centre to the periphery. The Nissl substance becomes much less prominent and appears to dissolve away: hence the term chromatolysis. Ultrastructural and histochemical alterations occur in the cell body. The severity of the reaction shown by the cell body is variable. In some cases chromatolysis ends in cell death, followed by degeneration of all its processes. The reaction is more severe when the injury to the axon is near the cell body. If the cell survives, the changes described above are reversed after a period of time.

It is sometimes observed that changes resulting from axonal injury are not confined to the injured neuron, but extend to other neurons with which the injured neuron synapses. This phenomenon is referred to as *transneuronal degeneration.* The degeneration can extend through several synapses (as demonstrated in the visual pathway).

Changes in the proximal part of the axon are confined to a short segment near the site of injury (Fig. 9.22). If the injury is sharp and clean the effects extend only up to one or two nodes of Ranvier proximal to the injury. If the injury is severe a longer segment of the axon may be affected. The changes in the affected part are exactly the same as described for the distal part of the axon. They are soon followed by active growth at the tip of the surviving part of the axon. This causes the terminal part of the axon to swell up (Fig. 9.22 F). It then gives off a number of fine branches. These branches grow into the connective tissue at the site of injury in an effort to reach the distal cut end of the nerve (Fig. 9.22 G.H). We have seen that the Schwann cells of the distal part of the nerve proliferate to form a series of tubes. When one of the regenerating axonal branches succeeds in reaching such a tube, it enters it and then grows rapidly within it. The tube serves as a guide to the growing fibre. Axonal branches that fail to reach one of the tubes degenerate. It often happens that more than one axonal branch enters the same tube. In that case the largest branch survives and the others

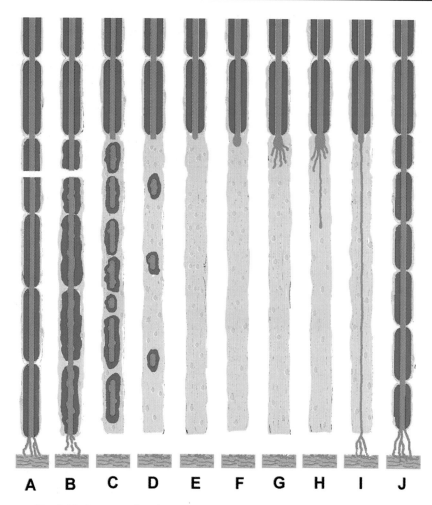

Fig. 9.22. Stages in the degeneration of a nerve fibre after injury (A to E)
and its subsequent regeneration (F to J). For explanation see text.

degenerate. The axon terminal growing through the Schwann cell tube ultimately reaches, and establishes contact with, an appropriate peripheral end organ. Failure to do so results in degeneration of the newly formed axon. The new axon formed in this way is at first very thin and devoid of a myelin sheath (Fig. 9.22 I). However, there is progressive increase in its thickness and a myelin sheath is formed around it. (Fig. 9.22 J).

From the above account it will be clear that chances of regeneration of a cut nerve are considerably increased if the two cut ends are

near each other, and if scar tissue does not intervene between them. It has been observed that tubes formed by Schwann cells begin to disappear if they are not invaded by axons for a long time.

Axons in the CNS do not regenerate as in peripheral nerves. However, it has been seen that if a peripheral nerve is implanted into the CNS, axons tend to grow into the nerve. This may provide a method by which regeneration of tracts could be achieved within the CNS. It appears probable that implanted peripheral nerves provide the necessary environment for regeneration of axons (which the CNS is itself unable to provide).

Peripheral Nerve Endings

We have seen that peripheral nerves contain afferent (or sensory) fibres, and efferent (or motor fibres). In relation to the peripheral endings of afferent nerve fibres there are *receptors* that respond to various kinds of stimuli. Most efferent nerve fibres supply muscle, and at the junction of a nerve fibre with muscle we see neuromuscular junctions. In this chapter we will study the structure of various kinds of sensory receptors, and of neuromuscular junctions

SENSORY RECEPTORS

Preliminary remarks about receptors and their classification

The peripheral terminations of afferent fibres are responsible for receiving stimuli and are, therefore, referred to as *receptors.* Receptors can be classified in various ways.

1. From a functional point of view receptors can be classified on the basis of the kind of information they provide. They may be of the following types.

(a)   *Cutaneous receptors* are concerned with touch, pain, temperature and pressure. These are also called *exteroceptive receptors* or *exteroceptors*.

(b)   *Proprioceptive receptors* (or *proprioceptors*) provide information about the state of contraction of muscles, and of joint movement and position. This information is necessary for precise control of movement and for maintenance of body posture. By and large these activities occur as a result of reflex action and the information from these receptors may or may not be consciously perceived.

(c)   *Interoceptive receptors* (or *interoceptors*) are located in thoracic and abdominal viscera and in blood vessels. These include specialized structures like the carotid sinus and the carotid body.

(d)   The above three categories also include receptors that are stimulated by damaging influences which are perceived as pain, discomfort or irritation. Such receptors are referred to as *nociceptors.*

(e)   *Special sense receptors* of vision, hearing, smell and taste are present in the appropriate organs. As these receptors (like those from the skin) provide information about factors external to the body they are in a sense exteroceptors.

2. Receptors may also be classified on the basis of the manner in which they are stimulated as follows.

(a)   *Mechanoreceptors* are stimulated by mechanical deformation. These include receptors for touch, pressure, stretch etc. They also include end organs in the internal ear. After receiving a stimulus some receptors quickly return to the original state and are in a position to record repeated stimulation discretely. Such receptors are termed *fast adapting.* In contrast, *slow adapting* receptors record repeated stimuli as if there was one continuous stimulus (e.g., that of position sense at joints).

(b)   *Chemoreceptors* are stimulated by chemical influences e.g., receptors in taste buds, or in the carotid bodies.

(c)   *Photoreceptors* are stimulated by light e.g., rods and cones of the retina.

(d)   *Thermoreceptors* respond to alterations

in temperature.

(e) **Osmoreceptors** respond to changes in osmotic pressure.

Many receptors are **polymodal** in that they may respond to more than one kind of stimulus.

3. A third way of classifying receptors is on the basis of their structure. Essentially, most receptors consist of peripheral terminations of sensory nerve fibres that receive the sensory input directly. The somata of the neurons concerned are located in spinal ganglia. As the receptor element is part of a neuron the general term **neuronal receptor** is applied to them.

At some sites the sensory input is received by an epithelial cell which transmits the same to a peripheral nerve fibre. A synapse-like arrangement is seen at the junction of the epithelial cell with the axon terminal. In distinction to neuronal receptors these are termed **epithelial receptors**.

In the olfactory epithelium we have **neuroepithelial receptors**. Here the receptor cell is a modified neuron that lies within the epithelial lining and directly gives off neuronal processes that travel centrally towards the CNS.

Although the receptor element in a neuronal receptor is a nerve terminal such terminals are often intimately surrounded by epithelial elements as described below.

Depending upon the orientation of these epithelial elements many types of endings have been described, but only the better known of these are given below. In the past, efforts have been made to correlate structural variations with specific sensory modalities. However, it is now realized that one type of sensation may be perceived by more than one variety of receptor. At the same time the same type of ending may subserve different functions in different locations. Finally, it is possible that the same receptor may respond to different kinds of

stimuli under different circumstances. In spite of these reservations it appears reasonable to assume that some of the end organs described below are concerned predominantly with particular sensations. It must be remembered, however, that receptors act together and not in isolation and that it is the total pattern of impulses received by the nervous system that determines the nature of the sensations perceived.

For a sensation to be perceived through a receptor three essential steps are involved. Firstly, the receptor terminal has to receive an adequate stimulus. Secondly, the stimulus has to be translated to a change in electrical potential by depolarisation of membrane. Finally, this change in potential has to excite an action potential (in the nerve fibre concerned) that travels to the CNS.

We will now examine the structure of some sensory receptors.

These are illustrated in Fig.9.23.

EXTEROCEPTIVE RECEPTORS

Free Nerve Endings

When the terminals of sensory nerves do not show any particular specialization of structure they are called free nerve endings. Such endings are widely distributed in the body. They are found in connective tissue. They are also seen in relation to the epithelial lining of the skin, cornea, alimentary canal, and respiratory system.

Free nerve endings are particularly numerous in relation to hair follicles. They respond mainly to deformation of hair i.e., they are fast adapting mechanoreceptors. The abundance of free nerve endings in relation to hair follicles is to be correlated with the fact that hair increase the sensitivity of skin to touch. Free nerve endings

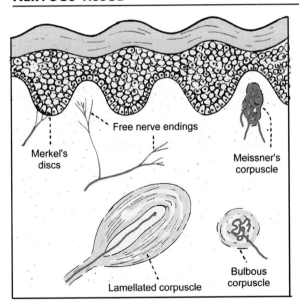

Fig. 9.23. Some sensory receptors present in relation to skin.

may also be thermoreceptors and nociceptors.

Some free nerve endings present in relation to hair follicles are described as *lanceolate endings*. These terminals are seen running along the hair root, below the opening of the sebaceous duct. The terminations of the nerve fibres are flattened with sharp edges that make direct contact with epithelial cells of the hair root.

Tactile Corpuscles (of Meissner)

These are small oval or cylindrical structures seen in relation to dermal papillae in the hand and foot, and in some other situations. These corpuscles are believed to be responsible for touch. They are slow adapting mechano-receptors.

Each corpuscle is about 80μm long and 30μm broad. It consists of an outer capsule and a central core. The capsule is made up of several layers of greatly folded cells and is continuous with the perineurium of nerves supplying the corpuscle. The core contains cells and nerve fibres. Each

corpuscle is supplied by several myelinated nerve fibres. Some unmyelinated fibres may also be present.

Lamellated Corpuscles (of Pacini)

Pacinian corpuscles are circular or oval structures. These are much larger than tactile corpuscles. They may be up to 2 mm in length, and up to 0.5 mm across. They are found in the subcutaneous tissue of the palm and sole, in the digits, and in various other situations. Lamellated corpuscles are believed to be fast adapting mechanoreceptors specially sensitive to vibration. They also respond to pressure.

Each corpuscle has a capsule, an intermediate zone, and a central core. The capsule is arranged in about thirty concentric layers (like the layers of an onion). The intermediate zone is cellular. The core consists of an outer layer of cells from which cytoplasmic lamellae project inwards and interdigitate with each other. In the centre of the core there is, generally, a single nerve fibre. The terminal part of the fibre is expanded into a bulb. Pacinian corpuscles are supplied by thick mye-linated nerve fibres (Type A).

Bulbous Corpuscles (of Krause)

These are spherical structures about 50 μm in diameter. They consist of a capsule within which a nerve fibre terminates in a club-shaped manner. Their significance is controversial. Some authorities regard them to be degenerating or regenerating terminals of nerve fibres rather than as specialized endings.

Tactile Menisci (Merkel cell receptors)

These are small disc-like structures seen in relation to specialized epithelial cells (Merkel cells) present in the stratum spinosum of the epidermis. The discs are expanded ends of nerve fibres. Merkel cells bear spine-like protrusions that interdigitate with surrounding epidermal cells. Tactile menisci are slow adapting mechanoreceptors sensitive to pressure. They are supplied by large myelinated nerve fibres. Apart from surface epithelium of the skin, Merkel cell receptors may be found in relation to the sheaths of hair follicles.

Ruffini endings

These are spindle-shaped structures present in the dermis of hairy skin. Some are also found in non-hairy skin. Similar receptors are also present in relation to joints, in the gums, and in the glans penis.

Within a fibrocellular sheath there are collagen fibres amongst which there are numerous unmyelinated endings of myelinated nerve fibres. Ruffini endings are slow adapting cutaneous mechanoreceptors responsive to stresses in dermal collagen. They resemble the Golgi tendon organs described below.

Summary of functions of cutaneous receptors.

We can summarize the functions of cutaneous receptors as follows.

(a) Merkel discs and Ruffini endings are slowly adapting mechanoreceptors.

(b) Pacinian corpuscles and some types of free nerve endings act as rapidly adapting mechanoreceptors.

(c) Other free nerve endings act as nociceptors and thermoreceptors.

(d) Pacinian corpuscles and Ruffini endings lie deep to skin in the dermis or in tissue deep to skin. Their receptive fields are large and sensations mediated through them are not accurately localized. Pacinian corpuscles are useful mainly for appreciation of vibration. Ruffini endings respond to stretching of the dermis.

(e) In contrast to Pacinian corpuscles and Ruffini endings, Merkel cell receptors and Meissner's corpuscles have small receptor fields (specially over the fingers) and allow good tactile localisation.

(f) Apart from their sensory functions afferent nerve fibres may play a role in inflammation and repair of tissue, probably by releasing peptides (in particular substance P) at their endings. However, these views are not fully established at present.

PROPRIOCEPTIVE RECEPTORS

Golgi Tendon Organs

They are also called the neurotendinous organs of Golgi. These organs are located at the junction of muscle and tendon. Each organ is about 500 μm long and about 100 μm in diameter. It consists of a capsule made up of concentric sheets of cytoplasm (Fig. 9.24). Inside the capsule there are small bundles of tendon fibres. The organ is innervated by one or more myelinated nerve fibres that divide to form several branches (spray-like arrangement). These receptors are stimulated by pull upon the tendon during active contraction of the muscle, and to a lesser degree by passive stretching.

In the past Golgi tendon organs have been considered to be involved in myotactic reflexes that prevent the development of excessive tension in muscle. However, it is now believed that their role is mainly in providing proprioceptive information; and that they are slow adapting receptors.

Similar endings are also present in ligaments of joints. At this site they serve as slow adapting, high threshold, receptors. Impulses from them lead to reflex inhibition of adjacent muscles, preventing excessive stresses on ligaments.

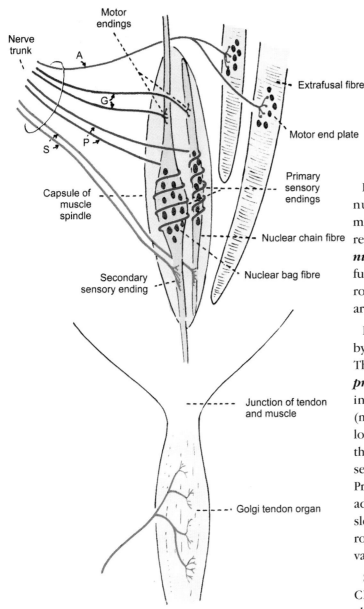

Fig. 9.24. Scheme to show the structure of a muscle spindle and of a Golgi tendon organ.

Muscle Spindles

These are spindle-shaped sensory end organs located within striated muscle (Fig.9.24). The spindle is bounded by a fusiform connective tissue covering (forming an external capsule) within which there are a few muscle fibres of a special kind. These are called **intrafusal fibres** in contrast to **extrafusal fibres** that constitute the main bulk of the muscle. Each spindle contains six to fourteen intrafusal fibres. Each intrafusal fibre is surrounded by an internal capsule of flattened fibroblasts and collagen.

Intrafusal fibres contain several nuclei that are located near the middle of the fibre. In some fibres this region is dilated into a bag: these are **nuclear bag fibres**. In other intra-fusal fibres the nuclei lie in a single row, there being no dilatation: these are **nuclear chain fibres**.

Each muscle spindle is innervated by sensory as well as motor nerves. The sensory endings are of two types, **primary** and **secondary.** The motor innervation of intrafusal fibres is (mainly) by axons of gamma neurons located in the ventral grey column of the spinal cord (Also see below). The sensory endings respond to stretch. Primary sensory endings are rapidly adapting while secondary endings are slow adapting. However, the precise role of these receptors is complex and varies in different types of fibres.

Spindles provide information to the CNS about the extent and rate of changes in length of muscle. Nuclear bag fibres are stimulated by rapid changes, while nuclear chain fibres react more slowly. Contraction of intrafusal fibres makes the spindle more sensitive to stretch.

Some further details about muscle spindles are as follows.

1. The nuclear bag fibres are considerably larger

than the nuclear chain fibres. They extend beyond the capsule and gain attachment to the endomysium of extrafusal fibres. The nuclear chain fibres, on the other hand, remain within the capsule to which their ends are attached. On the basis of their ultrastructure and physiological properties nuclear bag fibres are divided into two types. Bag$_1$ (or dynamic bag$_1$) fibres respond to rapid changes in muscle length. Bag$_2$ (or static bag$_2$) fibres are less responsive to such changes.

The various types of intrafusal fibres differ from extrafusal fibres, and from each other, in ultrastructure and in some features of histochemistry.

2. The primary sensory fibres wind spirally around the nuclear region of intrafusal fibres and are, therefore, referred to as *annulospiral endings.* The secondary endings (also called *flower spray endings)* are seen mostly on nuclear chain fibres and are located away from the nuclear region. Both primary and secondary nerve fibres are derived from large myelinated axons, but are themselves unmyelinated.

3. The motor endings on intrafusal fibres of muscle spindles are of three types.

(a) Terminals of gamma-efferents that end on the equator of the nuclear bag, and do not show typical end plates.

(b) Gamma-efferents ending some distance away from the equator of the nuclear bag and having typical end plates. These are also called P$_2$ endings.

(c) Terminals of delta-efferents (equivalent to beta-efferents of some species), which are collaterals of alpha-fibres supplying extrafusal muscle fibres. These terminals are located near the ends of nuclear bag fibres. They are also called P$_1$ endings.

The motor nerve fibres innervating intrafusal fibres are thin but are myelinated. Those ending over nuclear bags do not show end plates. The P$_2$ endings show typical end plates. P$_1$ endings show en grappe end plates (see page 161).

Receptors present in relation to joints

Four types of receptors have been demonstrated in relation to joints.

1. Type I. These resemble Ruffini endings. They are innervated by myelinated nerve fibres, and serve as slowly adapting mechanoreceptors. These receptors are responsible for the sense of joint position and sense of movement.

2. Type II. These are similar to Pacinian corpuscles. They are fast adapting mechanoreceptors, supplied by myelinated nerve fibres.

3. Type III. These are similar to neurotendinous organs of Golgi. Impulses arising in them are probably responsible for reflex inhibition of muscle contraction, thus preventing excessive movement.

4. Type IV. These are free nerve endings, probably responsible for pain.

NEUROMUSCULAR JUNCTIONS

We have seen that skeletal muscle fibres are supplied by ramifications of somatic efferent neurons. We have also seen that axonal branches arising from one neuron may innervate a variable number of muscle fibres (that constitute a motor unit).

Each skeletal muscle fibre receives its own direct innervation. The site where the nerve ending comes into intimate contact with the muscle fibre is a *neuromuscular (or myoneural) junction*. Details of these junctions vary in different skeletal muscle fibres as follows.

1. Motor end plates or 'en plaque' endings:
In most neuromuscular junctions the nerve terminal comes in contact with a specialized area

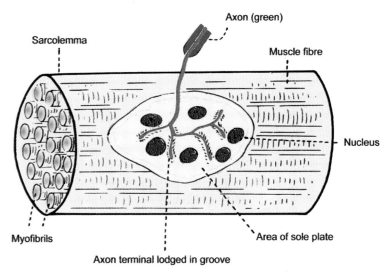

Fig. 9.25. Motor end plate seen in relation to a muscle fibre (surface view). Schwann cell cytoplasm covering the nerve terminal has not been shown for sake of clarity.

near the middle of the muscle fibre. This area is roughly oval or circular, and is referred to as the **sole plate**. The sole plate plus the axon terminal constitute the ***motor end plate***. Motor end plates are considered in detail below.

2. 'En Grappe' endings:

On reaching a muscle fibre some axon terminals divide into a number of small ramifications each ending in an expansion applied to the surface of the muscle fibre. These are referred to as 'en grappe' endings.

3. Trail endings:

In some cases the nerve fibre runs for some distance along the length of the muscle fibre giving off several ramifications that come in contact with the latter.

'En grappe' and trail endings are seen mainly in relation to intrafusal muscle fibres (present in muscle spindles).

Structure of a typical Motor end Plate:

In the region of the motor end plate axon terminals are lodged in grooves in the sarcolemma covering the sole plate. Between the axolemma (over the axon) and the sarcolemma (over the muscle fibre) there is a narrow gap (about 40 nm) occupied by various proteins that form a basal lamina. It follows that there is no continuity between axoplasm and sarcoplasm.

Axon terminals are lodged in grooves in the sarcolemma covering the sole plate. In section (Fig. 9.26) this groove is seen as a semicircular depression. This depression is the ***primary cleft***. The sarcolemma in the floor of the primary cleft is thrown into numerous small folds resulting in the formation of ***secondary (or subneural) clefts.***

In the region of the sole plate the sarcoplasm of the muscle fibre is granular. It contains a number of nuclei and is rich in mitochondria, endoplasmic reticulum and Golgi complexes.

Axon terminals are also rich in mitochondria. Each terminal contains vesicles similar to those seen in presynaptic boutons. The vesicles contain the neurotransmitter acetyl choline. Acetyl choline is released when nerve impulses reach the neuromuscular junction. It initiates a wave of depolarisation in the sarcolemma resulting in contraction of the entire muscle fibre. Thereafter the acetyl choline is quickly destroyed by the enzyme acetyl choline esterase. The presence of acetyl choline receptors has been demonstrated in the sarcolemma of the sole plate.

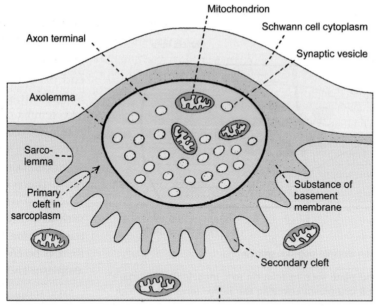

Fig. 9.26. Neuromuscular junction. This figure is a section across one of the axon terminals (and related structures) shown in Fig. 9.25. These details are seen only by EM.

Nerve endings on smooth muscle

Nerve fibres innervating smooth muscle are unmyelinated. They end a short distance away from the myocyte surface. (In other words axolemma and sarcolemma do not come into contact). At most places, the nerve fibres are covered by Schwann cell cytoplasm. However, at places this cytoplasm is retracted exposing a segment of the axon. This segment of the axon shows the presence of vesicles. Neurotransmitter released from the vesicles diffuses to the myocytes.

In sympathetic terminals the vesicles contain catecholamines (usually noradrenaline). Monamine oxidases present in relation to sympathetic endings destroy catecholamines and thus regulate sympathetic activity. At parasympathetic terminals the vesicles in axon terminals are clear. They contain acetyl choline.

Recently it has been shown that some autonomic terminals contain neither noradrenaline nor acetyl choline. These are described as ***non-adrenergic non-cholinergic endings***. The neurotransmitter present at these endings is probably a purine (adenosine triphosphate). Such fibres have been demonstrated in the walls of the alimentary and urinary tracts, and also in the CNS. These endings are believed to be predominantly inhibitory.

Other effector endings:

Apart from muscle, effector endings are present in relation to glands (secretomotor endings), to myoepithelial cells, and to adipose tissue.

GANGLIA

Introductory Remarks

We have seen (page 146) that aggregations of cell bodies of neurons, present outside the brain and spinal cord are known as ganglia. Ganglia are of two main types: sensory, and autonomic.

Sensory ganglia are present on the dorsal nerve roots of spinal nerves, where they are called dorsal nerve root ganglia or spinal ganglia. They are also present on the 5th, 7th, 8th, 9th and 10th cranial nerves. We have seen that the neurons in these ganglia are of the unipolar type (except in the case of ganglia associated with the vestibulo-cochlear nerve in which they are bipolar). The peripheral process of each neuron forms an afferent (or sensory) fibre of a peripheral nerve. The central process enters the spinal cord or brain stem. (For further details of the connections of these neurons see the author's Textbook of Human Neuroanatomy).

Autonomic ganglia are concerned with the nerve supply of smooth muscle or of glands. The pathway for this supply always consists of two neurons: preganglionic and postganglionic. The cell bodies of preganglionic neurons are always located within the spinal cord or brainstem. Their axons leave the spinal cord or brainstem and terminate by synapsing with postganglionic neurons, the cell bodies of which are located in autonomic ganglia. Autonomic ganglia are, therefore, aggregations of the cell bodies of postganglionic neurons. These neurons are multipolar. Their axons leave the ganglia as postganglionic fibres to reach and supply smooth muscle or gland. Autonomic ganglia are subdivisible into two major types: sympathetic and parasympathetic. Sympathetic ganglia are located on the right and left sympathetic trunks. Parasympathetic ganglia usually lie close to the viscera supplied through them. (For further details of the connections of sympathetic and parasympathetic ganglia see the author's Textbook of Human Neuroanatomy).

Structure of Sensory Ganglia

In haematoxylin and eosin stained sections the neurons of sensory ganglia are seen to be large and arranged in groups chiefly at the periphery of the ganglion (Fig. 9.28). The groups of cells are separated by groups of myelinated nerve fibres.

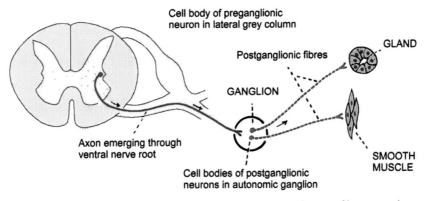

Fig. 9.27. Scheme to show the arrangement of visceral nerve fibres supplying glands and smooth muscle.

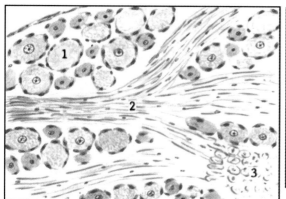

Fig. 9.28. Section through a sensory ganglion. Note large neurons arranged in groups separated by bundles of nerve fibres.

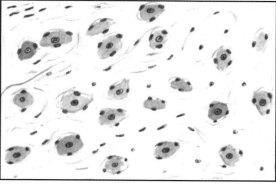

Fig. 9.30. Section through an autonomic ganglion. The neurons are not arranged in groups but are scattered amongst nerve fibres.

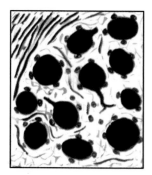

Fig. 9.29. Section of sensory ganglion stained by silver impregnation and viewed at high magnification. Note that the neurons are unipolar.

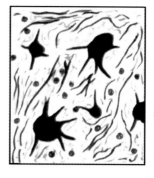

Fig. 9.31. Section through autonomic ganglion stained by silver impregnation and viewed at high magnification. Note that the neurons are multipolar.

The cell body of each neuron is surrounded by a layer of flattened capsular cells or satellite cells. Outside the satellite cells there is a layer of delicate connective tissue. (The satellite cells are continuous with the Schwann cells covering the processes arising from the neuron. The connective tissue covering each neuron is continuous with the endoneurium).

The entire ganglion is pervaded by fine connective tissue. The ganglion is covered on the outside by a connective tissue capsule.

In sections stained by silver impregnation the neurons can be seen to be unipolar (Fig. 9.29).

Structure of Autonomic Ganglia

The neurons of autonomic ganglia are smaller than those in sensory ganglia (Fig. 9.30). With silver impregnation they are seen to be multipolar (Fig. 9.31). The neurons are not arranged in definite groups as in sensory ganglia, but are scattered throughout the ganglion. The nerve fibres are non-myelinated and thinner. They are, therefore, much less conspicuous than in sensory ganglia.

Satellite cells are present around neurons of autonomic ganglia, but they are not so well defined. The ganglion is permeated by connective tissue which also provides a capsule for it (just as in sensory ganglia).

The Nissl substance of the neurons is much

better defined in autonomic ganglia than in sensory ganglia. In sympathetic ganglia the neuronal cytoplasm synthesizes catechol-amines; and in parasympathetic ganglia it synthesizes acetylcholine. These neurotransmitters travel down the axons to be released at nerve terminals.

NEUROGLIA

In addition to neurons, the nervous system contains several types of supporting cells. These are:

(i) *Neuroglial cells*, found in the parenchyma of the brain and spinal cord.

(ii) *Ependymal cells*, lining the ventricular system.

(iii) *Schwann cells*, forming sheaths for axons of peripheral nerves. They are also called *lemnocytes* or *peripheral glia.*

(iv) *Capsular cells* (also called *satellite cells* or *capsular gliocytes*) that surround neurons in peripheral ganglia.

(v) Various types of supporting cells found in relation to motor and sensory terminals of nerve fibres.

Some workers use the term neuroglia for all these categories while others restrict the term only to supporting cells present within the brain and spinal cord. The latter convention is used in the description that follows.

Neuroglial cells may be divided into two major categories.

1. MACROGLIA (or large glial cells)
These are of two types.

(i) *Astrocytes,* which may be subdivided into *fibrous* and *protoplasmic* astrocytes.

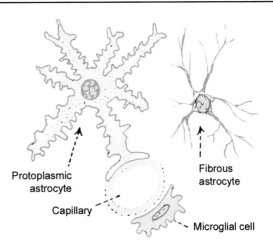

Fig. 9.32. Astrocytes and microglial cells.

(ii) *Oligodendrocytes.*

2. MICROGLIA (or small glial cells)
Macroglial cells are derived from ectoderm of the neural tube. Microglial cells are, on the other hand, of mesodermal origin.

All neuroglial cells are much smaller in size than neurons. However, they are far more numerous. It is interesting to note that the number of glial cells in the brain and spinal cord is ten to fifty times as much as that of neurons. Neurons and neuroglia are separated by a very narrow extracellular space.

In ordinary histological preparations only the nuclei of neuroglial cells are seen. Their processes can be demonstrated by special techniques.

Astrocytes
These are small star-shaped cells that give off a number of processes (Fig. 9.32). The processes are often flattened into leaf-like laminae that may partly surround neurons and separate them from other neurons. The processes frequently end in expansions in relation to blood vessels or in relation to the surface of the brain. Small swellings called *gliosomes* are present on the processes of astrocytes. These swellings are rich in mitochondria. Fibrous astrocytes are seen mainly

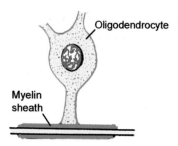

Fig. 9.33. Oligodendrocyte giving off a process that forms a segment of the myelin sheath of an axon.

in white matter . Their processes are thin and are asymmetrical. Protoplasmic astrocytes are, on the other hand, seen mainly in grey matter. Their processes are thicker than those of fibrous astrocytes and are symmetrical. Intermediate forms between fibrous and protoplasmic astrocytes are also present. Protoplasmic extensions of astrocytes surround nodes of Ranvier, but the significance of this is not understood.

The processes of astrocytes are united to those of other astrocytes through gap junctions. Astrocytes communicate with one another through calcium channels. Such communication is believed to play a role in regulation of synaptic activity, and metabolism of neurotransmitters and of neuro-modulators.

Astrocytes play a role in maintenance of the blood brain barrier. Substances secreted by end feet of astrocytes probably assist in maintaining a membrane, the **glia limitans externa**, that covers the exposed surfaces of the brain. They also help to maintain the basal laminae of blood vessels that they come in contact with.

Oligodendrocytes

These cells have rounded or pear-shaped bodies with relatively few processes (olig = scanty). These cells provide myelin sheaths to nerve fibres that lie within the brain and spinal cord. Their relationship to nerve fibres is basically similar to that of Schwann cells to peripheral nerve fibres (page 138).

However, in contrast to a Schwann cell that

ensheaths only one axon, an oligodendrocyte may enclose several axons. Oligodendrocytes are classified into several types depending on the number of neurons they provide sheaths to. As a rule oligodendrocytes present in relation to large diameter axons provide sheaths to fewer axons than those related to axons of small diameter. The plasma membranes of oligodendrocytes comes into contact with axolemma at nodes of Ranvier.

The composition and structure of myelin sheaths formed by oligodendrocytes show differences from those formed by Schwann cells. The two are different in protein content and can be distinguished by immunocytochemical methods. As damage to neurons within the central nervous system is not followed by regeneration, oligodendrocytes have no role to play in this respect.

Microglia

These are the smallest neuroglial cells. The cell body is flattened. The processes are short. These cells are frequently seen in relation to capillaries. As already stated they differ from other neuroglial elements in being mesodermal in origin. They are probably derived from monocytes that invade the brain during fetal life. They are more numerous in grey matter than in white matter. They become active after damage to nervous tissue by trauma or disease and act as phagocytes.

FUNCTIONS OF NEUROGLIA

The following are the functions of neuroglia.

(i) They provide mechanical support to neurons.

(ii) In view of their non-conducting nature they serve as insulators and prevent neuronal impulses from spreading in unwanted directions.

(iii) They are believed to help neuronal function by playing an important role in maintaining a suitable metabolic environment for the neurons. They can absorb neurotransmitters from synapses thus terminating their action. It has been held that they play a role in maintaining the blood-brain barrier, but this view is open to question.

(iv) They are responsible for repair of damaged areas of nervous tissue. Neuroglial cells proliferate in such regions (gliosis). These cells (specially microglia) may act as macrophages.

(Macrophages are cells that can engulf and destroy unwanted material).

(v) As mentioned above, oligodendrocytes provide myelin sheaths to nerve fibres within the central nervous system.

(vi) Ependymal cells are concerned in exchanges of material between the brain and the cerebrospinal fluid.

10

The Cardiovascular System

The cardiovascular system consists of the heart and of blood vessels. The blood vessels that take blood from the heart to various tissues are called *arteries*. The smallest arteries are called *arterioles*. Arterioles open into a network of *capillaries* that pervade the tissues. Exchanges of various substances between the blood and the tissues take place through the walls of capillaries. In some situations capillaries are replaced by slightly different vessels called *sinusoids*. Blood from capillaries (or from sinusoids) is collected by small *venules* which join to form *veins*. The veins return blood to the heart.

Endothelium

The inner surfaces of the heart and of all blood vessels are lined by flattened *endothelial cells* or *endotheliocytes*. On surface view the cells are polygonal, and elongated along the length of the vessel. Cytoplasm is sparse.

The cytoplasm contains endoplasmic reticulum and mitochondria. Microfilaments and intermediate filaments are also present, and these provide mechanical support to the cell. Many endothelial cells show invaginations of cell membrane (on both internal and external surfaces). Sometimes the inner and outer invaginations meet to form channels passing right across the cell (seen typically in small arterioles). These features are seen in situations where vessels are highly permeable.

Adjoining endothelial cells are linked by tight junctions, and also by gap junctions. Externally, they are supported by a basal lamina.

Apart from providing a smooth internal lining to blood vessels and to the heart, endothelial cells perform a number of other functions as follows.

1. Endothelial cells are sensitive to alterations in blood pressure, in blood flow, and in oxygen tension in blood.

2. They secrete various substances that can produce vasodilation by influencing the tone of muscle in the vessel wall.

3. They produce factors that control coagulation of blood. Under normal conditions clotting is inhibited. When required, coagulation can be facilitated.

4. Under the influence of adverse stimuli (e.g., by cytokines: page 81) endothelial cells undergo changes that facilitate passage of lymphocytes through the vessel wall. In acute inflammation, endothelium allows neutrophils to pass from blood into surrounding tissues.

5. Under the influence of histamine (produced in allergic states: page 75) endothelium becomes highly permeable, allowing proteins and fluid to diffuse from blood into tissues. The resultant accumulation of fluid in tissues is called *oedema*.

Changes in properties of endothelium described above take place rapidly (within minutes).

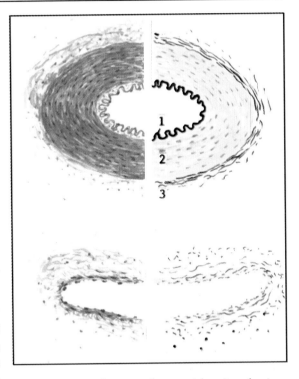

ARTERIES

Basic Structure of Arteries

The histological structure of an artery varies considerably with its diameter. However, all arteries have some features in common which are as follows (10.1 A, B).

The wall of an artery is made up of three layers.

(1) The innermost layer is called the ***tunica intima*** (tunica = coat). It consists of (a) an endothelial lining; (b) a thin layer of glycoprotein which lines the external aspect of the endothelium and is called the ***basal lamina***; (c) a delicate layer of subendothelial connective tissue; and (d) of a membrane formed by elastic fibres called the ***internal elastic lamina***.

(2) Outside the tunica intima there is the ***tunica media*** or middle layer. The media may

Fig. 10.1B. Medium sized artery (above) and vein (below). The left half of the figure shows the appearance as seen with haematoxylin and eosin staining. The right half shows appearance when elastic fibres are stained black (Verheoff's method). 1-Internal elastic lamina. 2-Tunica media. 3-Tunica adventitia

consist predominantly of elastic tissue or of smooth muscle. Some connective tissue is usually present. On the outside the media is limited by a membrane formed by elastic fibres: this is the external elastic lamina.

(3) The outermost layer is called the ***tunica adventitia***. This coat consists of connective tissue in which collagen fibres are prominent. This layer prevents undue stretching or distension of the artery.

It is of interest to note that the fibrous elements in the intima and the adventitia (mainly collagen) run longitudinally (i.e., along the length of the vessel), whereas those in the media (elastic tissue

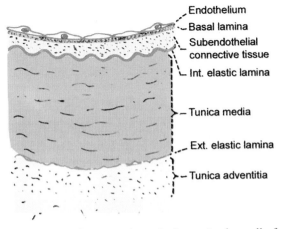

Endothelium
Basal lamina
Subendothelial connective tissue
Int. elastic lamina

Tunica media

Ext. elastic lamina

Tunica adventitia

Fig. 10.1A. Scheme to show the layers in the wall of a typical artery.

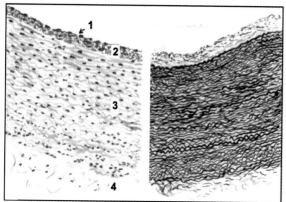

Fig. 10.1C. Section through an elastic artery. Staining is as in Fig. 10.1B. 1-Endothelial lining. 2-Tunica intima. 3-Tunica media. 4-Tunica adventitia.

or muscle) run circularly. Elastic fibres, including those of the internal and external elastic laminae are often in the form of fenestrated sheets. (fenestrated = having holes in it).

Elastic and Muscular Arteries

On the basis of the kind of tissue that predominates in the tunica media, arteries are often divided into elastic arteries and muscular arteries. Elastic arteries include the aorta and the large arteries supplying the head and neck (carotids) and limbs (subclavian, axillary, iliac). The remaining arteries are muscular.

Although all arteries carry blood to peripheral tissues, elastic and muscular arteries play differing additional roles. When the left ventricle of the heart contracts, and blood enters the large elastic arteries with considerable force, these arteries distend significantly. They are able to do so because of much elastic tissue in their walls. During diastole (i.e., relaxation of the left ventricle) the walls of the arteries come back to their original size because of the elastic recoil of their walls. This recoil acts as an additional force that pushes the blood into smaller arteries. It is because of this fact that blood flows continuously through arteries (but with fluctuation of pressure

during systole and diastole). In contrast a muscular artery has the ability to alter the size of its lumen by contraction or relaxation of smooth muscle in its wall. Muscular arteries can, therefore, regulate the amount of blood flowing into the regions supplied by them.

Details of the differences in structure of elastic and muscular arteries are given below.

Differences between Elastic and Muscular Arteries

(a) The main difference in structure of elastic and muscular arteries is in the constitution of the tunica media. In elastic arteries the media is made up mainly of elastic tissue. The elastic tissue is in the form of a series of concentric membranes that are frequently fenestrated. In the aorta (which is the largest elastic artery) there may be as many as fifty layers of elastic membranes. Between the elastic membranes there is some loose connective tissue. Some smooth muscle cells may be present. On the contrary in muscular arteries the media is made up mainly of smooth muscle. This muscle is arranged circularly. Between groups of muscle fibres some connective tissue is present: this may contain some elastic fibres.

Longitudinally arranged muscle is present in the media of arteries that undergo repeated stretching or bending. Examples of such arteries are the coronary, carotid, axillary and palmar arteries.

The transition from elastic to muscular arteries is not abrupt. In proceeding distally along the artery there is a gradual reduction in elastic fibres and increase in smooth muscle content in the media.

(b) There is not much difference in the intima of elastic and muscular arteries, except that the subendothelial connective tissue contains more elastic fibres in the former. In elastic arteries the internal elastic lamina is not distinct from the media as it has the same structure as the elastic membranes of the media. It, however, stands out distinctly from the muscular media of smaller arteries.

(c) The adventitia also does not show significant differences in elastic and muscular arteries. It is relatively thin in large arteries, in which a greater proportion of elastic fibres are present. These fibres merge with the external elastic lamina.

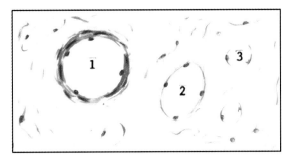

Fig. 10.2A. Section showing an arteriole (1), a venule (2), and a capillary (3). 20–10,

Atheroma

The most common disease of arteries is *atheroma*, in which the intima becomes infiltrated with fat and collagen. The thickenings formed are *atheromatous plaques*. Atheroma leads to narrowing of the arterial lumen, and consequently to reduced blood flow. Damage to endothelium can induce coagulation of blood forming a *thrombus* which can completely obstruct the artery. This leads to death of the tissue supplied. When this happens in an artery supplying the myocardium (*coronary thrombosis*) it leads to *myocardial infarction* (manifesting as a *heart attack*). In the brain (*cerebral thrombosis*) it leads to a *stroke* and paralysis. An artery weakened by atheroma may undergo dilation (*aneurysm*), or may even rupture.

diameter (Fig. 10.2A). Arterioles less than 50 μm in diameter are called *terminal arterioles.* Muscular arterioles can be distinguished from true arteries (i) by their small diameter, and (ii) by the fact that they do not have an internal elastic lamina. They have a few layers of smooth muscle in their media. Terminal arterioles can be distinguished from muscular arterioles as follows.

(a) As stated above they have a diameter less than 50 μm, the smallest terminal arterioles having a diameter as small as 12 μm. 50–12.

(b) They have only a thin layer of muscle in their walls.

(c) They give off lateral branches (called meta-arterioles) to the capillary bed.

The initial segment of each lateral branch is surrounded by a few smooth muscle cells. These muscle cells constitute the *precapillary sphincter* (See page 175). The adventitia of arterioles is formed by a thin network of collagen fibres.

ARTERIOLES *Internal elastic lamina is absent?*

When traced distally, muscular arteries progressively decrease in calibre till they have a diameter of about 100 μm. They then become continuous with arterioles. The larger or *muscular arterioles* are 100 to 50 μm in

Fig. 10.2B. Longitudinal section through a vein to show a valve made up of two cusps.

VEINS

The basic structure of veins is similar to that of arteries. The tunica intima, media and adventitia can be distinguished specially in large veins. The structure of veins differs from that of arteries in the following respects (Fig. 10.1B).

1. The wall of a vein is distinctly thinner than that of an artery having the same sized lumen.

2. The tunica media contains a much larger quantity of collagen than in arteries. The amount of elastic tissue or of muscle is much less.

3. Because of the differences mentioned above, the wall of a vein is easily compressed. After death veins are usually collapsed. In contrast arteries retain their patency.

4. In arteries the tunica media is usually thicker than the adventitia. In contrast the adventitia of veins is thicker than the media (specially in large veins). In some large veins (e.g., the inferior vena cava) the adventitia contains a considerable amount of elastic and muscle fibres which run in a predominantly longitudinal direction. These fibres facilitate elongation and shortening of the vena cava with respiration. This is also facilitated by the fact that collagen fibres in the adventitia form a meshwork that spirals around the vessel.

5. A clear distinction between the tunica intima, media and adventitia cannot be made out in small veins as all these layers consist predominantly of fibrous tissue. Muscle is conspicuous by its complete absence in venous spaces of erectile tissue, in veins of cancellous bone, dural venous sinuses, retinal veins, and placental veins.

Valves of Veins

Most veins contain valves that allow the flow of blood towards the heart, but prevent its regurgitation in the opposite direction. Typically each valve is made up of two semilunar cusps (Fig. 10.2B). Each cusp is a fold of endothelium within which there is some connective tissue that is rich in elastic fibres. Valves are absent in very small veins; in veins within the cranial cavity, or within the vertebral canal; in the venae cavae; and in some other veins.

Flow of blood through veins is assisted by contractions of muscle in their walls. It is also assisted by contraction of surrounding muscles specially when the latter are enclosed in deep fascia.

VENULES

The smallest veins, into which capillaries drain, are called venules (Fig. 10.2A). They are 20-30 μm in diameter. Their walls consist of endothelium, basal lamina, and a thin adventitia consisting of longitudinally running collagen fibres. Flattened or branching cells called **pericytes** may be present outside the basal laminae of small venules (called **post-capillary venules**), while some muscle may be present in larger vessels (**muscular venules**).

Functionally, venules have to be distinguished from true veins. The walls of venules (specially those of postcapillary venules) have considerable permeability and exchanges between blood and surrounding tissues can take place through them. In particular venules are the sites at which lymphocytes and other cells may pass out of (or into) the blood stream.

CAPILLARIES

We have seen that terminal arterioles (page 171) are continued into a capillary plexus which pervades the tissue supplied. The arrangement of the capillary plexus and its density varies from tissue to tissue, the density being greatest in tissues having high metabolic activity. Exchanges (of oxygen, carbon dioxide, fluids and various molecules) between blood and tissue take place through the walls of the capillary plexus (and through postcapillary venules).

The average diameter of a capillary is $8\,\mu$m. The wall of a capillary is formed essentially by endothelial cells which are lined on the outside by a basal lamina (glycoprotein). Overlying the basal lamina there may be isolated branching perivascular cells (pericytes), and a delicate network of reticular fibres and cells.

Some variations in the structure of the capillary wall are seen in different tissues. Typically, the edges of endothelial cells fuse completely with those of adjoining cells to form a continuous wall. Such capillaries are called ***continuous capillaries***. As such capillaries are seen most typically in muscle they are also called ***muscular capillaries*** (a highly misleading term as the capillaries have no muscle in their walls). In some organs the walls of capillaries appear to have apertures in their endothelial lining: these are, therefore, called ***fenestrated capillaries***. The 'apertures' are, however, always closed by a thin diaphragm (which may represent greatly thinned out cytoplasm of an endothelial cell, or only the basal lamina).

Some fenestrations represent areas where endothelial cell cytoplasm has pores passing through the entire thickness of the cell.

In continuous capillaries exchanges of material between blood and tissue take place through the cytoplasm of endothelial cells. This is suggested

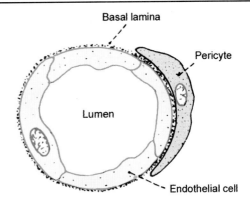

Fig. 10.3. Diagram to show the structure of a continuous capillary.

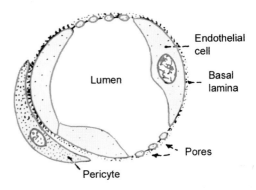

Fig. 10.4. Diagram to show the structure of a fenestrated capillary.

by the presence of numerous pinocytotic vesicles in the cytoplasm; and by the presence of numerous depressions (***caveolae***) on the cell surfaces, which may represent pinocytotic vesicles in the process of formation. Apart from transport through the cytoplasm, substances may also pass through the intercellular material separating adjoining endothelial cells.

In the case of fenestrated capillaries diffusion of substances takes place through the numerous fenestrae in the capillary wall.

Continuous capillaries are seen in the skin, connective tissue, muscle, lungs and brain. Fenestrated capillaries are seen in renal glomeruli, intestinal villi, endocrine glands, and pancreas.

SINUSOIDS *Bone marrow, Spleen, lymph nodes*

In some tissues the 'exchange' network is made up of vessels that are somewhat different from capillaries, and are called sinusoids. The main differences between capillaries and sinusoids are as follows.

(1) The wall of a sinusoid consists only of endothelium supported by a thin layer of connective tissue. The wall may be incomplete at places, so that blood may come into direct contact with tissue cells. Deficiency in the wall may be in the form of fenestrations (*fenestrated sinusoids*) or in the form of long slits (*discontinuous sinusoids*, as in the spleen).

(2) At some places the wall of the sinusoid consists of phagocytic cells instead of endothelial cells (Fig. A73).

(3) Sinusoids have a broader lumen (about 20 μm) than capillaries. The lumen may be irregular. Because of this fact blood flow through them is relatively sluggish.

Sinusoids are found typically in organs that are made up of cords or plates of cells. These include the liver, the adrenal cortex, the hypophysis cerebri, and the parathyroid glands. Sinusoids are also present in the spleen, in the bone marrow, and in the carotid body.

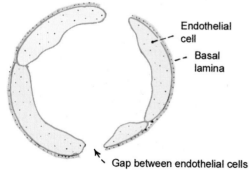

Endothelial cell

Basal lamina

Gap between endothelial cells

Fig. 10.5. Diagram to show the structure of a sinusoid.

MECHANISMS CONTROLLING BLOOD FLOW THROUGH THE CAPILLARY BED

The requirements of blood flow through a tissue may vary considerably at different times. For example, a muscle needs much more blood when engaged in active contraction, than when relaxed. Blood flow through intestinal villi needs to be greatest when there is food to be absorbed. The mechanisms that adjust blood flow through capillaries are considered below.

Blood supply to relatively large areas of tissue is controlled by contraction or relaxation of smooth muscle in the walls of muscular arteries and arterioles. Control of supply to smaller areas is effected through arteriovenous anastomoses, precapillary sphincters, and thoroughfare channels as described below.

Arteriovenous Anastomoses

In many parts of the body small arteries and veins are connected by direct channels that constitute arteriovenous anastomoses. These channels may be straight or coiled. Their walls have a thick muscular coat which is richly supplied with sympathetic nerves. When the anastomoses are patent blood is short circuited from the artery to the vein so that very little blood passes through the capillary bed. However, when the muscle in the wall of the anastomosing channel contracts its lumen is occluded so that all blood now passes through the capillaries. Arteriovenous anastomoses are found in the skin specially in that of the nose, lips and external ear; and in the mucous membrane of the alimentary canal and nose. They are also seen in the tongue, in the thyroid, in sympathetic ganglia, and in the erectile tissues of sex organs.

Arteriovenous anastomoses in the skin help in regulating body temperature, by increasing blood flow through capillaries in warm weather; and decreasing it in cold weather to prevent heat loss.

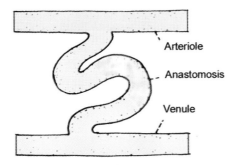

Fig. 10.6. Diagram to show an arteriovenous anastomosis (glomus).

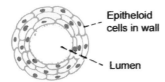

Fig. 10.7. Section across the connecting channel of an arteriovenous anastomosis.

In some regions we see arteriovenous anastomoses of a special kind. The vessels taking part in these anastomoses are in the form of a rounded bunch covered by connective tissue. This structure is called a *glomus*. Each glomus consists of an afferent artery; one or more coiled (S-shaped) connecting vessels; and an efferent vein. Blood flow through the glomus is controlled in two different ways. Firstly, the wall of the afferent artery has a number of elevations that project into the lumen; and probably have a valvular function. These projections are produced partly by endothelium, and partly by muscle. Secondly the connecting vessels have thick muscular walls in which the muscle fibres are short and thick with central nuclei. These cells have some resemblance to epithelial cells and are, therefore, termed *epitheloid cells.* They have similarities to pericytes present around capillaries. The lumen

of the connecting channel can be occluded by contraction (or swelling) of epitheloid cells.

Glomera are found in the skin at the tips of the fingers and toes (specially in the digital pads and nail beds); in the lips; the tip of the tongue; and in the nose. They are concerned with the regulation of the circulation in these areas in response to changes in temperature.

Arteriovenous anastomoses are few and inefficient in the new-born. In old age again, arteriovenous anastomoses of the skin decrease considerably in number. These observations are to be correlated with the fact that temperature regulation is not efficient in the new-born as well as in old persons.

Precapillary Sphincters & Thoroughfare Channels

Arteriovenous anastomoses described above control blood flow through relatively large segments of the capillary bed. Much smaller segments can be individually controlled as follows.

We have seen that capillaries arise as side branches of terminal arterioles; and that the initial segment of each such branch is surrounded by a few smooth muscle cells that constitute a *precapillary sphincter*. Blood flow

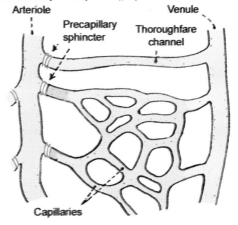

Fig. 10.8. Diagram to show precapillary sphincters and thoroughfare channels.

through any part of the capillary bed can be controlled by the precapillary sphincter.

> In many situations arterioles and venules are connected (apart from capillaries) by some channels that resemble capillaries, but have a larger calibre. These channels run a relatively direct course between the arteriole and venule. Isolated smooth muscle fibres may be present on their walls. These are called *thoroughfare channels*. At times when most of the precapillary sphincters in the region are contracted (restricting flow through capillaries), blood is short circuited from arteriole to venule through the thoroughfare channels. A thoroughfare channel and the capillaries associated with it are sometimes referred to as a *microcirculatory unit*.

BLOOD VESSELS, LYMPHATICS & NERVES SUPPLYING BLOOD VESSELS

The walls of small blood vessels receive adequate nutrition by diffusion from blood in their lumina. However, the walls of large and medium sized vessels are supplied by small arteries called *vasa vasorum* (literally 'vessels of vessels': singular = *vas vasis*). These vessels supply the adventitia and the outer part of the media. These layers of the vessel wall also contain many lymphatic vessels.

Blood vessels have a fairly rich supply by autonomic nerves (sympathetic). The nerves are unmyelinated. Most of the nerves are vasomotor and supply smooth muscle. Their stimulation causes vasoconstriction in some arteries, and vasodilatation in others. Some myelinated sensory nerves are also present in the adventitia.

THE HEART

There are three layers in the wall of the heart.

(a) The innermost layer is called the *endocardium*. It corresponds to the tunica intima of blood vessels. It consists of a layer of endothelium that rests on a thin layer of delicate connective tissue. Outside this there is a thicker *subendocardial layer* of connective tissue.

(b) The main thickness of the wall of the heart is formed by a thick layer of cardiac muscle. This is the *myocardium*. The structure of cardiac muscle has already been described (page 128).

> It has been shown that atrial myocardial fibres secrete a *natriuretic hormone* when they are excessively stretched (as in some diseases). The hormone increases renal excretion of water, sodium and potassium. It inhibits the secretion of renin (by the kidneys), and of aldosterone (by the adrenal glands) thus reducing blood pressure.

(c) The external surface of the myocardium is covered by the *epicardium* (or *visceral layer of serous pericardium*). It consists of a layer of connective tissue which is covered, on the free surface, by a layer of flattened mesothelial cells.

At the junction of the atria and ventricles, and around the openings of large blood vessels there are rings of dense fibrous tissue. Similar dense fibrous tissue is also present in the interventricular septum. These masses of dense fibrous tissue constitute the 'skeleton' of the heart. They give attachment to fasciculi of heart muscle.

The *valves of the heart* are folds of endocardium that enclose a plate like layer of dense fibrous tissue.

> The *conducting system of the heart* is made up of a special kind of cardiac muscle. The *Purkinje fibres* of this system are chains of cells.

The cells are united by desmosomes. Intercalated discs are absent. These cells have a larger diameter, and are shorter, than typical cardiac myocytes. Typically each cell making up a Purkinje fibre has a central nucleus surrounded by clear cytoplasm containing abundant glycogen. Myofibrils are inconspicuous and are confined to the periphery of the fibres. Mitochondria are numerous and the sarcoplasmic reticulum is prominent. **Nodal myocytes** (present in the AV node and the SA node) are narrow, rounded, cylindrical or polygonal cells with single nuclei. They are responsible for pace-maker functions. **Transitional myocytes** are present in the nodes, and in the stem and main branches of the AV bundle. They are similar to cardiac myocytes except that they are narrower. Conduction through them is slow.

In the SA node and the AV node the muscle fibres are embedded in a prominent stroma of connective tissue. This tissue contains many blood vessels and nerve fibres.

11

Lymphatics and Lymphoid Tissue

Introductory Remarks

When circulating blood reaches the capillaries part of its fluid content passes into the surrounding tissues as tissue fluid. Most of this fluid re-enters the capillaries at their venous ends. Some of it is, however, returned to the circulation through a separate system of *lymphatic vessels* (usually called *lymphatics*). The fluid passing through the lymphatic vessels is called *lymph*. The smallest lymphatic (or lymph) vessels are lymphatic capillaries which join together to form larger lymphatic vessels. The largest lymphatic vessel in the body is the *thoracic duct*. It drains lymph from the greater part of the body. The thoracic duct ends by joining the left subclavian vein at its junction with the internal jugular vein. On the right side there is the *right lymphatic duct* which has a similar termination.

Scattered along the course of lymphatic vessels there are numerous small bean-shaped structures called *lymph nodes* that are usually present in groups. Lymph nodes are masses of lymphoid tissue described below. As a rule lymph from any part of the body passes through one or more lymph nodes before entering the blood stream. (There are some exceptions to this rule. For example, some lymph from the thyroid gland drains directly into the thoracic duct). Lymph nodes act as filters removing bacteria and other particulate matter from lymph. Lymphocytes are added to lymph in these nodes.

Each group of lymph nodes has a specific area of drainage. For the location of various groups of lymph nodes, and the areas of the body drained by them see a book on gross anatomy.

Aggregations of lymphoid tissue are also found at various other sites. Two organs, the thymus and the spleen are almost entirely made up of lymphoid tissue. Prominent aggregations of lymphoid tissue are present in close relationship to the lining epithelium of the gut. Such aggregations present in the region of the pharynx constitute the *tonsils*. Isolated nodules of lymphoid tissue, and larger aggregations called *Peyer's patches* are present in the mucosa and submucosa of the small intestines (specially the ileum). The mucosa of the vermiform appendix contains abundant lymphoid tissue. Lymphoid tissue is seen in the mucosa of the large intestines. Collections of lymphoid tissue are also to be seen in the walls of the trachea and larger bronchi, and in relation to the urinary tract.

Lymph

Lymph is a transudate from blood and contains the same proteins as in plasma, but in smaller amounts, and in somewhat different proportions. Suspended in lymph there are cells that are chiefly lymphocytes. Most of these lymphocytes are added to lymph as it passes through lymph nodes, but some are derived from tissues drained by the nodes.

Large molecules of fat (chylomicrons) that are absorbed from the intestines enter lymph vessels. After a fatty meal these fat globules may be so numerous that lymph becomes milky (and is then called *chyle*). Under these conditions the lymph vessels can be seen easily as they pass through the mesentery.

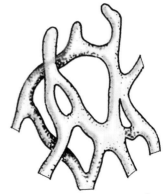

Fig. 11.1. Diagram to show part of a network of lymphatic capillaries.

Lymph capillaries are present in most tissues of the body. They are absent in avascular tissues (e.g., the cornea, hair, nails); in the splenic pulp; and in the bone marrow. It has been held that lymphatics are not present in nervous tissue, but we now know that some vessels are present.

LYMPHATIC VESSELS

Lymph Capillaries

Lymph capillaries (or lymphatic capillaries) begin blindly in tissues where they form a network. The structure of lymph capillaries is basically similar to that of blood capillaries, but is adapted for much greater permeability. There is an inner lining of endothelium. The basal lamina is absent or poorly developed. Pericytes or connective tissue are not present around the capillary.

As compared to blood capillaries, much larger molecules can pass through the walls of lymph capillaries. These include colloidal material, fat droplets, and particulate matter such as bacteria. It is believed that these substances pass into lymph capillaries through gaps between endothelial cells lining the capillary; or by pinocytosis.

Larger Lymph Vessels

The structure of the thoracic duct and of other larger lymph vessels is similar to that of veins. A tunica intima, media and adventitia can be distinguished. Elastic fibres are prominent and can be seen in all three layers. The media, and also the adventitia contains some smooth muscle. In most vessels, the smooth muscle is arranged

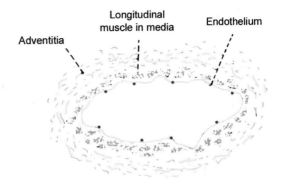

Fig. 11.2. Transverse section across the thoracic duct.

circularly, but in the thoracic duct the muscle is predominantly longitudinal.

Numerous valves, similar to those in veins, are present in small as well as large lymphatic vessels. They are more numerous than in veins. The valves often give lymph vessels a beaded appearance.

Acute inflammation of lymph vessels is called *lymphangitis*. When this happens in vessels of the skin, the vessels are seen as red lines that are painful.

LYMPH NODES

Each lymph node consists of a connective tissue framework; and of numerous lymphocytes, and other cells, that fill the interstices of the network. The entire node is bean-shaped, the concavity constituting a hilum through which blood vessels enter and leave the node. Several lymph vessels

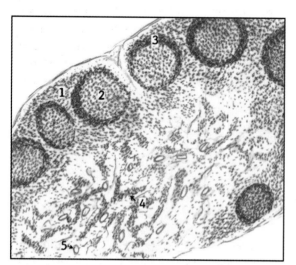

Fig.11.3. Section through a lymph node. 1-Cortex. 2, 3-Germinal center and outer zone of lymphatic follicle. 4-Medulla. 5-Blood vessel.

enter the node on its convex aspect. Usually, a single lymph vessel leaves the node through its hilum.

When a section through a lymph node is examined (at low magnification) it is seen that the node has an outer zone which contains densely packed lymphocytes, and therefore stains darkly: this part is the *cortex*. The cortex does not extend into the hilum. Surrounded by the cortex, there is a lighter staining zone in which lymphocytes are fewer: this area is the *medulla* (Fig. 11.3).

Within the cortex there are several rounded areas that are called *lymphatic follicles* or *lymphatic nodules*. Each nodule has a paler staining *germinal centre* surrounded by a zone of densely packed lymphocytes.

Within the medulla, the lymphocytes are arranged in the form of branching and anastomosing cords.

We will now consider some of these constituents in greater detail.

The Connective Tissue Framework

The lymph node is covered by a *capsule* consisting mainly of collagen fibres. Some elastic fibres and some smooth muscle may be present. A number of *septa* (or *trabeculae*) extend into the node from the capsule and divide the node into lobules. The hilum is occupied by a mass of dense fibrous tissue.

The remaining space within the node is filled by a delicate network of reticular fibres. Associated with the network there are reticular cells that have traditionally been regarded as macrophages. However, it is now believed that they are fibroblasts and do not have phagocytic properties.

The Cells of Lymph Nodes

Lymphocytes

The cell population of a lymph node is made up (overwhelmingly) of lymphocytes. The structure, origin and functions of these cells have been considered on pages 76 to 81: these pages should be re-read at this stage.

Lymphocytes enter lymph nodes from blood. Some enter through lymph. The general arrangement of lymphocytes within a node has been considered above. Studies using immunofluorescent staining have revealed that both B-lymphocytes and T-lymphocytes are present in lymph nodes. The lymphatic nodules

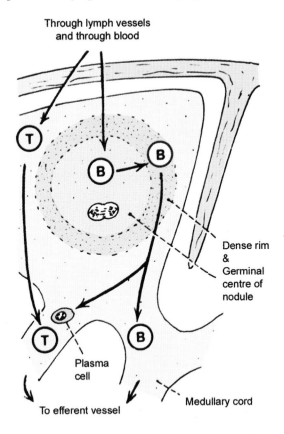

Fig. 11.4. Scheme to show the circulation of B-lymphocytes and of T-lymphocytes through a lymph node.

(which constitute the **cortex proper**) are composed of B-lymphocytes. The cells in the paler germinal centres of the nodules are mainly lymphoblasts. It is believed that they represent B-lymphocytes that have been stimulated, by antigens, to enlarge and undergo multiplication.

The lymphocytes divide repeatedly and give rise to more B-lymphocytes aggregations of which form the dark staining 'rims' around the germinal centres. These B-lymphocytes mature into plasma cells (page 65) which are seen mainly in the medullary cords. Because of this location, antibodies produced by them pass easily into efferent lymph vessels, and from there into the blood stream.

B-lymphocytes entering a lymph node from blood can behave in two ways. (a) If stimulated by antigens they proliferate and produce plasma cells. Such lymphocytes remain in lymph nodes for prolonged periods as **memory cells**. (b) If not stimulated lymphocytes return to the blood stream (via lymph) after spending just a few hours in the node.

The diffuse lymphoid tissue intervening between nodules (often called the **paracortex** or **thymus dependent cortex**) is made up mainly of T-lymphocytes. T-lymphocytes are also present in medullary cords. Note that the medullary cords contain both B-lymphocytes and T-lymphocytes.

T-cells enter lymph nodes from blood. After a few hours they leave the node via efferent lymph vessels. When activated by antigens they multiply to form a large number of activated T-cells that are sensitive to the particular antigen. These T-cells reach various tissues through the circulation.

Some workers describe the germinal centres of lymphatic follicles as **zone 3**, and the dark rims of the follicles as **zone 2**. The term **zone 1** is applied to the region immediately around the follicle containing loosely packed lymphocytes, plasma cells and macrophages. Zone I becomes continuous with the medullary cords.

Cells other than lymphocytes

Apart from lymphocytes and plasma cells various other cells are present in a lymph node as follows.

1. In association with the framework of reticular fibres, there are numerous fibroblasts (previously called reticular cells. See page 61).

2. Numerous macrophages are present in the lymph sinuses (see below) and around germinal centres. They are more numerous in the medulla than in the cortex. Some of them lie along the walls of lymph sinuses.

Macrophages play an important role in the immune response by phagocytosis of antigens,

and by presenting these antigens to lymphocytes (*antigen presenting function*). Macrophages are, therefore, referred to as *immunologic accessory cells*. Several functional types of such cells can be recognized. Dendritic antigen presenting cells (page 88) are present in the paracortex.

3. Lining the blood vessels of the node there are endothelial cells. The lymph sinuses (see below) are also lined by endothelial cells. Pericytes (page 172) and smooth muscle cells are also present around blood vessels.

Circulation of Lymph through Lymph nodes

We have seen that the entire lymph node is pervaded by a reticular network. Most of the spaces of this network are packed with lymphocytes. At some places, however, these spaces contain relatively few cells, and form channels through which lymph circulates. These channels are lined by endothelium, but their walls allow free movement of lymphocytes into and out of the channels.

Afferent lymphatics reaching the convex outer surface of the node enter an extensive

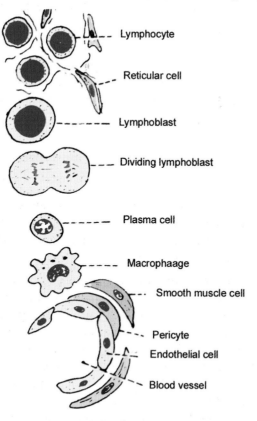

Fig. 11.5. Diagram to show various types of cells that may be seen in a lymph node.

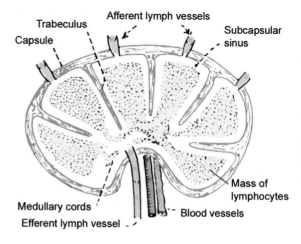

Fig. 11.6. Scheme to show some features of the structure of a lymph node.

subcapsular sinus (Fig.11.6). From this sinus a number of radial cortical sinuses run through the cortex towards the medulla. Reaching the medulla the sinuses join to form larger medullary sinuses. In turn the medullary sinuses join to form (usually) one, or more than one, efferent lymph vessel through which lymph leaves the node. Note that afferent vessels to a lymph node enter the cortex, while the efferent vessel emerges from the medulla. The sinuses are lined by endothelium.

Lymph passing through the system of sinuses comes into intimate contact with macrophages present in the node. Bacteria and other particulate matter are removed from lymph by these cells. Lymphocytes freely enter or leave the node through these channels. Lymphocytes also enter the node from blood by passing through postcapillary venules. (For circulation of lymphocytes see page 76).

Blood Supply of Lymph Nodes

Arteries enter a lymph node at the hilum. They pass through the medulla to reach the cortex where they end in arterioles and capillaries. These arterioles and capillaries are arranged as loops that drain into venules. Postcapillary venules in lymph nodes are unusual in that they are lined by cuboidal endothelium. (They are, therefore, called **high endothelial venules**). This 'high' endothelium readily allows the passage of lymphocytes between the blood stream and the surrounding tissue. These endothelial cells bear receptors that are recognized by circulating lymphocytes. Contact with these receptors facilitates passage of lymphocytes through the vessel wall.

Summary of Functions of Lymph Nodes

From what has been said in the preceding paragraphs it will be obvious that lymph nodes perform the following major functions.

1. They are centres of lymphocyte production. Both B-lymphocytes and T-lymphocytes are produced here by multiplication of preexisting lymphocytes. These lymphocytes (which have been activated) pass into lymph and thus reach the blood stream.

2. Bacteria and other particulate matter are removed from lymph through phagocytosis by macrophages. Antigens thus carried into these cells are 'presented' to lymphocytes stimulating their proliferation. In this way lymph nodes play an important role in the immune response to antigens.

3. Plasma cells (representing fully mature B-lymphocytes) produce antibodies against invading antigens, while T-lymphocytes attack cells that are 'foreign' to the host body (see page 78).

Applied Anatomy

Infection in any part of the body can lead to enlargement and inflammation of lymph nodes draining the area. Inflammation of lymph nodes is called **lymphadenitis**.

Carcinoma (cancer) usually spreads from its primary site either by growth of malignant cells along lymph vessels, or by 'loose' cancer cells passing through lymph to nodes into which the area drains. This leads to enlargement of the lymph nodes of the region. Examination of lymph nodes gives valuable information about the spread of cancer. In surgical excision of cancer lymph nodes draining the region are usually removed.

THE SPLEEN

Connective Tissue Basis

The spleen is the largest lymphoid organ of the body (Fig. 11.7). Except at the hilum, the surface of the spleen is covered by a layer of peritoneum (referred to as the *serous coat*. Deep to the serous layer the organ is covered by a *capsule*. *Trabeculae* arising from the capsule extend into the substance of the spleen. As they do so the trabeculae divide into smaller divisions which form a network. The capsule and trabeculae are made up of fibrous tissue in which elastic fibres are abundant. In some animals they contain much smooth muscle, but this is not a prominent feature of the human spleen.

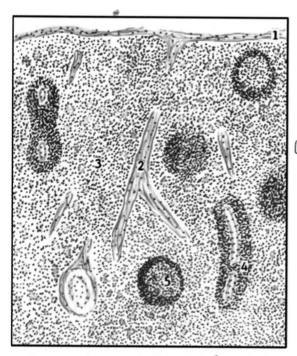

Fig. 11.7. Section through spleen. 1-Capsule. 2-Septum. 3-Red pulp. 4, 5-Cords of densely packed lymphocytes around arteriole.

The spaces between the trabeculae are pervaded by a network formed by reticular fibres embedded in an amorphous matrix. Fibroblasts (reticular cells) and macrophages are also present in relation to the reticulum. The interstices of the reticulum are pervaded by lymphocytes, blood vessels and blood cells, and by macrophages. To understand further details of the arrangement of these tissues it is necessary to first consider some aspects of the circulation through the spleen.

Circulation through the Spleen

On reaching the hilum of the spleen the splenic artery divides into about five branches that enter the organ independently. Each branch divides and subdivides as it travels through the trabecular network. Arterioles arising from this network leave the trabeculae to pass into the inter-trabecular spaces. For some distance each arteriole is surrounded by a dense sheath of lymphocytes. These lymphocytes constitute the *white pulp* of the spleen. The arteriole then divides into a number of straight vessels that are called *penicilli*. Each of the penicilli shows a localized thickening of its wall that is called an *ellipsoid*. The ellipsoid consists of concentric lamellae formed by aggregation of fibroblasts and macrophages. The lumen of each penniculus is much narrowed at the ellipsoid.

Distal to the ellipsoid the vessel dilates to form an *ampulla* the walls of which become continuous with the reticular framework. As a result blood flows into spaces lined by reticular cells, coming into direct contact with lymphocytes there. The part of splenic tissue which is infiltrated with blood in this way is called the *red pulp*. The circulation in the red pulp of the spleen is thus an 'open' one in contrast to the 'closed' circulation in other organs. However, circulation in the white pulp, and in trabeculae,

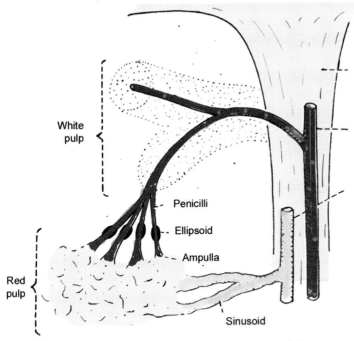

White
pulp

Red
pulp

Trabeculus

Trabecular
artery

Trabecular
vein

Penicilli

Ellipsoid

Ampulla

Sinusoid

Fig. 11.8. Scheme to show some features of the
splenic circulation.

The White pulp

We have seen that the white pulp is made up of lymphocytes that surround arterioles. As a result it is in the form of cord-like aggregations of lymphocytes that follow the branching pattern of the arterioles. The cords appear to be circular in transverse section. At places the cords are thicker than elsewhere and contain lymphatic nodules similar to those seen in lymph nodes. These nodules are called ***Malpighian bodies***. Each nodule has a germinal centre and a surrounding cuff of densely packed lymphocytes. The nodules are easily distinguished from those of lymph nodes because of the presence of an arteriole in each of them. The arteriole is placed eccentrically at the margin of the germinal centre (between it and the surrounding cuff of densely packed cells). More than one arteriole may be present in relation to one germinal centre.

The functional significance of the white pulp is similar to that of cortical tissue of lymph nodes. Most of the lymphocytes in white pulp are T-lymphocytes. Lymphatic nodules of the white pulp are aggregations of B-lymphocytes. The germinal centres are areas where B-lymphocytes are dividing.

The Red Pulp

The red pulp is like a sponge. It is permeated by spaces lined by reticular cells. The intervals between the spaces are filled by B-lymphocytes as well as T-lymphocytes, macrophages, and

is of the normal closed type. Blood from spaces of the red pulp is collected by wide sinusoids which drain into veins in the trabeculae.

The sinusoids of the spleen are lined by a somewhat modified endothelium. The endothelial cells here are elongated and are shaped like bananas. They are referred to as *stave cells*. With the EM a system of ultramicroscopic fibrils is seen to be present in their cytoplasm. The fibrils may help to alter the shape of the endothelial cells thus opening or closing gaps between adjoining cells.

The spleen acts as a filter for worn out red blood cells. Normal erythrocytes can change shape and pass easily through narrow passages in penicilli and ellipsoids. However, cells that are aged are unable to change shape and are trapped in the spleen where they are destroyed by macrophages.

blood cells. These cells appear to be arranged as cords (*splenic cords*, of Billroth). The cords form a network.

The zone of red pulp immediately surrounding white pulp is the *marginal zone*. This zone has a rich network of sinusoids. Numerous antigen presenting cells are found close to the sinusoids. This region seems to be specialized for bringing antigens confined to circulating blood (eg., some bacteria) into contact with lymphocytes in the spleen so that an appropriate immune response can be started against the antigens. (Such contact does not take place in lymph nodes. Antigens reach lymph nodes from tissues, through lymph). Surgical removal of the spleen (splenectomy) reduces the ability of the body to deal with blood borne infections.

Lymph Vessels of the Spleen

Traditionally, it has been held that in the spleen lymph vessels are confined to the capsule and trabeculae. Recent studies have shown, however, that they are present in all parts of the spleen. Lymphocytes produced in the spleen reach the blood stream mainly through the lymph vessels.

FUNCTIONS OF THE SPLEEN

1. Like other lymphoid tissues the spleen is a centre where both B-lymphocytes and T-lymphocytes multiply, and play an important role in immune responses (see page 78). As stated above, the spleen is the only site where an immune response can be started against antigens present in circulating blood (but not present in tissues).

2. The spleen contains the largest aggregations of macrophages of the mononuclear phagocyte system. In the spleen the main function of these cells is the destruction of red blood corpuscles that have completed their useful life. This is facilitated by the intimate contact of blood with the macrophages because of the presence of an open circulation. Macrophages also destroy worn out leucocytes, and bacteria.

3. In fetal life the spleen is a centre for production of *all* blood cells. In later life only lymphocytes are produced here.

4. The spleen is often regarded as a store of blood which can be thrown into the circulation when required. This function is much less important in man than in some other species.

In conditions calling for increased lymphocyte production (leukaemias); or conditions in which there is increased phagocytosis by macrophages (as in any infection); and in conditions involving increased destruction of erythrocytes (e.g., malaria) there may be enlargement of the spleen. The condition is called *splenomegaly*.

THE THYMUS

The thymus is an organ that is a hazy entity for most students. This is because of the fact that the organ is not usually seen in dissection hall cadavers (because of atrophy in old people, and because of rapid autolysis after death). The organ is also not accessible for clinical examination (as it lies deep to the manubrium sterni). At birth the thymus weighs 10-15 g. The weight increases to 30-40 g at puberty. Subsequently, much of the organ is replaced by fat. However, the thymus is believed to produce T-lymphocytes throughout life.

The thymus consists of right and left lobes that are joined together by fibrous tissue. Each lobe

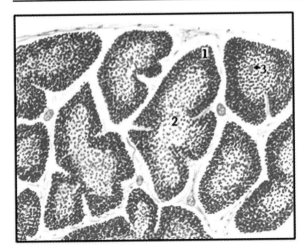

Fig. 11.9. Thymus (low power view). Note masses of lymphocytes arranged in the form of lobules. 1-Cortex. 2-Medulla. 3-Hassal's corpuscle.

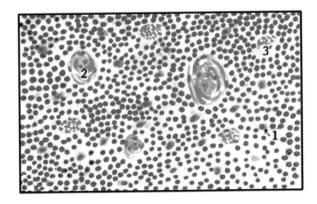

Fig. 11-10. Thymus. (High power view). 1- Epithelial cell. 2-Hassal's corpuscle. 3-Capillary.

has a connective tissue capsule. Connective tissue septa passing inwards from the capsule incompletely subdivide the lobe into a large number of lobules (Figs. 11.9, 11.10)).

Each lobule is about 2 mm in diameter. It has an outer cortex and an inner medulla. Both the cortex and medulla contain cells of two distinct lineages as described below. The medulla of adjoining lobules is continuous.

The thymus has a rich blood supply. It does not receive any lymph vessels, but gives off efferent vessels.

Epithelial Cells (Epitheliocytes)

Embryologically these cells are derived from endoderm lining the third pharyngeal pouch. (It is possible that some of them may be of ectodermal origin). The cells lose all contact with the pharyngeal wall. In the fetus their epithelial origin is obvious. Later they become flattened and may branch. The cells join to form sheets that cover the internal surface of the capsule, the surfaces of the septa, and the surfaces of blood vessels. The epithelial cells lying deeper in the lobule develop processes that join similar processes of other cells to form a reticulum. It may be noted that this reticulum is cellular, and has no similarity to the reticulum formed by reticular fibres (and associated fibroblasts) in lymph nodes and spleen. Epithelial cells of the thymus are not phagocytic.

It has been suggested that the sheets of epithelial cells present deep to the capsule, around septa, and around blood vessels form an effective **blood-thymus barrier** that prevents antigens (present in blood) from reaching lymphocytes present in the thymus. Epitheliocytes also promote T-cell differentiation and proliferation.

On the basis of structural differences several types of epitheliocytes are recognized. Type 1 epitheliocytes line the inner aspect of the capsule, the septa and blood vessels. These are the cells forming the partial haemothymic barrier mentioned above. Type 2 and type 3 cells are present in the outer and inner parts of the cortex respectively. Type 4 cells lie in the deepest parts of the cortex, and also in the medulla. They form a network containing spaces which are occupied by lymphocytes. Type 5 cells are present around corpuscles of Hassall (see below).

Cortical epitheliocytes are also described as **thymic nurse cells**. They destroy lymphocytes that react against self antigens.

Lymphocytes of the thymus (Thymocytes)

In the cortex of each lobule of the thymus the reticulum formed by epithelial cells is densely packed with lymphocytes. Stem cells formed in bone marrow travel to the thymus. Here they come to lie in the superficial part of the cortex, and divide repeatedly to form small lymphocytes. Lymphatic nodules are not present in the normal thymus.

The medulla of each lobule also contains lymphocytes, but these are less densely packed than in the cortex. As a result the epithelial reticulum is more obvious in the medulla than in the cortex. As thymocytes divide they pass deeper into the cortex, and into the medulla. Ultimately, they leave the thymus by passing into blood vessels and lymphatics. For further details of thymic lymphocytes see below.

Macrophages

Apart from epithelial cells and lymphocytes the thymus contains a fair number of macrophages (belonging to the mononuclear phagocyte system). They are present subjacent to the capsule, at the cortico-medullary junction, and in the medulla. The subcapsular macrophages are highly phagocytic. Deeper lying macrophages are dendritic cells (page 88). Their significance is considered below.

Corpuscles of Hassall

These are small rounded structures present in the medulla of the thymus. Each corpuscle has a central core formed by epithelial cells that have undergone degeneration. These cells ultimately form a pink staining hyaline mass. Around this mass there is a wall formed by concentrically arranged epithelial cells. These cells also stain bright pink with haematoxylin and eosin. The central mass of the corpuscle may also contain degenerating macrophages. The functional significance of the corpuscles of Hassall is not understood.

FUNCTIONS OF THE THYMUS

1. The role of the thymus in lymphopoiesis has been discussed on page 76. Stem cells (from bone marrow) that reach the superficial part of the cortex divide repeatedly to form smaller lymphocytes. It has been postulated that during these mitoses the DNA of the lymphocytes undergoes numerous random mutations, as a result of which different lymphocytes acquire the ability to recognize a very large number of different proteins, and to react to them. As it is not desirable for lymphocytes to react against the body's own proteins, all lymphocytes that would react against them are destroyed. It is for this reason that 90% of lymphocytes formed in the thymus are destroyed within three to four days. The remaining lymphocytes, that react only against proteins foreign to the body, are thrown into the circulation as circulating, immunologically competent T-lymphocytes. They lodge themselves in secondary lymph organs like lymph nodes, spleen etc., where they multiply to form further T-lymphocytes of their own type when exposed to the appropriate antigen.

From the above it will be understood why the thymus is regarded as a *primary lymphoid organ* (along with bone marrow). It has been held that, within the thymus, lymphocytes are not allowed to come into contact with foreign antigens, because of the presence of the blood-thymic barrier. It has also been said that because of this thymocytes do not develop into large lymphocytes or into plasma cells, and do not form lymphatic nodules. While these views may hold as far as the thymic cortex is concerned, they do not appear to be correct in respect of the medulla. Recently it has been postulated that the medulla of the thymus (or part of it) is a separate 'compartment'. After thymocytes move into this compartment they probably come into contact with antigens presented to them through dendritic macrophages. Such contact may be a necessary step in making T-lymphocytes competent to distinguish between foreign antigens and proteins of the body itself.

2. The proliferation of T-lymphocytes and their conversion into cells capable of reacting to antigens, probably takes place under the influence of hormones produced by epithelial cells of the thymus. T-lymphocytes are also influenced by direct cell contact with epitheliocytes. Hormones produced by the thymus may also influence lymphopoiesis in peripheral lymphoid organs. This influence appears to be specially important in early life, as lymphoid tissues do not develop normally if the thymus is removed. Thymectomy has much less influence after puberty as the lymphoid tissues have fully developed by then.

A number of hormones produced by the thymus have now been identified as follows. They are produced by epitheliocytes.

(a) *Thymulin* enhances the function of various types of T-cells (page 79), specially that of suppresser cells.

(b) *Thymopoietin* stimulates the production of cytotoxic T-cells. The combined action of thymulin and thymopoietin allows precise balance of the activity of cytotoxic and suppresser cells.

(c) *Thymosin alpha 1* stimulates lymphocyte production, and also the production of antibodies.

(b) *Thymosin beta 4* is produced by mononuclear phagocytes.

(e) *Thymic humoral factor* controls the multiplication of helper and suppresser T-cells.

Apart from their actions on lymphocytes, hormones (or other substances) produced in the thymus probably influence the adenohypophysis and the ovaries. In turn, the activity of the thymus is influenced by hormones produced by the adenohypophysis, by the adrenal cortex, and by sex hormones.

Thymus and Myasthenia gravis

Enlargement of the thymus is often associated with a disease called myasthenia gravis. In this condition there is great weakness of skeletal muscle. In many such cases the thymus is enlarged and there may be a tumour in it. Removal of the thymus may result in considerable improvement in some cases.

Myasthenia gravis is now considered to be a disturbance of the immune system. There are some proteins to which acetyl choline released at motor end plates gets attached. In myasthenia gravis antibodies are produced against these proteins rendering them ineffective. Myasthenia gravis is, thus, an example of a condition in which the immune system begins to react against one of the body's own proteins. Such conditions are referred to as *autoimmune diseases*.

MUCOSA ASSOCIATED LYMPHOID TISSUE

We have seen that the main masses of lymphoid tissue in the body are the lymph nodes, the spleen and the thymus. Small numbers of lymphocytes may be present almost anywhere in the body, but significant aggregations are seen in relation to the mucosa of the respiratory, alimentary and urogenital tracts. These aggregations are referred to as *mucosa associated lymphoid tissue (MALT)*. The total volume of MALT is more or less equal to that of the lymphoid tissue present in lymph nodes and spleen. Mucosa associated aggregations of lymphoid tissue have some features in common as follows.

1. These aggregations are in the form of one or more lymphatic follicles (nodules) having a structure similar to nodules of lymph nodes. Germinal centres may be present. Diffuse lymphoid tissue (termed the *parafollicular zone*) is present in the intervals between the nodules. The significance of the nodules and of the diffuse aggregations of lymphocytes are the same as already described in the case of lymph nodes. The nodules consist predominantly of B-lymphocytes, while the diffuse areas contain T-lymphocytes.

2. These masses of lymphoid tissue are present in very close relationship to the lining epithelium of the mucosa in the region concerned, and lie in the substantia propria. Larger aggregations extend into the submucosa. Individual lymphocytes may infiltrate the epithelium and may pass through it into the lumen.

3. The aggregations are not surrounded by a capsule, nor do they have connective tissue septa. A supporting network of reticular fibres is present.

4. As a rule these masses of lymphoid tissue do not receive afferent lymph vessels, and have no lymph sinuses. They do not, therefore, serve as filters of lymph. However, they are centres of lymphocyte production. Lymphocytes produced here pass into lymph nodes of the region through efferent lymphatic vessels. Some lymphocytes pass through the overlying epithelium into the lumen.

Apart from B-lymphocytes and T-lymphocytes, phagocytic macrophages and dendritic phagocytes are present. The post capillary venules have a structure similar to that in lymph nodes.

Mucosa Associated Lymphoid Tissue in the Respiratory System

In the respiratory system the aggregations are relatively small and are present in the walls of the trachea and large bronchi. The term *bronchial associated lymphoid tissue* (*BALT*) is applied to these aggregations.

Mucosa Associated Lymphoid Tissue in the Alimentary System

This is also called *gut associated lymphoid tissue* (GALT). In the alimentary system the aggregations of lymphoid tissue are as follows.

(a) Near the junction of the oral cavity with the pharynx there are a number of collections of lymphoid tissue that are referred to as *tonsils*. The largest of these are the right and left *palatine tonsils*, present on either side of the oropharyngeal isthmus. (In common usage the word tonsils refers to the palatine tonsils). Another midline collection of lymphoid tissue, the *pharyngeal tonsil,* is present on the posterior wall of the pharynx. Smaller collections are present on the dorsum of the posterior part of the tongue (*lingual tonsils*), and around the pharyngeal openings of the auditory tubes (*tubal*

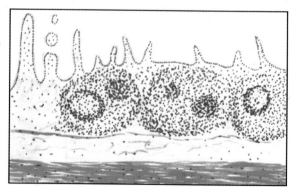

Fig. 11.11. Section through ileum showing an aggregated lymphatic follicle (Peyer's patch) in the submucosa.

tonsils). The structure of the palatine tonsils is described below.

(b) Small collections of lymphoid tissue, similar in structure to the follicles of lymph nodes, may be present anywhere along the length of the gut. They are called **solitary lymphatic follicles**. Larger aggregations of lymphoid tissue, each consisting of 10 to 200 follicles are also present in the small intestine. They are called **aggregated lymphatic follicles** or **Peyer's patches**. These patches can be seen by naked eye, and about 200 of them can be counted in the human gut. The mucosa overlying them may be devoid of villi or may have rudimentary villi. Peyer's patches always lie along the antemesenteric border of the intestine and measure 2 cm to 10 cm. Both solitary and aggregated follicles increase in number and size in proceeding caudally along the small intestine, being most numerous and largest in the terminal ileum (Fig. 11.11). In addition to lymphoid follicles, a large number of lymphocytes and plasma cells are present in the connective tissue of the gut wall.

It has been held that gut associated lymphoid tissue may possibly have a role to play in the processing of B-lymphocytes (similar to that of T-lymphocytes in the thymus), but at present there is not much evidence to support this view.

Keeping in view the fact that respiratory and alimentary epithelia come in contact with numerous organisms, and other antigens, lymphatic tissue in relation to these epithelia is probably concerned in defence mechanisms against such antigens. In this connection it is interesting to note that special phagocytic cells (called **follicle associated epithelial cells**, **FAE**, or **M-cells**) have been demonstrated in epithelia overlying lymphoid follicles. They may ingest antigens present in the lumen (of the gut), then pass through the epithelium and carry the antigens into lymphoid tissue. In this way these cells could help in stimulating immune responses against the antigens.

B-lymphocytes present in the gut wall mature into plasma cells which produce antibodies. A form of IgA (called secretory IgA) is secreted into the gut lumen where it can destroy pathogens before they have a chance to invade the gut wall.

The Palatine Tonsils

Each palatine tonsil (right or left) consists of diffuse lymphoid tissue in which lymphatic nodules are present. The lymphoid tissue is covered by stratified squamous epithelium continuous with that of the mouth and pharynx. This epithelium extends into the substance of the tonsil in the form of several **tonsillar crypts**. Numerous mucous glands open into the crypts. The lumen of a crypt usually contains some lymphocytes that have travelled into it through the epithelium. Desquamated epithelial cells and bacteria are also frequently present in the lumen of the crypt (Fig. 11.12).

The palatine tonsils are often infected (**tonsillitis**). This is a common cause of sore throat. Frequent infections can lead to

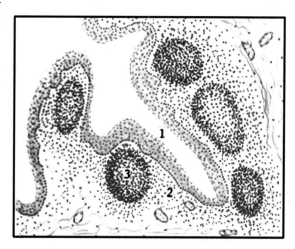

Fig. 11.12. Section through palatine tonsil. 1-Crypt. 2-Diffuse lymphoid tissue. 3- Lymphatic nodule.

considerable enlargement of the tonsils specially in children. Such enlarged tonsils may become a focus of infection and their surgical removal (*tonsillectomy*) may then become necessary.

The Pharyngeal Tonsil

This is a mass of lymphoid tissue present on the posterior wall of the nasopharynx, in the midline. It is covered by epithelium. In children the pharyngeal tonsil may hypertrophy and is then referred to as the *adenoids*. The resulting swelling may be a cause of obstruction to normal breathing. The child tends to breathe through the mouth, and this may in turn lead to other abnormalities.

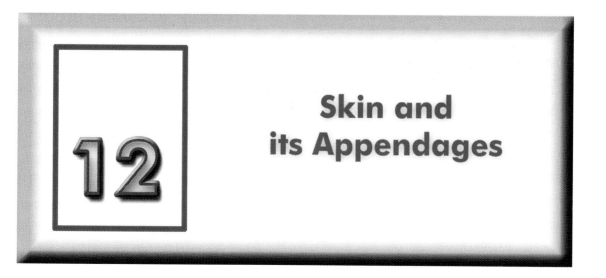

Skin and its Appendages

BASIC FACTS ABOUT SKIN STRUCTURE

The skin consists of a superficial layer the *epidermis*, made up of stratified squamous epithelium; and a deeper layer, the *dermis*, made up of connective tissue (Fig. 12.1A). The dermis rests on subcutaneous tissue (*subcutis*). This is sometimes described as a third layer of skin.

In sections through the skin the line of junction of the two layers is not straight, but is markedly wavy because of the presence of numerous finger-like projections of dermis upwards into the epidermis. These projections are called *dermal papillae*. The downward projections of the epidermis (in the intervals between the dermal papillae) are sometimes called *epidermal papillae*.

The surface of the epidermis is also often marked by elevations and depressions. These are most prominent on the palms and ventral surfaces of the fingers, and on the corresponding surfaces of the feet. Here the elevations form characteristic *epidermal ridges* that are responsible for the highly specific finger prints of each individual.

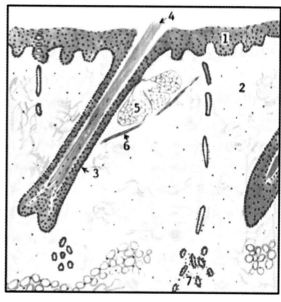

Fig. 12.1A. Section through skin. 1-Epidermis. 2-Dermis. 3-Hair follicle. 4-Hair. 5-Sebaceous gland. 6- Arrector pili. 7-Sweat gland.

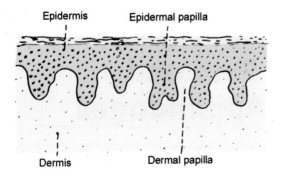

Fig. 12.1B. Dermal and epidermal papillae.

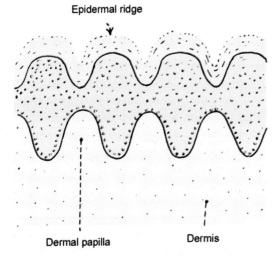

Fig. 12.2. Scheme to show epidermal ridges.

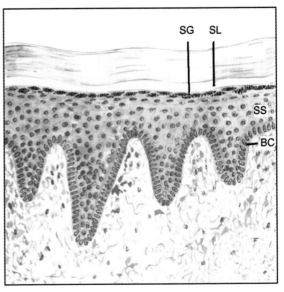

Fig. 12.3A. Section through skin showing the layers of the epidermis. SC-Stratum corneum. SL-Stratum lucidum. SG-Stratum granulosum. SS-Stratum spinosum. BC-Basal cell layer.

The Epidermis

The epidermis consists of stratified epithelium in which the following layers can be recognized (Fig. 12.3A).

(a) The deepest or ***basal layer*** (***stratum basale***) is made up of a single layer of columnar cells that rest on a basal lamina.

The basal layer contains stem cells that undergo mitosis to give off cells called ***keratinocytes***. Keratinocytes form the more superficial layers of the epidermis described below. The basal layer is, therefore, also called the ***germinal layer*** (***stratum germinativum***).

(b) Above the basal layer there are several layers of polygonal keratinocytes that constitute the ***stratum spinosum*** (or ***Malpighian layer***). The cells of this layer are attached to one another by numerous desmosomes. During routine preparation of tissue for sectioning the cells often retract from each other except at the desmosomes. As a result the cells appear to have a number of 'spines': this is the reason for calling this layer the stratum spinosum. For the same reason the keratinocytes of this layer are also called ***prickle cells***. The cytoplasm of cells in the stratum spinosum is permeated with fibrils (made up of bundles of keratin filaments). The fibrils are attached to the cell wall at desmosomes.

Some mitoses may be seen in the deeper cells of the stratum spinosum. Because of this fact the stratum spinosum is included, along with the basal cell layer, in the ***germinative zone*** of the epidermis.

(c) Overlying the stratum spinosum there are a few (1 to 5) layers of flattened cells that are

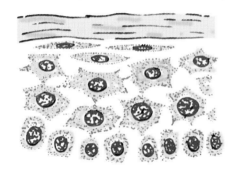

Fig. 12.3B. Cells of the stratum spinosum showing typical spines.

characterized by the presence of deeply staining granules in their cytoplasm. These cells constitute the **stratum granulosum**. The granules in them consist of a protein called **keratohyalin**. The nuclei of cells in this layer are condensed and dark staining (pyknotic).

With the EM it is seen that, in the cells of this layer, keratin filaments (already mentioned in relation to the stratum spinosum) have become much more numerous, and are arranged in the form of a thick layer. The fibres lie in a meshwork formed by keratohyalin granules. Further details about keratinocytes are given on page 196.

(d) Superficial to the stratum granulosum there is the **stratum lucidum** (lucid = clear). This layer is so called because it appears homogeneous, the cell boundaries being extremely indistinct. Traces of flattened nuclei are seen in some cells.

(e) The most superficial layer of the epidermis is called the **stratum corneum**. This layer is acellular. It is made up of flattened scale like elements (squames) containing keratin filaments embedded in protein. The squames are held together by a glue like material containins lipids and carbohydrates. The presence of lipid makes this layer highly resistant to permeation by water.

The thickness of the stratum corneum is greatest where the skin is exposed to maximal friction e.g., on the palms and soles. The superficial layers of the epidermis are being constantly shed off, and are replaced by proliferation of cells in deeper layers.

The stratum corneum, the stratum lucidum, and the stratum granulosum are collectively referred to as the **zone of keratinization**, or as the **cornified zone** (in distinction to the germinative zone described above). The stratum granulosum and the stratum lucidum are well formed only in thick non-hairy skin (e.g., on the palms). They are usually absent in thin hairy skin.

Some further details about the epidermis are given below.

The Dermis

The dermis is made up of connective tissue. Just below the epidermis the connective tissue is dense and constitutes the **papillary layer**. Deep to this there is a network of thick fibre bundles that constitute the **reticular layer** of the dermis.

The papillary layer includes the connective tissue of the dermal papillae. These papillae are best developed in the thick skin of the palms and soles. Each papilla contains a capillary loop. Some papillae contain tactile corpuscles (page 157).

The reticular layer of the dermis consists mainly of bundles of collagen fibres. It also contains considerable numbers of elastic fibres. Intervals between the fibre bundles are usually occupied by adipose tissue. The dermis rests on the superficial fascia through which it is attached to deeper structures. For some further details about the dermis see page 198.

ADDITIONAL DETAILS ABOUT SKIN STRUCTURE

Although the epidermis is, by tradition, described as a stratified squamous epithelium, it has been pointed out that the majority of cells in it are not squamous (flattened). The stratum corneum is not cellular at all.

Some details about Keratinocytes

1. Apart from **stem cells**, the basal layer also contains some keratinocytes formed from stem cells.

2. After entering the stratum spinosum some keratinocytes may undergo further mitoses. Such cells are referred to as **intermediate stem cells**. Thereafter, keratinocytes do not undergo further cell division.

3. Essential steps in the formation of keratin are as follows.

(a) Basal cells of the epidermis contain numerous intermediate filaments. These are called **cytokeratin filaments** or **tonofibrils**. As basal cells move into the stratum spinosum the proteins forming the tonofibrils undergo changes that convert them to **keratin filaments**.

(b) When epidermal cells reach the stratum granulosum, they synthesize **keratohyalin granules**. These granules contain specialized proteins (which are rich in sulphur containing amino acids e.g., histidine, cysteine).

(c) Keratin consists of keratin filaments embedded in keratohyalin. Cells of the superficial layers of the stratum granulosum are packed with keratin. These cells die leaving behind the keratin mass in the form of an acellular layer of thin flakes.

(d) Cells in the granular layer also show membrane bound, circular, granules that contain glycophospholipids. These granules are referred to as **lamellated bodies**, or **keratosomes**. When these cells die the material in these granules is released and acts as a glue that hold together flakes of keratin. The lipid content of this material makes the skin resistant to water. However, prolonged exposure to water causes the material to swell. This is responsible for the altered appearance of the skin after prolonged exposure to water (more so if the water is hot, or contains detergents).

4. The time elapsing between the formation of a keratinocyte in the basal layer of the epidermis, and its shedding off from the surface of the epidermis is highly variable. It is influenced by many factors including skin thickness, and the degree of friction on the surface. On the average it is 40-50 days.

5. In some situations it is seen that flakes of keratin in the stratum corneum are arranged in regular columns (one stacked above the other). It is believed that localized areas in the basal layer of the epidermis contain groups of keratinocytes all derived from a single stem cell. It is also believed that all the cells in the epidermis overlying this region are derived from the same stem cell. Such groups of cells, all derived from a single stem cell, and stacked in layers passing from the basal layer to the surface of the epidermis, constitute **epidermal proliferation units**. One dendritic cell (see below) is present in close association with each such unit.

Pigmentation of the Skin

The cells of the basal layer of the epidermis, and the adjoining cells of the stratum spinosum contain a brown pigment called **melanin**. The pigment is much more prominent in dark skinned individuals. The cells actually responsible for synthesis of melanin are called **melanocytes** (See note below). Melanocytes are derived from melanoblasts that arise from the neural crest. They may be present amongst the cells of the germinative zone, or at the junction of the epidermis and the dermis. Each melanocyte gives off many processes each of

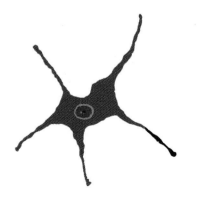

Fig. 12.4. Melanocyte showing dendritic processes.

the manner in which most cells of the germinative zone acquire their pigment.

The colour of skin is influenced by the amount of melanin present. It is also influenced by some other pigments present in the epidermis; and by pigments (haemoglobin and oxyhaemoglobin) present in blood circulating through the skin. The epidermis is sufficiently translucent for the colour of blood to show through, specially in light skinned individuals. That is why the skin becomes pale in anaemia; blue when oxygenation of blood is insufficient; and pink while blushing.

which is applied to a cell of the germinative zone. Melanin granules formed in the melanocyte are transferred to surrounding non-melanin-producing cells through these processes. Because of the presence of processes melanocytes are also called *dendritic cells* (to be carefully distinguished from the dendritic macrophages described below).

Melanin (*eumelanin*) is derived from the amino acid tyrosine. Tyrosine is converted into dihydroxy-phenylalanine (DOPA) which is in turn converted into melanin. Enzymes responsible for transformation of DOPA into melanin can be localized histochemically by incubating sections with DOPA which is converted into melanin. This is called the DOPA reaction. It can be used to distinguish between true melanocytes and other cells that only store melanin. (In the past the term melanocyte has sometimes been applied to epithelial cells that have taken up melanin produced by other cells. However, the term is now used only for cells capable of synthesizing melanin).

With the EM melanin granules are seen to be membrane bound organelles that contain pigment. These organelles are called *melanosomes*. Melanosomes bud off from the Golgi complex. They enter the dendrites of the melanocytes. At the ends of the dendrites melanosomes are shed off from the cell and are engulfed by neighbouring keratinocytes. This is

Other Cells present in Epidermis

Dendritic cells of Langherhans

Apart from keratinocytes and dendritic melanocytes the stratum spinosum also contains other dendritic cells that are quite different in function from the melanocytes. These are the dendritic cells of Langherhans. These cells belong to the mononuclear phagocyte system. The dendritic cells of Langherhans originate in bone marrow. They are believed to play an important role in protecting the skin against viral and other infections. It is believed that the cells take up antigens in the skin and transport them to lymphoid tissues where the antigens stimulate T-lymphocytes. Under the EM dendritic cells are seen to contain characteristic elongated vacuoles that have been given the name *Langherhans bodies*, or *Birbeck bodies*. The contents of these vacuoles are discharged to the outside of the cell through the cell membrane.

The dendritic cells of Langherhans also appear to play a role in controlling the rate of cell division in the epidermis. They increase in number in chronic skin disorders, specially those resulting from allergy.

Cells of Merkel

The basal layer of the epidermis also contains specialized sensory cells called the cells of Merkel (page 156). Sensory nerve endings are present in relation to these cells.

Further facts about the Dermis

The fibre bundles in the reticular layer of the dermis mostly lie parallel to one another. In the limbs the predominant direction of the bundles is along the long axis of the limb; while on the trunk and neck the direction is transverse. The lines along which the bundles run are often called *cleavage lines* as they represent the natural lines along which the skin tends to split when penetrated. The cleavage lines are of importance to the surgeon as incisions in the direction of these lines gape much less than those at right angles to them.

We have seen that the dermis contains considerable amounts of elastic fibres. Atrophy of elastic fibres occurs with age and is responsible for loss of elasticity and wrinkling of the skin.

If for any reason the skin in any region of the body is rapidly stretched, fibre bundles in the dermis may rupture. Scar tissue is formed in the region and can be seen in the form of prominent white lines. Such lines may be formed on the anterior abdominal wall in pregnancy: they are known as *linea gravidarum.*

Blood Supply of the Skin

Blood vessels to the skin are derived from a number of arterial plexuses. The deepest plexus is present over the deep fascia. There is another plexus just below the dermis (*rete cutaneum* or *reticular plexus*); and a third plexus just below the level of the dermal papillae (*rete subpapillare*, or *papillary plexus*). Capillary loops arising from this plexus pass into each dermal papilla.

Blood vessels do not penetrate into the epidermis. The epidermis derives nutrition entirely by diffusion from capillaries in the dermal papillae. Veins from the dermal papillae drain (through plexuses present in the dermis) into a venous plexus lying on deep fascia.

A special feature of the blood supply of the skin is the presence of numerous arterio-venous anastomoses that regulate blood flow through the capillary bed and thus help in maintaining body temperature. The structure of arteriovenous anastomoses has been described on page 174.

Nerve Supply of the Skin

The skin is richly supplied with sensory nerves. Dense networks of nerve fibres are seen in the superficial parts of the dermis. Sensory nerves end in relation to various types of specialized terminals that have been described on page 155.

In contrast to blood vessels some nerve fibres do penetrate into the deeper parts of the epidermis.

Apart from sensory nerves the skin receives autonomic nerves which supply smooth muscle in the walls of blood vessels; the arrectores pilorum muscles; and myoepithelial cells present in relation to sweat glands. They also provide a secretomotor supply to sweat glands. In some regions (nipple, scrotum) nerve fibres innervate smooth muscle present in the dermis.

FUNCTIONS OF THE SKIN

1. The skin provides mechanical protection to underlying tissues. In this connection we have noted that the skin is thickest over areas exposed to greatest friction.

The skin also acts as a physical barrier against

entry of microorganisms and other substances. However, the skin is not a perfect barrier and some substances, both useful (e.g., ointments) or harmful (poisons), may enter the body through the skin.

2. The skin prevents loss of water from the body. The importance of this function is seen in persons who have lost extensive areas of skin through burns. One important cause of death in such cases is water loss.

3. The pigment present in the epidermis protects tissues against harmful effects of light (specially ultraviolet light). This is to be correlated with the heavier pigmentation of skin in races living in the tropics; and with increase in pigmentation after exposure to sunlight. However, some degree of exposure to sunlight is essential for synthesis of vitamin D.

4. The skin offers protection against damage of tissues by chemicals, by heat, and by osmotic influences.

5. The skin is a very important sensory organ, containing receptors for touch and related sensations. The presence of relatively sparse and short hair over most of the skin increases its sensitivity.

6. The skin plays an important role in regulating body temperature. Blood flow through capillaries of the skin can be controlled by numerous arterio-venous anastomoses present in it. In cold weather blood flow through capillaries is kept to a minimum to prevent heat loss. In warm weather the flow is increased to promote cooling. In extreme cold, when some peripheral parts of the body (like the digits, the nose and the ears) are in danger of being frozen the blood flow through these parts increases to keep them warm.

In warm climates cooling of the body is facilitated by secretion of sweat and its evaporation. Sweat glands also act as excretory organs.

APPENDAGES OF THE SKIN

The appendages of the skin are the hairs, nails, sebaceous glands and sweat glands. The mammary glands may be regarded as highly specialized appendages of the skin.

Hairs

Hairs are present on the skin covering almost the whole body. The sites where they are not present include the palms, the soles, the ventral surface and sides of the digits, and some parts of the male and female external genitalia.

Differences in the length and texture of hairs over different parts of the body, and the differences in distribution of hairs in the male and female, are well known and do not need description. It has to be emphasized, however, that many areas that appear to be hairless (e.g., the eyelids) have very fine hairs, some of which may not even appear above the surface of the skin.

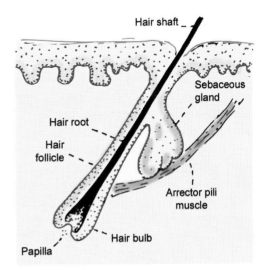

Fig. 12.5 Basic structure of a hair follicle.
Also see Fig. 12.1A.

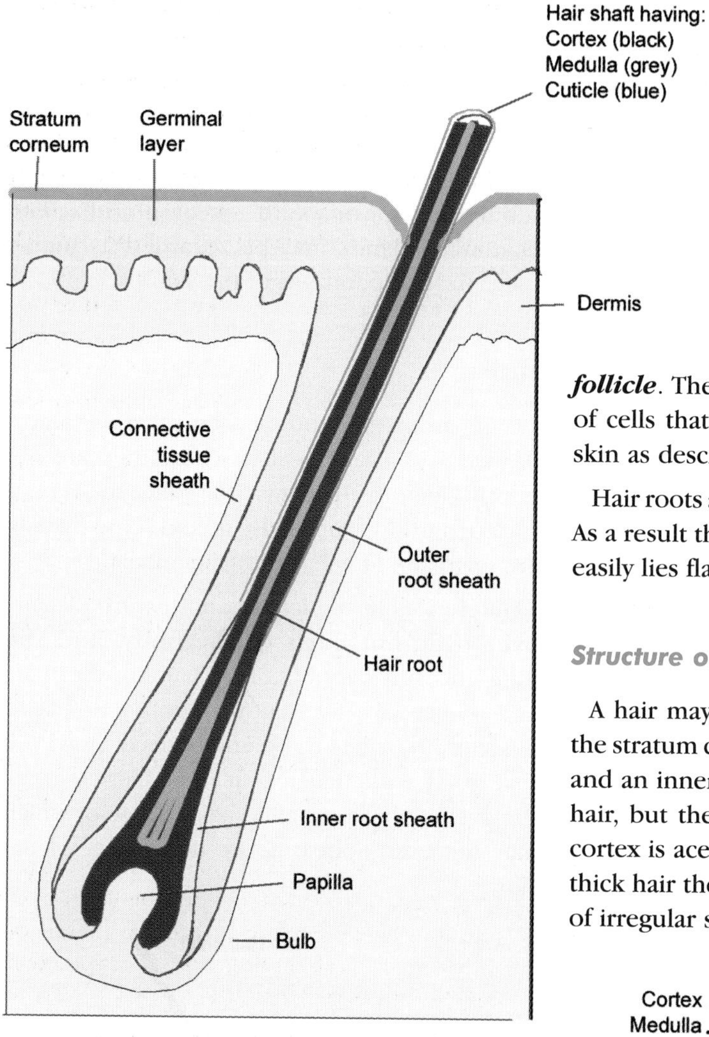

Hair shaft having:
Cortex (black)
Medulla (grey)
Cuticle (blue)

Stratum
corneum

Germinal
layer

Dermis

Connective
tissue
sheath

Outer
root sheath

Hair root

Inner root sheath

Papilla

Bulb

Fig. 12.6. Scheme to show some details of
a hair follicle.

part anchored in the thickness of the skin. The visible part is called the *shaft*, and the embedded part is called the *root*. The root has an expanded lower end called the *bulb*. The bulb is invaginated from below by part of the dermis that constitutes the *hair papilla*. The root of each hair is surrounded by a tubular sheath called the *hair follicle*. The follicle is made up of several layers of cells that are derived from the layers of the skin as described below.

Hair roots are always attached to skin obliquely. As a result the emerging hair is also oblique and easily lies flat on the skin surface.

Structure of Hair Shaft

A hair may be regarded as a modified part of the stratum corneum of the skin. An outer cortex and an inner medulla can be made out in large hair, but there is no medulla in thin hair. The cortex is acellular and is made up of keratin. In thick hair the medulla consists of cornified cells of irregular shape.

In animals with a thick coat of hair (fur) the hair help to keep the animal warm. In man this function is performed by subcutaneous fat. The relative hairlessness of the human skin is an adaptation to make the skin a more effective sensory surface. The presence of short, sparsely distributed hairs, with a rich nerve supply of their roots, increases the sensitivity of the skin.

Each hair consists of a part (of variable length) that is seen on the surface of the body; and a

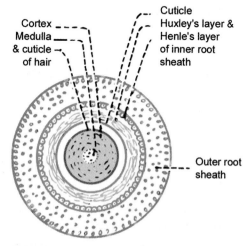

Cortex
Medulla
& cuticle
of hair

Cuticle
Huxley's layer &
Henle's layer
of inner root
sheath

Outer root
sheath

Fig. 12.7. Diagram to show the various layers to be
seen in a hair follicle.

The surface of the hair is covered by a thin membrane called the **cuticle**, which is formed by flattened cornified cells. Each of these cells has a free edge (directed distally) that overlaps part of the next cell. The cornified elements making up the hair contain melanin which is responsible for their colour. Both in the medulla and in the cortex of a hair minute air bubbles are present: they influence its colour. The amount of air present in a hair increases with age and, along with loss of pigment, is responsible for greying of hair.

Structure of Hair Follicle

The hair follicle may be regarded as a part of the epidermis that has been invaginated into the dermis around the hair root. Its innermost layer, that immediately surrounds the hair root is, therefore, continuous with the surface of the skin; while the outermost layer of the follicle is continuous with the dermis. The wall of the follicle consists of three main layers. Beginning with the innermost layer they are:

(**a**) The **inner root sheath** present only in the lower part of the follicle.

(**b**) The **outer root sheath** which is continuous with the stratum spinosum.

(**c**) A connective tissue sheath derived from the dermis.

The inner root sheath is further divisible into the following (Fig.12.7).

(**1**) The innermost layer is called the **cuticle**. It lies against the cuticle of the hair, and consists of flattened cornified cells.

(**2**) Next there are one to three layers of flattened nucleated cells that constitute **Huxley's layer**, or the **stratum epitheliale granuloferum**. Cells of this layer contain large eosinophilic granules (**trichohyaline granules**).

(**3**) The outer layer (of the inner root sheath) is made up of a single layer of cubical cells with flattened nuclei. This is called **Henle's layer**, or the **stratum epitheliale pallidum**.

The outer root sheath is continuous with the stratum spinosum of the skin, and like the latter it consists of living, rounded and nucleated cells. When traced towards the lower end of the follicle the cells of this layer become continuous with the hair bulb (at the lower end of the hair root). The cells of the hair bulb also correspond to those of the stratum spinosum, and constitute the **germinative matrix**. These cells show great mitotic activity. Cells produced here pass superficially and undergo keratinization to form the various layers of the hair shaft already described. They also give rise to cells of the inner root sheath. The cells of the papilla are necessary for proper growth in the germinative matrix. The outermost layer of cells of the outer root sheath, and the lowest layer of cells of the hair bulb (that overlie the papilla) correspond to the basal cell layer of the skin.

The outer root sheath is separated from the connective tissue sheath by a basal lamina which appears structureless and is, therefore, called the **glassy membrane**. (This membrane is strongly eosinophilic and PAS positive).

The **connective tissue sheath** is made up of tissue continuous with that of the dermis. The tissue is highly vascular, and contains numerous nerve fibres that form a basket-like network round the lower end of the follicle.

Present in close association with hair follicles there are sebaceous glands (described below). One such gland normally opens into each follicle near its upper end. The arrector pili muscles (described below), pass obliquely from the lower part of the hair follicle towards the junction of the epidermis and dermis.

Some other terms used in relation to the hair follicle may be mentioned here. Its lower expanded end is the **fundus**. The region above the opening of the sebaceous duct is the **infundibulum**. Below the infundibulum the **isthmus** extends up to the attachment of the arrector pili. The part of the follicle below this point is the **inferior segment**.

Arrector Pili Muscles

These are bands of smooth muscle attached at one end to the dermis, just below the dermal papillae; and at the other end to the connective tissue sheath of a hair follicle. It lies on that side of the hair follicle which forms an obtuse angle with the skin surface (Fig. 12.1A). A sebaceous gland (see below) lies in the angle between the hair follicle and the arrector pili. Contraction of the muscle has two effects. Firstly, the hair follicle becomes almost vertical (from its original oblique position) relative to the skin surface). Simultaneously the skin surface overlying the attachment of the muscle becomes depressed while surrounding areas become raised. These reactions are seen during exposure to cold, or during emotional excitement, when the 'hair stand on end' and the skin takes on the appearance of 'goose flesh'. The second effect of contraction of the arrector pili muscle is that the sebaceous gland is pressed upon and its secretions are squeezed out into the hair follicle. The arrector pili muscles receive a sympathetic innervation.

Sebaceous Glands

As mentioned above sebaceous glands are seen most typically in relation to hair follicles. Each gland consists of a number of alveoli that are connected to a broad duct that opens into a hair follicle (Figs. 12.1A, 12.8). Each alveolus is pear shaped. It consists of a solid mass of polyhedral cells and has hardly any lumen. The outermost cells are small and rest on a basement membrane. The inner cells are larger, more rounded, and filled with lipid. This lipid is discharged by disintegration of the innermost cells which are replaced by proliferation of outer cells. The sebaceous glands are, therefore, examples of holocrine glands (See page 53). The secretion of sebaceous glands is called *sebum*. Its oily nature

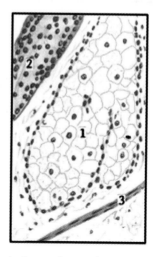

Fig. 12.8. Sebaceous gland (high power view). 1-Sebaceous gland. 2-Part of hair follicle. 3-Arrector pili.

helps to keep the skin and hair soft. It helps to prevent dryness of the skin and also makes it resistant to moisture. Sebum contains various lipids including triglycerides, cholesterol, cholesterol esters and fatty acids.

In some situations sebaceous glands occur independently of hair follicles. Such glands open directly on the skin surface. They are found around the lips, and in relation to some parts of the male and female external genitalia. The tarsal (Meibomian) glands of the eyelid are modified sebaceous glands. Montgomery's tubercles present in the skin around the nipple (areola) are also sebaceous glands. Secretion by sebaceous glands is not under nervous control.

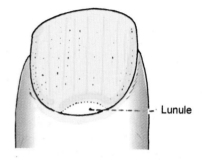

Fig. 12.9. Drawing to show the lunule of a nail.

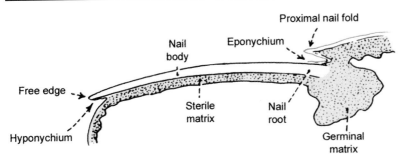

Fig. 12.10A. Parts of a nail and some related structures as seen in a longitudinal section.

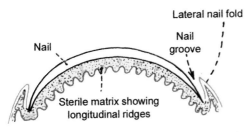

Fig. 12.10B. Transverse section across a nail.

Nails

Nails are present on fingers and toes. The main part of a nail is called its **body**. The body has a free distal edge. The proximal part of the nail is implanted into a groove on the skin and is called the **root** (or **radix**). The tissue on which the nail rests is called the **nail bed**. The nail bed is highly vascular, and that is why the nails look pink in colour.

The nail represents a modified part of the zone of keratinization of the epidermis. It is usually regarded as a much thickened continuation of the stratum lucidum, but it is more like the stratum corneum in structure. The nail substance consists of several layers of dead, cornified, 'cells' filled with keratin.

When we view a nail in longitudinal section (Fig. 12.9) it is seen that the nail rests on the cells of the germinative zone (stratum spinosum and stratum basale). The germinative zone is particularly thick near the root of the nail where

it forms the **germinal matrix**. The nail substance is formed mainly by proliferation of cells in the germinal matrix. However, the superficial layers of the nail are derived from the proximal nail fold. When viewed from the surface (i.e., through the nail substance) the area of the germinal matrix appears white (in comparison to the pink colour of the rest of the nail). Most of this area is overlapped by the fold of skin (**proximal nail fold**) covering the root of the nail, but just distal to the nail fold a small semilunar white area called the **lunule** is seen. The lunule is most conspicuous in the thumb nail. The germinal matrix is connected to the underlying bone (distal phalanx) by fibrous tissue.

The germinative zone underlying the body of the nail (i.e., the nail bed) is much thinner than the germinal matrix. It does not contribute to the growth of the nail; and is, therefore, called the **sterile matrix**. As the nail grows it slides distally over the sterile matrix. The dermis that lies deep to the sterile matrix does not show the usual dermal papillae. Instead it shows a number of parallel, longitudinal ridges. These ridges look like very regularly arranged papillae in transverse sections through a nail (Fig.12.10).

We have seen that the root of the nail is overlapped by a fold of skin called the proximal nail fold. The greater part of each lateral margin of the nail is also overlapped by a skin fold called the **lateral nail fold**. The groove between the lateral nail fold and the nail bed (in which the lateral margin of the nail lies) is called the **lateral nail groove**.

The stratum corneum lining the deep surface

of the proximal nail fold extends for a short distance on to the surface of the nail. This extension of the stratum corneum is called the **eponychium**. The stratum corneum lining the skin of the finger tip is also reflected onto the undersurface of the free distal edge of the nail: this reflection is called the **hyponychium**.

The dermis underlying the nail bed is firmly attached to the distal phalanx. It is highly vascular and contains arteriovenous anastomoses. It also contains numerous sensory nerve endings.

Nails undergo constant growth by proliferation of cells in the germinal matrix. Growth is faster in hot weather than in cold. Finger nails grow faster than toe nails. Nail growth can be disturbed by serious illness or by injury over the nail root, resulting in transverse grooves or white patches in the nails. These grooves or patches slowly grow towards the free edge of the nail. If a nail is lost by injury a new one grows out of the germinal matrix if the latter is intact.

Nails have evolved from the claws of animals. Their main function in man is to provide a rigid support for the finger tips. This support increases the sensitivity of the finger tips and increases their efficiency in carrying out delicate movements.

Sweat Glands

Sweat glands produce sweat or perspiration. They are present in the skin over most of the body. Apart from typical sweat glands there are atypical ones present at some sites.

Typical Sweat Glands

As described on page 53, exocrine glands discharge their secretions in various ways and are accordingly classified as merocrine (or eccrine), apocrine and holocrine. Typical sweat glands are of the merocrine variety. Their number and size varies in the skin over different parts of

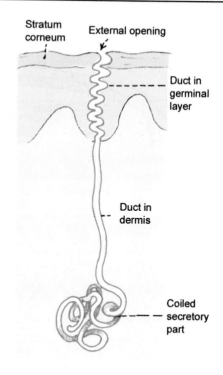

Fig. 12.11. Diagrammatic representation of the parts of a typical sweat gland.

the body. They are most numerous in the palms and soles, the forehead and scalp, and the axillae.

The entire sweat gland consists of a single long tube. The lower end of the tube is highly coiled on itself and forms the **body** (or **fundus**) or the gland. The body is made up of the secretory part of the gland. It lies in the reticular layer of the dermis, or sometimes in subcutaneous tissue. The part of the tube connecting the secretory element to

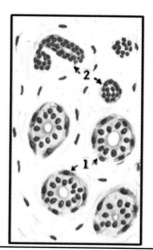

Fig. 12.12. Sweat gland (high power view). 1- Sections through secretory part. 2-Sections through duct.

the skin surface is the ***duct***. It runs upwards through the dermis to reach the epidermis. Within the epidermis the duct follows a spiral course to reach the skin surface. The orifice is funnel shaped. On the palms, soles and digits the openings of sweat glands lie in rows on epidermal ridges (page 190).

The wall of the tube making up the gland consists of an inner epithelial lining, its basal lamina, and a supporting layer of connective tissue.

In the secretory part the epithelium is made up of a single layer of cubical or polygonal cells. Sometimes the epithelium may appear to be pseudostratified).

EM studies have shown that the lining cells are of two types, dark and clear. The bodies of ***dark cells*** are broad next to the lumen and narrow near the basement membrane. In contrast the ***clear cells*** are broadest next to the basement membrane and narrow towards the lumen. The dark cells are rich in RNA and in mucopolysaccharides (which are PAS positive). Their secretion is mucoid. The clear cells contain much glycogen. Their cytoplasm is permeated by canaliculi that contain microvilli. The secretion of clear cells is watery.

In larger sweat glands flattened contractile, ***myoepithelial cells*** are present between the epithelial cells and their basal lamina. They probably help in expressing secretion out of the gland. (See page 133).

In the duct the lining epithelium consists of two or more layers of cuboidal cells (constituting a stratified cuboidal epithelium). As the duct passes through the epidermis its wall is formed by the elements that make up the epidermis.

As is well known the secretion of sweat glands has a high water content. Evaporation of this water plays an important role in cooling the body (page 196). Sweat glands (including the myoepithelial cells) are innervated by cholinergic nerves.

Atypical Sweat Glands

We have seen that typical sweat glands are merocrine. In contrast sweat glands in some parts of the body are of the apocrine variety. In other words the apical parts of the secretory cells are shed off as part of their secretion. Apocrine sweat glands are confined to some parts of the body including the axilla, the areola and nipple, the perianal region, the glans penis, and some parts of the female external genitalia. Apart from differences in mode of secretion apocrine sweat glands have the following differences from typical (merocrine) sweat glands.

1. Apocrine sweat glands are much larger in size. However, they become fully developed only after puberty.

2. The tubes forming the secretory parts of the glands branch and may form a network.

3. Their ducts open not on the skin surface, but into hair follicles.

4. The lumen of secretory tubules is large. The lining epithelium is of varying height: it may be squamous, cuboidal or columnar. When the cells are full of stored secretion they are columnar. With partial shedding of contents the cells appear to be cuboidal, and with complete emptying they become flattened. (Some workers describe a layer of flattened cells around the inner cuboidal cells). Associated with the apocrine mode of secretion (involving shedding of the apical cytoplasm) the epithelial surface is irregular, there being numerous projections of protoplasm on the luminal surface of the cells. Cell discharging their secretions in a merocrine or holocrine manner may also be present.

5. The secretions of apocrine sweat glands are viscous and contain proteins. They are odourless, but after bacterial decomposition they give off body odours that vary from person to person.

6. Conflicting views have been expressed regarding the innervation of apocrine sweat glands. According to some authorities the glands are not under nervous control. Others describe an adrenergic innervation (in contrast to cholinergic innervation of typical sweat glands); while still others describe both adrenergic and cholinergic innervation.

Wax producing *ceruminous glands* of the external acoustic meatus, and *ciliary glands* of the eyelids are modified sweat glands.

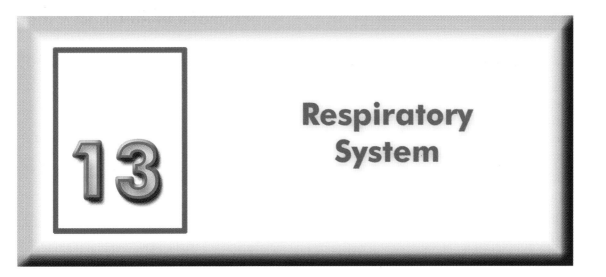

Respiratory System

13

The respiratory system consists of the lungs, and the passages through which air reaches them. These passages are the nasal cavities, the pharynx, the trachea, the bronchi and their intrapulmonary continuations. With regard to the pharynx, it should be noted that this organ consists of nasal, oral and laryngeal parts. The nasal part is purely respiratory in function, but the oral and laryngeal parts are more intimately concerned with the alimentary system.

The passages in question all have some features in common. Their walls have a skeletal basis made up variably of bone, cartilage, and connective tissue. The skeletal basis keeps the passages always patent. Smooth muscle present in the walls of the trachea and bronchi enables some alterations in the size of the lumen. The interior of the passages is lined over most of its extent by pseudostratified, ciliated, columnar epithelium. The epithelium is kept moist by the secretions of numerous serous glands. Numerous goblet cells and mucous glands cover the epithelium with a protective mucoid secretion which serves to trap dust particles present in inhaled air. This mucous (along with the dust particles in it) is constantly moved towards the pharynx by action of cilia. When excessive mucous accumulates it is brought out by

coughing, or is swallowed. Deep to the mucosa there are numerous blood vessels that serve to warm the inspired air. With this brief introduction we will now consider the histology of some parts of the respiratory passages.

THE NASAL CAVITIES

Histologically, the wall of each half of the nasal cavity is divisible into three distinct regions.

(1) The *vestibule* of the nasal cavity is lined by skin continuous with that on the exterior of the nose. Hair and sebaceous glands are present.

(2) Apart from their respiratory function the nasal cavities serve as end organs for smell. Receptors for smell are located in the *olfactory mucosa* which is confined to a relatively small area on the superior nasal concha, and on the adjoining part of the nasal septum. It is described below.

(3) The rest of the wall of each half of the nasal cavity is covered by *respiratory mucosa* lined by pseudostratified ciliated columnar epithelium.

Respiratory Mucosa

As stated above, this mucosa is lined by a pseudostratified ciliated columnar epithelium resting on a basal lamina. Apart from the predominant ciliated columnar cells the following cells are present (Fig.13.1).

(a) *Goblet cells* scattered in the epithelium produce mucous.

(b) *Non-ciliated columnar cells* with microvilli on the free surface probably secrete a serous fluid which keeps the mucosa moist.

(c) *Basal cells* lying near the basal lamina probably give rise to ciliated cells to replace those lost.

At places the respiratory mucosa may be lined by a simple ciliated columnar epithelium, or even a cuboidal epithelium.

Deep to the basal lamina supporting the epithelium lining, the mucosa contains a layer of fibrous tissue, through which the mucosa is firmly connected to underlying periosteum or perichondrium. The fibrous tissue may contain numerous lymphocytes. It also contains mucous and serous glands that open on to the mucosal surface. Some serous cells contain basophilic granules, and probably secrete amylase. Others with eosinophilic granules produce lysozyme.

The deeper parts of the mucosa contain a rich capillary network that constitutes a *cavernous tissue*. Blood flowing through the network warms inspired air. Variations in blood flow can cause swelling or shrinkage of the mucosa.

Respiratory mucosa also lines the paranasal air sinuses. Here it is closely bound to underlying periosteum forming a *mucoperiosteum*.

The lamina propria of nasal mucosa contains lymphocytes, plasma cells, macrophages, a few neutrophils and eosinophils. Eosinophils increase greatly in number in persons suffering from allergic rhinitis.

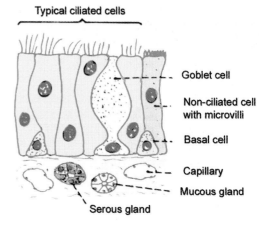

Fig. 13.1. Structure of respiratory part of nasal mucosa.

Olfactory Mucosa

This is yellow in colour, in contrast to the pink colour of the respiratory mucosa. It consists of a lining epithelium and a lamina propria.

The *olfactory epithelium* is pseudostratified. It is much thicker than the epithelium lining the respiratory mucosa (about 100 μm). Within the epithelium there is a superficial zone of clear cytoplasm below which there are several rows of nuclei (Fig. 13.2). Using special methods three types of cells can be recognized in the epithelium (Fig. 13.3).

(1) The *olfactory cells* are modified neurons. Each cell has a central part containing a rounded nucleus. Two processes, distal and proximal, arise from this central part. The distal process (representing the dendrite) passes towards the surface of the olfactory epithelium. It ends in a thickening (called the *rod* or *knob*) from which a number of non-motile olfactory cilia arise and project into a layer of fluid covering the epithelium. [Some of them pass laterally in between the microvilli of adjacent sustentacular cells]. The proximal process of each olfactory cell represents the axon. It passes into the subjacent connective tissue where it forms one fibre of the

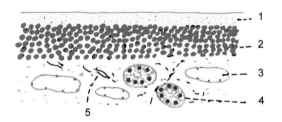

Fig. 13.2A. Olfactory mucosa seen in section stained by routine methods. 1. Clear zone of cytoplasm. 2. Several layers of nuclei. 3. Capillary. 4. Bowman's gland. 5. Nerve fibre.

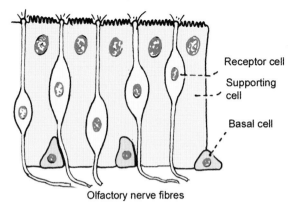

Olfactory nerve fibres

Fig. 13.2B. Cells to be seen in olfactory epithelium. RC- receptor cell. SC- supporting cell. BC-basal cell

olfactory nerve. The nuclei of olfactory cells lie at various levels in the basal two-thirds of the epithelium.

In vertebrates, olfactory cells are unique in being the only neurons that have cell bodies located in an epithelium.

Olfactory cells are believed to have a short life. Dead olfactory cells are replaced by new cells produced by division of basal cells (see below). This is the only example of regeneration of neurons in mammals.

(2) The *sustentacular cells* support the olfactory cells. Their nuclei are oval, and lie near the free surface of the epithelium. The free surface of each cell bears numerous microvilli (embedded in overlying mucous). The cytoplasm contains yellow pigment (lipofuscin) which gives olfactory mucosa its yellow colour. In addition

to their supporting function sustentacular cells may be phagocytic, and the pigment in them may represent remnants of phagocytosed olfactory cells.

(3) The *basal cells* lie deep in the epithelium and do not reach the luminal surface. They divide to form new olfactory cells to replace those that die. Some basal cells have a supporting function.

The lamina propria, lying deep to the olfactory epithelium consists of connective tissue within which blood capillaries, lymphatic capillaries and olfactory nerve bundles are present. It also contains serous glands (of Bowman) the secretions of which constantly 'wash' the surface of the olfactory epithelium. This fluid may help in transferring smell carrying substances from air to receptors on olfactory cells. The fluid may also offer protection against bacteria.

THE PHARYNX

The wall of the pharynx is fibro-muscular. (For details see a book on gross anatomy). In the nasopharynx the epithelial lining is ciliated columnar, or pseudostratified ciliated columnar. Over the inferior surface of the soft palate, and over the oropharynx and laryngo-pharynx the epithelium is stratified squamous (as these parts come in contact with food during swallowing). Subepithelial aggregations of lymphoid tissue are present specially on the posterior wall of the nasopharynx, and around the orifices of the auditory tubes, forming the nasopharyngeal and tubal tonsils (page 192). The palatine tonsils, present in relation to the oropharynx have been described on page 191. Numerous mucous glands are present in the submucosa, including that of the soft palate.

THE LARYNX

The wall of the larynx has a complex structure made up of a number of cartilages, membranes and muscles. (For details of these and of subdivisions of the larynx see a book on gross anatomy).

The Mucous Membrane

The epithelium lining the mucous membrane of the larynx is predominantly pseudostratified ciliated columnar. However, over some parts that come in contact with swallowed food the epithelium is stratified squamous. These parts include the epiglottis (anterior surface and upper part of the posterior surface: Fig. 13.3), and the upper parts of the aryepiglottic folds. The vocal folds do not come in contact with swallowed food, but their lining epithelium is exposed to considerable stress during vibration of the folds. These folds are also covered with stratified squamous epithelium.

Numerous goblet cells and subepithelial mucous glands provide a mucous covering to the epithelium. Mucous glands are specially numerous over the epiglottis; in the lower part of the aryepiglottic folds (where they are called **arytenoid glands**); and in the saccule. The glands in the saccule provide lubrication to the vocal folds. Serous glands and lymphoid tissue are also present.

EM studies have shown that epithelial cells lining the vocal folds bear microvilli and ridge-like foldings of the surface plasma membrane (called **microplicae**). It is believed that these help to retain fluid on the surface of the cells keeping them moist.

The connective tissue subjacent to the epithelial lining of vocal folds is devoid of lymph vessels.

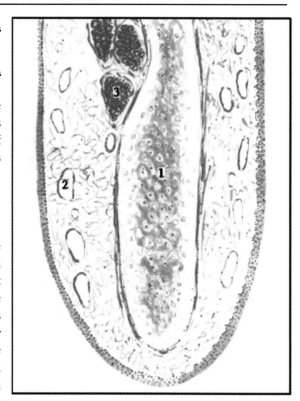

Fig. 13.3. Epiglottis. Its surface is covered all over by stratified squamous epithelium. 1-Elastic cartilage. 2-Blood vessels. 3-Glands.

This factor shows down lymphatic spread of cancer arising in the epithelium of the vocal folds.

Cartilages of the Larynx

Most of the cartilages of the larynx are made of hyaline cartilage. The cartilage of the epiglottis, the corniculate cartilage, the cuneiform cartilage, and the apical part of the arytenoid cartilage are made up of elastic cartilage (page 92). With advancing age, calcification may occur in hyaline cartilage, but not in elastic cartilage.

THE EPIGLOTTIS

The epiglottis is considered separately because sections through it are usually included in sets of class slides. The epiglottis has a central core of elastic cartilage, the structure of which has been described on page 92. Overlying the cartilage there is mucous membrane. The greater part of the mucous membrane is lined by stratified squamous epithelium (non-keratinizing). The mucous membrane over the lower part of the posterior surface of the epiglottis is lined by pseudostratified ciliated columnar epithelium. This part of the epiglottis does not come in contact with swallowed food as it is overlapped by the aryepiglottic folds. Some taste buds are present in the epithelium of the epiglottis. Their structure is considered in Chapter 14. (A few taste buds may be seen in the epithelium elsewhere in the larynx).

Numerous glands, predominantly mucous, are present in the mucosa deep to the epithelium. Some of them lie in depressions present on the epiglottic cartilage.

THE TRACHEA & PRINCIPAL BRONCHI

Trachea

The skeletal basis of the trachea is made up of 16 to 20 tracheal cartilages. Each of these is a C-shaped mass of hyaline cartilage. The open end of the 'C' is directed posteriorly. Occasionally, adjoining cartilages may partly fuse with each other or may have Y-shaped ends. The intervals between the cartilages are filled by fibrous tissue that becomes continuous with the perichondrium covering the cartilages. The gaps between the cartilage ends, present on the posterior aspect, are filled in by smooth muscle and fibrous tissue. The connective tissue in the wall of the trachea contains many elastic fibres.

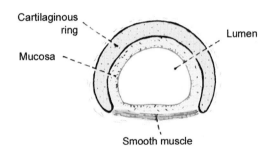

Fig. 13.4A. Low power view of a section through the trachea.

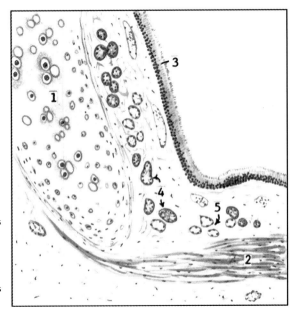

Fig. 13.4B. Section through trachea (posterior part). 1-Cartilage. 2-Smooth muscle. 3-Mucous membrane lined by pseudostratified columnar epithelium. 4-Serous gland. 5-Mucous gland.

The lumen of the trachea is lined by mucous membrane which consists of a lining epithelium and an underlying layer of connective tissue. The lining epithelium is pseudostratified ciliated columnar. It contains numerous goblet cells, and basal cells that lie next to the basement membrane. Numerous lymphocytes are seen in deeper parts of the epithelium.

The subepithelial connective tissue contains numerous elastic fibres. It contains serous glands that keep the epithelium moist; and mucous glands that provide a covering of mucous in which dust particles get caught. The mucous is continuously moved towards the larynx by ciliary action. Numerous aggregations of lymphoid tissue are present in the subepithelial connective tissue. Eosinophil leucocytes are also present.

Principal bronchi

The right and left principal bronchi (primary or main bronchi) have a structure similar to that of the trachea described above. The intrapulmonary bronchi are described with the lung (see below).

THE LUNGS

The structure of the lungs has to be understood keeping in mind their function of oxygenation of blood. The following features are essential for this purpose.

(1) A surface at which air (containing oxygen) can be brought into close contact with circulating blood. The barrier between air and blood has to be very thin to allow oxygen (and carbon dioxide) to pass through it. The surface has to be extensive enough to meet the oxygen requirements of the body.

(2) A system of tubes to convey air to and away from the surface at which exchanges take place.

(3) A rich network of blood capillaries present in intimate relationship to the surface at which exchanges take place.

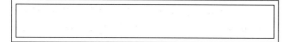

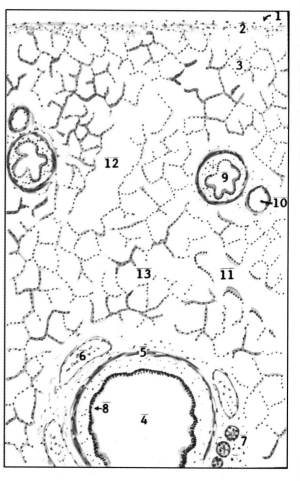

Fig. 13.5A. Section through part of a lung. 1, 2-Pleura. 3-Alveolus. 4-Bronchus. 5-Smooth muscle. 6-Cartilage. 7-Glands. 8-Epithelium of bronchus. 9-Bronchiole. 10-Artery. 11-Respiratory bronchiole. 12-Alveolar duct. 13-Atrium.

Intrapulmonary Passages

On entering the lung the principal bronchus divides into secondary, or *lobar bronchi* (one for each lobe). Each lobar bronchus divides into tertiary, or *segmental bronchi* (one for each segment of the lobe). (For precise details of the pattern of segmental bronchi consult a book on gross anatomy). The segmental bronchi divide into smaller and smaller bronchi, which ultimately end in *bronchioles*. The lung

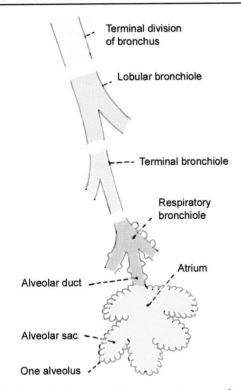

Terminal division
of bronchus

Lobular bronchiole

Terminal bronchiole

Respiratory
bronchiole

Atrium

Alveolar duct

Alveolar sac

One alveolus

Fig. 13.5B. Scheme to show some terms used to describe the terminal ramifications of the bronchial tree.

substance is divided into numerous lobules each of which receives a *lobular bronchiole*. The lobular bronchiole gives off a number of *terminal bronchioles* (Fig.13.5). As indicated by their name the terminal bronchioles represent the most distal parts of the conducting passage. Each terminal bronchiole ends by dividing into *respiratory bronchioles*. These are so called because they are partly respiratory in function as some air sacs (see below) arise from them. Each respiratory bronchiole ends by dividing into a few *alveolar ducts*. Each alveolar duct ends in a passage, the *atrium*, which leads into a number of rounded *alveolar sacs*. Each alveolar sac is studded with a number of air sacs or *alveoli*. The alveoli are blind sacs having very thin walls through which oxygen passes from air into blood, and carbon dioxide passes from blood into air.

The structure of the larger intrapulmonary bronchi is similar to that of the trachea. As these bronchi divide into smaller ones the following changes in structure are observed.

(1) The cartilages in the walls of the bronchi become irregular in shape, and are progressively smaller. Cartilage is absent in the walls of bronchioles: this is the criterion that distinguishes a bronchiole from a bronchus.

(2) The amount of muscle in the bronchial wall increases as the bronchi become smaller. The presence of muscle in the walls of bronchi is of considerable clinical significance. Spasm of this muscle constricts the bronchi and can cause difficulty in breathing. This is specially likely to occur in allergic conditions and leads to a disease called *asthma*.

(3) Subepithelial lymphoid tissue increases in quantity as bronchi become smaller. [The significance of this mucosa associated lymphoid tissue has been discussed on page 189]. Glands become fewer, and are absent in the walls of bronchioles.

(4) We have seen that the trachea and larger bronchi are lined by pseudostratified ciliated columnar epithelium. As the bronchi become smaller the epithelium first becomes simple ciliated columnar, then non-ciliated columnar, and finally cuboidal (in respiratory bronchioles). The cells contain lysosomes and numerous mitochondria.

EM studies have shown that apart from typical ciliated columnar cells, various other types of cells are to be seen in the epithelium lining the air passages. Details of their structure are beyond the scope of this book. Some of the cells encountered are as follows (Fig. 13.6).

(a) Goblet cells are numerous. They provide mucous which helps to trap dust entering the passages and is moved by ciliary action towards the larynx and pharynx.

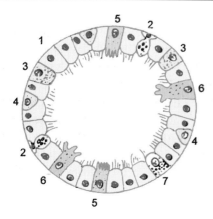

Fig. 13.6. Scheme to show the various types of cells to be seen lining the respiratory passages.
1. Typical ciliated columnar. 2. Goblet. 3. Serous. 4. Basal. 5. Brush, 6. Clara, 7. Argyrophile.

(b) Non-ciliated serous cells secrete fluid which keeps the epithelium moist.

(c) Basal cells multiply and transform into other cell types to replace those that are lost.

(d) Some non-ciliated cells present predominantly in terminal bronchioles (see below) produce a secretion which spreads over the alveolar cells forming a film that reduces surface tension. These include the *cells of Clara*.

Some other functions attributed to cells of Clara include:

1. Protection against harmful substances that are inhaled.

2. Protection against development of emphysema by opposing the action of substances (proteases) that tend to destroy walls of lung alveoli.

3. Stem cell function.

(e) Cells similar to diffuse endocrine cells of the gut, and containing argyrophil granules are present. They secrete hormones and active peptides including serotonin and bombesin.

(f) Lymphocytes and other leucocytes may be present in the epithelium. They migrate into the epithelium from surrounding tissues.

Structure Of Alveolar Wall

Each alveolus has a very thin wall. The wall is lined by an epithelium consisting mainly of flattened squamous cells. The epithelium rests on a basement membrane. Deep to the basement membrane there is a layer of delicate connective tissue through which pulmonary capillaries run. These capillaries have the usual endothelial lining that rests on a basement membrane. The barrier between air and blood is made up of the epithelial cells and their basement membrane; by endothelial cells and their basement membrane; and by intervening connective tissue. At many places the two basement membranes fuse greatly reducing the thickness of the barrier.

EM studies have shown that the cells forming the lining epithelium of alveoli (*pneumocytes*) are of various types.

(1) The most numerous cells are the squamous cells already referred to . They are called *type I alveolar epithelial cells*. Except in the region of the nucleus, these cells are reduced to a very thin layer (0.05 to 0.2 μm). The edges of adjoining cells overlap and are united by tight junctions (preventing leakage of blood from capillaries into the alveolar lumen). They form the lining of 90% of the alveolar surface.

(2) Scattered in the epithelial lining there are rounded secretory cells bearing microvilli on their free surfaces. These are designated *type II alveolar epithelial cells*. Their cytoplasm

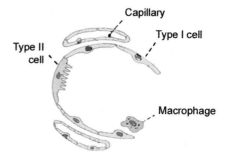

Fig. 13.7. Some cells to be seen in relation to an alveolus.

contains secretory granules that appear to be made up of several layers (and are, therefore, called *multilamellar bodies*). These cells are believed to produce a secretion which forms a film over the alveolar epithelium. This film or *pulmonary surfactant* reduces surface tension and prevents collapse of the alveolus during expiration.

Surfactant contains phospholipids, proteins and glycosaminoglycans produced in type II cells. (A similar fluid is believed to be produced by the cells of Clara present in bronchial passages).

Type II cells may multiply to replace damaged type I cells.

(3) *Type III alveolar cells*, or *brush cells*, of doubtful function, have also been described.

The connective tissue in the wall of the alveolus contains collagen fibres and numerous elastic fibres continuous with those of bronchioles. Fibroblasts, histiocytes, mast cells, lymphocytes and plasma cells may be present. Pericytes are present in relation to capillaries. Some macrophages enter the connective tissue from blood and pass through the alveolar epithelium to reach its luminal surface. Dust particles phagocytosed by them are seen in their cytoplasm. They are therefore called *dust cells*. These dust cells are expelled to the outside through the respiratory passages. In congestive heart failure (in which pulmonary capillaries become overloaded with blood) these macrophages phagocytose erythrocytes that escape from capillaries. The cells, therefore, acquire a brick red colour and are then called *heart failure cells*. Macrophages also remove excessive surfactant, and secrete several enzymes.

The endothelial cells lining the alveolar capillaries are remarkable for their extreme thinness. With the EM they are seen to have numerous projections extending into the capillary lumen. These projections greatly increase the surface of the cell membrane that is exposed to blood and is, therefore, available for exchange of gases. We have already seen that at many places the basement membrane of the endothelium fuses with that of the alveolar epithelium greatly reducing the thickness of the barrier between blood and air in alveoli.

There are about 200 million alveoli in a normal lung. The total area of the alveolar surface of each lung is extensive. It has been estimated to be about 75 square meters. The total capillary surface area available for gaseous exchanges is about 125 square meters.

Connective Tissue Basis of the Lung

The greater part of the surface of the lung is covered by a serous membrane, the visceral pleura. This membrane consists of a layer of flattened mesothelial cells, supported on a layer of connective tissue.

Deep to the pleura there is a layer of subserous connective tissue. This connective tissue extends into the lung substance along bronchi and their accompanying blood vessels, and divides the lung into lobules. Each lobule has a lobular bronchiole and its ramifications, blood vessels, lymphatics and nerves.

The epithelial lining of air passages is supported by a basal lamina deep to which there is the connective tissue of the lamina propria. Both in the basal lamina and in the lamina propria there are numerous elastic fibres. These fibres run along the length of respiratory passages and ultimately become continuous with elastic fibres present in the walls of air sacs. This elastic tissue plays a very important role by providing the physical basis for elastic recoil of lung tissue. This recoil is an important factor in expelling air from the lungs during expiration. Elastic fibres passing between lung parenchyma and pleura prevent collapse of alveoli and small bronchi during expiration.

Pleura

The pleura is lined by flat mesothelial cells that are supported by loose connective tissue rich in elastic fibres, blood vessels, nerves and lymphatics. There is considerable adipose tissue under parietal pleura.

Vessels & Nerves of the Lung

The lungs receive deoxygenated blood from the right ventricle of the heart through pulmonary arteries. Within the lung the arteries end in an extensive capillary network in the walls of alveoli. Blood oxygenated here is returned to the left atrium of the heart through pulmonary veins.

Oxygenated blood required for nutrition of the lung itself reaches the lungs through bronchial arteries. They are distributed to the walls of bronchi as far as the respiratory bronchioles. Blood reaching the lung through these arteries is returned to the heart partly through bronchial veins, and partly through the pulmonary veins.

Plexuses of lymph vessels are present just deep to the pleura and in the walls of bronchi. For details of the lymphatic drainage of the lungs see a book on gross anatomy.

The lungs receive autonomic nerves, both sympathetic and parasympathetic, and including both afferent and efferent fibres. Efferent fibres supply the bronchial musculature. Vagal stimulation produces bronchoconstriction. Efferent fibres also innervate bronchial glands. Afferent fibres are distributed to the walls of bronchi and of alveoli. Afferent impulses from the lungs play an important role in control of respiration through respiratory reflexes.

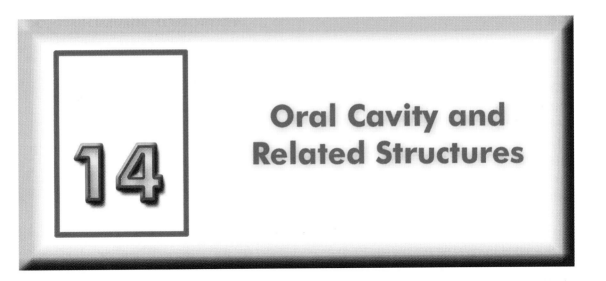

Oral Cavity and Related Structures

In this chapter we begin consideration of the histology of structures that form part of the alimentary or digestive system. This is an extensive system consideration of which will be continued in Chapters 15 and 16.

In ordinary English the word 'alimentary' means 'pertaining to nourishment'. In anatomical terminology the alimentary system includes all those structures that are concerned with eating, and with the digestion and absorption of food. The system consists of an *alimentary canal* which starts at the mouth, and ends at the anus. The alimentary canal includes the oral cavity, pharynx, oesophagus, stomach, small intestines, and large intestines (in that order).

The abdominal part of the alimentary canal (consisting of the stomach and intestines) is often referred to as the *gastrointestinal tract*. Closely related to the alimentary canal there are several accessory organs that form part of the alimentary system. These include the teeth, the tongue, the salivary glands, the liver and the pancreas.

In this chapter we shall consider the histology of some structures present in relation to the oral cavity. The pharynx has been described on page 209.

Oral Cavity

The wall of the oral cavity is made up partly of bone (jaws, hard palate), and partly of muscle and connective tissue (lips, cheeks, soft palate, and floor of mouth). These structures are lined by mucous membrane. The mucous membrane is lined by stratified squamous epithelium which rests on connective tissue, similar to that of the dermis.

The epithelium differs from that on the skin in that it is not keratinized (i.e., the stratum corneum, lucidum and granulosum are not present: See Fig. A9). Papillae of connective tissue (similar to dermal papillae) extend into the epithelium. The size of these papillae varies considerably from region to region. Over the alveolar processes (where the mucosa forms the gums), and over the hard palate, the mucous membrane is closely adherent to underlying periosteum. Elsewhere it is connected to underlying structures by loose connective tissue. In the cheeks, this connective tissue contains many elastic fibres and much fat (specially in children).

The Lips

The structure of the lips is considered separately as sections through them are commonly shown in classes.

The substance of each lip (upper or lower) is predominantly muscular (skeletal muscle). For details of the various muscles taking part in forming each lip see the author's TEXTBOOK OF ANATOMY. Each lip is usually said to have an 'external' surface lined by skin, and an 'internal' surface lined by mucous membrane. It must be noted, however, that part of the mucosal surface is 'free' and constitutes the region the lay person thinks of as the lip.

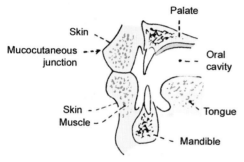

Fig. 14.1A. Diagram to show some relationships of the lips.

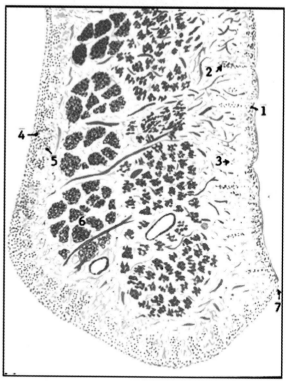

Fig. 14.1B. Section through lip. Its substance is formed by a mass of muscle. 1-Outer surface covered by skin. 2-Hair follicle. 4- Inner surface (mucosa) covered by thick stratified squamous epithelium. 6-Glands. 7-Junction of skin and mucosa.

This is a transitional zone, which is sometimes referred to as the ***vermilion***, because of its pink colour in fair skinned individuals. This part meets the skin along a distinct edge. The 'external' surface of the lip is lined by true skin in which hair follicles and sebaceous glands can be seen. The mucous membrane is lined by stratified squamous epithelium (as in the rest of the oral cavity). This epithelium is much thicker than that lining the skin (specially in infants). The epithelium has a well marked ***rete ridge system***.

The term rete ridges is applied to finger like projections of epithelium that extend into underlying connective tissue, just like the epidermal papillae: page 193. This arrangement anchors the epithelium to underlying connective tissue, and enables it to withstand friction. A similar arrangement is seen in the mucosa over the palate.

Subjacent to the epithelium the mucosa has a layer of connective tissue (corresponding to the dermis), and a deeper layer of loose connective tissue. The latter contains numerous mucous glands. Sebaceous glands, not associated with hair follicles, may be present. Their secretions prevent dryness and cracking of the exposed part of the mucosa.

THE TEETH

General Structure

A tooth consists of an 'upper' part, the **crown**, which is seen in the mouth; and of one or more **roots** which are embedded in sockets in the jaw bone (mandible or maxilla). The greater part of the tooth is formed by a bone-like material called **dentine**. In the region of the crown the dentine is covered by a much harder white material called the **enamel**. Over the root the dentine is covered by a thin layer of **cement**. The cement is united to the wall of the bony socket in the jaw by a layer of fibrous tissue that is called the **periodontal ligament**. The external surface of the alveolar process is covered by the gum which normally overlaps the lower edge of the crown. Within the dentine there is a **pulp canal** (or **pulp cavity**) which contains a mass of cells, blood vessels, and nerves which constitute the **pulp**. The blood vessels and nerves enter the pulp canal through the **apical foramen** which is located at the apex of the root .

The Enamel

The enamel is the hardest material in the body. It is made up almost entirely (96%) of inorganic salts. These salts are mainly in the form of complex crystals of hydroxyapatite (as in bone: See page 101). The crystals contain calcium phosphate and calcium carbonate. Some salts are also present in amorphous form. The crystals of hydroxyapatite are arranged in the form of rod-shaped **prisms**, which run from the deep surface of the enamel (in contact with dentine) to its superficial (or free) surface.

Prisms are separated by **interprismatic material**. There is no essential difference in the structure of prisms and of interprismatic material,

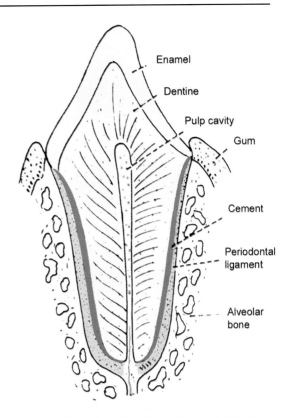

Fig. 14.2. Vertical section through a typical tooth.

the two appearing different only because of differing orientation of the hydroxyapatite crystals in them. The most superficial part of the enamel is devoid of prisms.

During development, enamel is laid down in the form of layers. When seen in section these layers can be distinguished as they are separated by lines running more or less parallel to the surface of the enamel. These lines are called the **incremental lines** or the **lines of Retzius**. In some teeth, in which enamel formation takes place partly before birth and partly after birth (e.g., in milk teeth), one of the incremental lines is particularly marked. It represents the junction of enamel formed before birth with that formed after birth, and is called the **neonatal line**.

At places, the enamel is penetrated by extraneous material. Projections entering the enamel from the dentine-enamel junction are called **enamel tufts**;

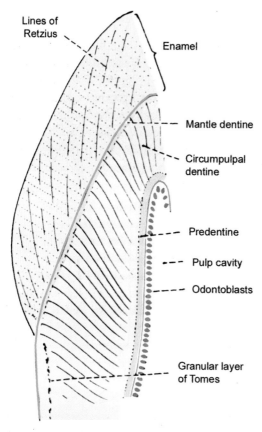

Fig. 14.3. Part of a tooth to show some features of the structure of enamel and of dentine.

and some projections entering it from the free surface are called *enamel lamellae* (because of their shape). Dentinal tubules (see below) may extend into the enamel forming *enamel spindles*.

The Dentine

Dentine is a hard material having several similarities to bone. It is made up basically of calcified ground substance (glycosaminoglycans) in which there are numerous collagen fibres (type 1). The calcium salts are mainly in the form of hydroxyapatite (page 101). Amorphous salts are also present. The inorganic salts account for 70% of the weight of dentine. Like bone, dentine is

laid down in layers that are parallel to the pulp cavity. The layers may be separated by less mineralized tissue that forms the *incremental lines of Von Ebner*. Dentine is permeated by numerous fine canaliculi that pass radially from the pulp cavity towards the enamel (or towards cement). These are the *dentinal tubules*. The tubules may branch specially near the enamel-dentine junction. We have seen (above) that some dentinal tubules extend into the enamel as enamel spindles.

The ground substance of dentine is more dense (than elsewhere) immediately around the dentinal tubules, and forms the *peritubular dentine* or the *dentinal sheath* (of Newmann). Each dentinal tubule contains a protoplasmic process arising from cells called *odontoblasts*, that line the pulp cavity. These protoplasmic processes are called the *fibres of Tomes*.

Near the surface of the root of the tooth (i.e., just deep to the cement) the dentine contains minute spaces which give a granular appearance. This is the *granular layer of Tomes*.

Brief mention must be made of some terms used to describe different parts of dentine. At the junction of dentine with the pulp cavity there is a layer of *predentine* that is not mineralized. Dentine near the enamel-dentine junction is less mineralized (than elsewhere) and is called the *mantle dentine*. The main part of dentine (between predentine and mantle dentine) is called the *circumpulpal dentine*. Dentine formed before eruption of the tooth is called *primary dentine*, while that formed after eruption is called *secondary dentine*.

The Cement

The cement may be regarded as a layer of true bone that covers the roots of the tooth. It covers the entire dentine not covered by enamel (Fig.14.2), but in old people part of the cement may be lost, the dentine being then exposed. In some parts (specially towards the apex of the

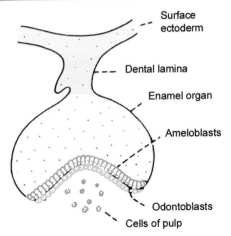

Fig. 14.4A. Formation of ameloblasts and odontoblasts.

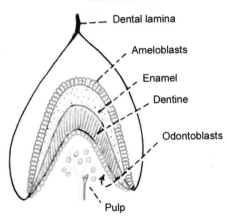

Fig. 14.4B. Formation of enamel and of dentine.

The Pulp

The dental pulp is made up of very loose connective tissue resembling embryonic mesenchyme. (See mucoid tissue, page 68). The ground substance is gelatinous and abundant. In it there are many spindle shaped and star shaped cells. Delicate collagen fibres, numerous blood vessels, lymphatics and nerve fibres are present. The nerve fibres are partly sensory and partly sympathetic.

Odontoblasts and Ameloblasts

Apart from the connective tissue cells of the pulp and of the periodontal membrane, and the cementocytes in cement, there are two main types of cells present in association with teeth. These are dentine forming *odontoblasts*, and enamel forming *ameloblasts*. To understand their significance brief reference has to be made to the development of teeth.

Each tooth may be regarded as a highly modified form of the stratified squamous epithelium covering the developing jaw (alveolar process). A thickening of epithelium grows downwards into the underlying connective tissue and enlarges to form an *enamel organ*. The enamel organ is invaginated (from below) by a mass of mesenchymal cells: these mesenchymal cells form the dental papilla. As a result of this invagination the enamel organ becomes cup-shaped. The cells of the enamel organ are derived from ectoderm. Those cells that line the inner wall of its cup shaped lower end differentiate into columnar cells that are called ameloblasts. Mesodermal cells of the papilla, that are adjacent to the ameloblasts, become cuboidal and form an epithelium-like layer. The cells of this layer are odontoblasts.

Ameloblasts are enamel forming cells. Odontoblasts are dentine forming cells. Both

tooth) the cement contains lacunae and canaliculi as in bone. The lacunae are occupied by cells similar to osteocytes (*cementocytes*). Some parts of cement are acellular.

Cement is covered by a fibrous membrane called the *periodontal membrane* (or ligament). This membrane may be regarded as the periosteum of the cement. Collagen fibres from this membrane extend into the cement, and also into the alveolar bone (forming the socket in which the root lies) as fibres of Sharpey (page 103). The periodontal membrane fixes the tooth in its socket. It contains numerous nerve endings that provide sensory information.

ameloblasts and odontoblasts behave in a way very similar to that of osteoblasts (page 106) and lay down layer upon layer of enamel (in the case of ameloblasts), or of dentine (in the case of odontoblasts). As a result of the formation of layers of enamel and dentine the ameloblasts and odontoblasts become progressively separated by these layers. The original line at which enamel and dentine formation begins remains as the enamel-dentine junction. Ultimately, ameloblasts come to line the external aspect of the enamel, and are removed by surface friction after the tooth erupts. The odontoblasts persist as a lining for the pulp cavity. We have seen that cytoplasmic processes from these cells extend into the dentinal tubules. For further details of development of teeth see the author's HUMAN EMBRYOLOGY.

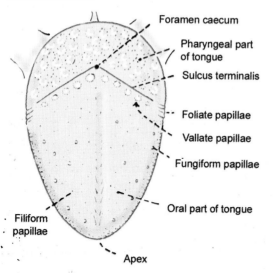

Fig. 14.5. Tongue as seen from above.

When examined by EM both ameloblasts and odontoblasts show the features typical of actively secreting cells. They have prominent Golgi complexes and abundant rough ER. The apical part of each cell is prolonged into a process. In the case of odontoblasts, the process runs into the proximal part of a dentinal tubule. In ameloblasts, the projection is called *Tomes process*. This process contains numerous

microtubules, and many secretory vesicles. Other smaller processes are present near the base of Tomes process. The organic matrix of enamel is released mainly by Tomes process, which also appears to be responsible for forming prisms of enamel.

THE TONGUE

The tongue lies on the floor of the oral cavity. It has a dorsal surface which is free; and a ventral surface that is free anteriorly, but is attached to the floor of the oral cavity posteriorly. The dorsal and ventral surfaces become continuous at the lateral margins, and at the tip (or apex) of the tongue.

Near its posterior end the dorsum of the tongue is marked by a V-shaped groove called the *sulcus terminalis*. The apex of the 'V' points backwards and is marked by a depression called the *foramen caecum*. The limbs of the sulcus terminalis run forwards and laterally. The sulcus terminalis divides the tongue into a larger (2/3) anterior, or oral, part; and a smaller (1/3) posterior, or pharyngeal, part.

The substance of the tongue is made up chiefly of skeletal muscle supported by connective tissue (Fig. 14.6A). The muscle is arranged in bundles that run in vertical, transverse and longitudinal directions. This arrangement of muscle permits intricate movements of the tongue associated with the chewing and swallowing of food, and those necessary for speech. The substance of the tongue is divided into right and left halves by a connective tissue septum.

The surface of the tongue is covered by mucous membrane lined by stratified squamous epithelium. The epithelium is supported on a

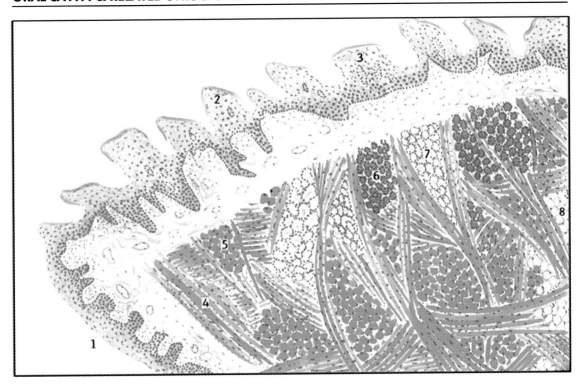

Fig. 14.6A. Tongue (Panoramic view). 2-Filiform papilla. 3-Fungiform papilla. 4, 5-Skeletal muscle. 6-Serous gland. 7-Mucous gland. 8-Adipose tissue.

layer of connective tissue. On the undersurface of the tongue the mucous membrane resembles that lining the rest of the oral cavity (page 217),

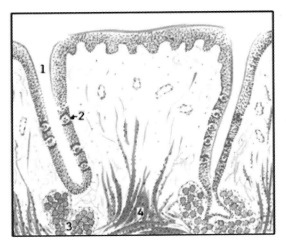

Fig. 14.6B. Vallate papilla. 1-Groove around papilla. 2-Taste bud. 3- Serous glands of Von Ebner). 4-Muscle extending into papilla.

and the epithelium is not keratinized. The mucous membrane covering the dorsum of the tongue is different over the anterior and posterior parts. Over the part lying in front of the sulcus terminalis the mucosa bears numerous projections or *papillae*. Each papilla consists of a lining of epithelium and a core of connective tissue. The epithelium over the papillae is partly keratinized.

The papillae are of various types as follows (Fig. 14.6A).

(a) The most numerous papillae are small and conical in shape. They are called *filiform papillae*. The epithelium at the tips of these papillae is keratinized. It may project in the form of threads.

(b) At the apex of the tongue, and along its lateral margins there are larger papillae with rounded summits and narrower bases. These are called *fungiform papillae*. Fungiform papillae bear taste buds (described below). In contrast to the filiform papillae the epithelium on fungiform papillae is (as a rule) not keratinized.

(c) The largest papillae of the tongue are called *circumvallate papillae*. They are arranged in a row just anterior to the sulcus terminalis. When viewed from the surface each papilla is seen to have a circular top demarcated from the rest of the mucosa by a groove. In sections through the papilla it is seen that the papilla has a circumferential 'lateral wall' that lies in the depth of the groove (Fig. 14.6B). Taste buds are present on this wall, and also on the 'outer' wall of the groove.

Another variety of papilla sometimes mentioned in relation to the tongue is the *papilla simplex*. Unlike the other papillae which can be seen by naked eye the papillae simplex are microscopic and are quite distinct from other papillae. They are not surface projections at all, but are projections of subjacent connective tissue into the epithelium. In other words these papillae are equivalent to dermal papillae of the skin.

The mucous membrane of the posterior (pharyngeal) part of the dorsum of the tongue bears numerous rounded elevations that are quite different from the papillae described above. These elevations are produced by collections of lymphoid tissue present deep to the epithelium. These collections of lymphoid tissue collectively form the *lingual tonsil*.

Numerous mucous and serous glands are present in the connective tissue deep to the epithelium of the tongue. Mucous glands are most numerous in the pharyngeal part, in relation to the masses of lymphoid tissue. They open into recesses of mucosa that dip into the masses of lymphoid tissue. The serous glands are present mainly in relation to circumvallate papillae, and open into the furrows surrounding the papillae. Serous glands also open in the

vicinity of other taste buds. It is believed that the secretions of these glands **(a)** dissolve the substance to be tasted and spread it over the taste bud; and **(b)** wash it away after it has been tasted.

The largest glands in the tongue are present on the ventral aspect of the apex. They contain both mucous and serous acini and are referred to as the *anterior lingual glands*.

Taste Buds

Taste buds are present in relation to circumvallate papillae, to fungiform papillae, and to leaf-like folds of mucosa (*folia linguae*) present on the posterolateral part of the tongue. Taste buds are also present on the soft palate, the epiglottis, the palatoglossal arches, and the posterior wall of the oropharynx.

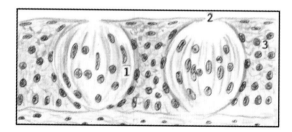

Fig. 14.7A. Taste buds. 1-Elongated cells. 2-Pore. 3-Stratified squamous epithelium.

Each taste bud is a piriform structure made up of modified epithelial cells (Fig. 14.7A). It extends through the entire thickness of the epithelium. Each bud has a small cavity that opens to the surface through a *gustatory pore*. The cavity is filled by a material rich in polysaccharides.

The cells present in taste buds are elongated and are vertically orientated, those towards the periphery being curved like crescents. Each cell has a central broader part containing the nucleus, and tapering ends. The cells are of two basic types. Some of them are *receptor cells* or *gustatory cells*. Endings of afferent nerves end

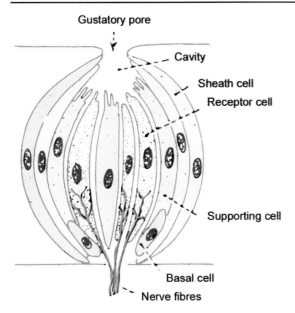

Fig. 14.7B. Scheme to show the cells in a taste bud.

in relation to them. Other cells perform a supporting function.

However, it is by no means easy to distinguish between receptor and supporter cells, the essential difference being the presence of innervation. Early observers using the light microscope found hairs at the tips of some cells and concluded that these were the receptor cells. However, this has not been confirmed by EM studies. The latter have shown that the 'hair' seen with the light microscope are microvilli which are more common on supporting cells rather on receptors. Two types of receptor cells can be distinguished on the basis of the vacuoles present in them.

Supporting cells are probably of three types. Some of them that lie at the periphery of the taste bud form a sheath for it. Those near the centre of the bud are truly supporting. They probably secrete a material that fills the cavity at the apex of the taste bud. Microvilli are often present at the tips of these cells. A third variety of supporting cell is seen in the basal part of the bud. These basal cells multiply and produce new supporting and

receptor cells to replace those that are worn out. This may be correlated with the fact that cells of taste buds have a short life and are continuously being replaced.

It has been held that taste buds in different parts of the tongue may respond best to particular modalities of taste. However, it is now known that the same taste bud can respond to different types of taste (sweet, sour, salt and bitter) and that taste is a complicated sensation depending upon the overall pattern of responses from taste buds all over the tongue. With this reservation in mind, we may note that sweet taste is best appreciated at the tip of the tongue, salt by the area just behind the tip and along the lateral border, and bitter taste by circumvallate papillae.

For development of the tongue see the author's HUMAN EMBRYOLOGY. For details of gross anatomy, blood supply, nerve supply and lymphatic drainage of the tongue see the author's TEXTBOOK OF ANATOMY.

SALIVARY GLANDS

These are the *parotid*, *submandibular* and *sublingual* glands, and numerous small glands situated in the mucous membrane of the lips (*labial glands*), cheeks (*buccal glands*), tongue (*lingual glands*), and palate (*palatine glands*). Some salivary gland tissue may be seen in the palatine and pharyngeal tonsils. The secretions of these glands help to keep the mouth moist, and provide a protective and lubricant coat of mucous. Some enzymes (amylase, lysozyme), and immunoglobulin IgA are also present in the secretions.

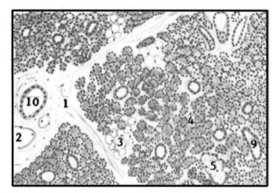

Fig. 14.8. Parotid gland. 1-Interlobular connective tissue.2-Blood vessel. 3-Adipose tissue. 4-Serous acini. 5-Mucous acini. 9-Intralobular duct. 10-Interlobular duct.

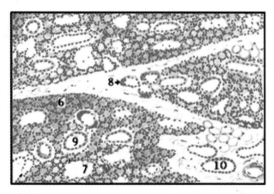

Fig. 14.9A. Submandibular gland (low power view). 6-Serous acini. 7-Mucous acini. 8-Demilune. 9-Intralobular duct. 10-Interlobular duct.

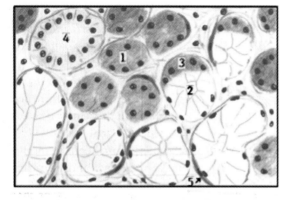

Fig. 14.9B. Submandibular gland (high power view). 1-Serous acini. 2-Mucous acini. 3-Demilune. 4-Ducts. 5-Myoepithelial cell.

Basic Histology

Salivary glands are compound tubulo-alveolar glands (racemose glands) (See page 51). Their secretory elements (also referred to as **end pieces** or as the **portio terminalis**) may be rounded (acini), pear shaped (alveoli), tubular, or a mixture of these (tubulo-acinar, tubulo-alveolar). The secretory elements lead into a series of ducts through which their secretions are poured into the oral cavity. In sections through salivary glands we see a large number of closely packed acini (or alveoli) with ducts scattered between them (Figs. 14.8, 14.9A). These elements are supported by connective tissue which also divides the glands into lobules, and forms capsules around them. Blood vessels, lymphatics and nerves run in the connective tissue which may at places contain some adipose tissue.

The cells lining the alveoli of salivary glands are usually described either as **serous** or **mucous**. In sections stained with haematoxylin and eosin serous cells stain darkly (because of the presence of zymogen granules: the colour varies from pink to dark purple). They have rounded nuclei that lie towards the base. In contrast mucous cells stain very lightly and, therefore, appear empty. The cells are in fact almost completely filled in by a mucoid material that stains very poorly Fig. 14.9B). This material pushes the nuclei towards the basement membrane. The nuclei are flattened. Further details of the structure of mucous and serous cells are considered below.

An alveolus is typically made up entirely of serous cells or of mucous cells. However, in some cases mucous alveoli are covered (on one or more sides) by groups of serous cells that are arranged in the form of **crescents** or **demilunes** (Fig. 14.9B). In the parotid gland the alveoli are almost entirely serous, only an occasional mucous alveolus being present (Fig. 14.8). In the

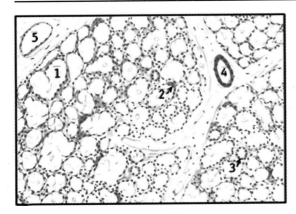

Fig. 14.10. Sublingual gland. 1- Mucous acini.
2-Demilune. 3-Duct.

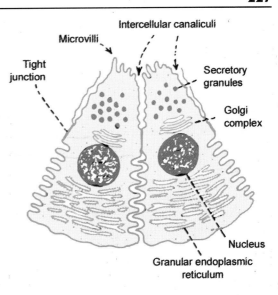

Fig. 14.11. Scheme to show some features of serous
cells in a salivary gland.

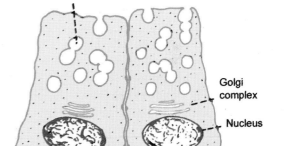

Fig. 14.12. Some features of the structure of
mucous cells in salivary glands.

submandibular gland some alveoli are serous and some are mucous, the latter being frequently capped by serous crescents (Fig. 14.9). The sublingual glands are made up predominantly of mucous alveoli, but a few serous demilunes may be present (Fig. 14.10).

A secretory unit, or gland, with only one type of cell (serous or mucous) is said to be *homocrine*. If it contains more than one variety of cell it is said to be *heterocrine*. From what has been said above it will be clear that all the three major salivary glands are heterocrine.

Secretions produced in alveoli pass along a system of ducts, different parts of which have differing structure. The smallest ducts are called *intercalated ducts*. They are lined by cuboidal or flattened cells. Intercalated ducts open into *striated ducts* lined by columnar cells. They are so called because the basal parts of the cells show vertical striations. Striated ducts open into *excretory ducts* which are lined by simple columnar epithelium.

Some Additional Details

1. Serous cells are usually arranged in the form of rounded acini. As a result each cell is roughly pyramidal having a broad base (towards the basement membrane) and a narrow apex (towards

the lumen). Some microvilli and pinocytotic vesicles are seen at the apex of the cell. The lumen of the acinus often extends for some distance between adjacent cells: these extensions are called *intercellular secretory canaliculi*. Deep to these canaliculi the cell membranes of adjoining cells are united by tight junctions (page 12). Deep to these junctions, the lateral cell margins show folds that interdigitate with those of adjoining cells. The apical cytoplasm contains secretory granules that are small, homogeneous, and electron dense. The cytoplasm also contains a well developed Golgi complex and abundant rough endoplasmic reticulum, both features indicating considerable synthetic activity. Mitochondria, lysosomes, and microfilaments are also present.

2. Mucous cells are usually arranged in the form of tubular secretory elements. Cresents present in relation to them are located at the ends of the tubules. The cells lining mucous cells tend to be columnar rather than pyramidal. Their secretory granules are large and ill defined. Rough endoplasmic reticulum and Golgi complex are similar to those in serous cells, but microvilli, foldings of plasma membrane, and intercellular canaliculi are not usually seen.

3. From the point of view of ultrastructure many cells of salivary glands are intermediate between serous and mucous cells. They are referred to as *seromucous cells*. Most of the cells identified as serous with light microscopy in the parotid and submandibular glands are really seromucous.

The secretions of all types of salivary secretory cells contain protein-carbohydrate complexes. Their concentration is lowest in cases of serous cells, very high in mucous cells, and with widely differing concentrations in seromucous cells.

4. We have seen that in the submandibular glands mucous acini are often capped by serous demilunes. The serous cells of a demilune drain into the lumen of the acinus through fine canaliculi passing through the intervals between mucous cells.

5. *Myoepithelial cells* are present in relation to alveoli and intercalated ducts of salivary glands (see page 133). They may also be seen in relation to larger ducts (intralobular and extralobular). These cells lie between the epithelial cells and their basement membrane. The myoepithelial cells located on alveoli are often branched (stellate) and

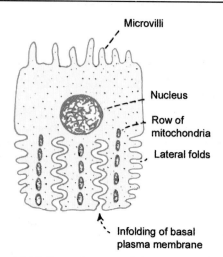

Fig. 14.14. Some features of the EM structure of a cell from a striated duct.

may form 'baskets' around the alveoli. Those located on the ducts are fusiform and run longitudinally along them.

With the EM myoepithelial cells are seen to contain the usual organelles. In addition they have conspicuous filaments that resemble myofilaments of smooth muscle cells. These filaments are numerous in processes arising from the cell. Cilia are present on some myoepithelial cells. It has been suggested that the cilia may subserve a sensory or chemoreceptor function.

Myoepithelial cells are contractile, their contraction helping to squeeze out secretion from alveoli. The cells receive an autonomic innervation (details of which are controversial).

6. The cells lining the striated ducts show an interesting ultrastructure. Their basal striations are seen to be due to the presence of numerous deep infoldings of the basal parts of the cell membranes. Numerous elongated mitochondria are present in the intervals between the folds. Similar cells are also present scattered in the epithelium of the excretory ducts. These cells are believed to play a role in regulating the water and electrolyte content of saliva to make it hypotonic. Immunoglobulin A, produced by plasma cells lying subjacent to the epithelium, passes into saliva through the cells lining the striated ducts.

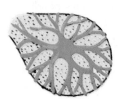

Fig. 14.13. Surface view of an alveolus showing a myoepithelial cell. Its processes form a basket around the alveolus.

Innervation of Salivary Glands

Secretion by salivary glands is under hormonal as well as neural control. A local hormone *plasmakinin* formed by secretory cells influences vasodilation. Salivary glands are innervated by autonomic nerves, both parasympathetic (cholinergic) and sympathetic (adrenergic). Parasympathetic nerves travel to secretory elements along ducts, while sympathetic nerves travel along arteries. Synaptic contacts between nerve terminals and effector cells form *neuro-effector junctions*.

Two types of junction, *epilemmal* and *hypolemmal*, are described. At epilemmal junctions the nerve terminal is separated from the secretory or effector cell by the basal lamina. At hypolemmal junctions the nerve terminal pierces the basal lamina and comes into direct contact with the effector cell. Nerve impulses reaching one effector cell spread to others through intercellular contacts. Classically, salivary secretion has been attributed to parasympathetic stimulation. While this is true, it is believed that sympathetic nerves can also excite secretion either directly, or by vasodilation. Autonomic nerves not only stimulate secretion, but also appear to determine its viscosity and other characteristics. Autonomic nerve terminals are also seen on myoepithelial cells and on cells lining the ducts of salivary glands. The latter probably influence reabsorption of sodium by cells lining the ducts. Salivary glands are sensitive to pain, and must therefore have a sensory innervation as well.

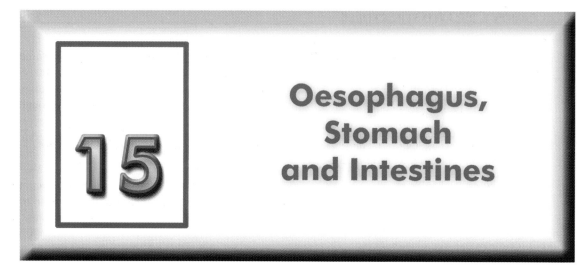

Oesophagus, Stomach and Intestines

15

BASIC PATTERN OF THE STRUCTURE OF THE ALIMENTARY CANAL

The structure of the alimentary canal, from the oesophagus up to the anal canal, shows several features that are common to all these parts. We shall consider these common features before examining the structure of individual parts of the canal.

While considering the structure of the oral cavity (page 217), and of the pharynx (page 209), we have seen that the walls of these parts of the alimentary canal are partly bony, and partly muscular. From the upper end of the oesophagus up to the lower end of the anal canal the alimentary canal has the form of a fibro-muscular tube. The wall of the tube is made up of the following layers (from inner to outer side).

A. The innermost layer is the ***mucous membrane*** which is made up of:

(**a**) A lining epithelium.

(**b**) A layer of connective tissue, the ***lamina propria***, that supports the epithelium.

(**c**) A thin layer of smooth muscle called the

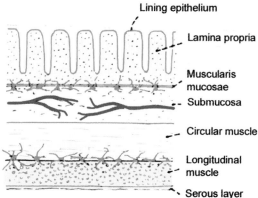

Fig. 15.1. Scheme to show the layers of the gut. Note the large blood vessels in the submucosa; the myenteric nerve plexus between the longitudinal and circular layers of muscle; and the subcutaneous nerve plexus near the muscularis mucosae.

muscularis mucosae.

B. The mucous membrane rests on a layer of loose areolar tissue called the ***submucosa***.

C. The gut wall derives its main strength and form because of a thick layer of muscle (***muscularis externa***) that surrounds the submucosa.

D. Covering the muscularis externa there is a ***serous layer*** or (alternatively) an ***adventitial layer***.

Some general features of these layers are briefly considered below.

It may be noted at the outset that the oesophagus and anal canal are merely transport passages. The part of the alimentary canal from the stomach to the rectum is the proper digestive tract, responsible for digestion and absorption of food. Reabsorption of secreted fluids is an important function of the large intestine.

The Lining Epithelium

The lining epithelium is columnar all over the gut; except in the oesophagus, and in the lower part of the anal canal, where it is stratified squamous. This stratified squamous epithelium has a protective function in these situations. The cells of the more typical columnar epithelium are either absorptive or secretory.

The epithelium of the gut presents an extensive absorptive surface. The factors contributing to the extent of the surface are as follows.

1. The *considerable length* of the alimentary canal, and specially that of the small intestine.

2. The presence of *numerous folds* involving the entire thickness of the mucous membrane. These folds can be seen by naked eye. The submucosa extends into the folds.

3. At numerous places the epithelium dips into the lamina propria forming *crypts* (see below).

4. In the small intestine the mucosa bears numerous finger-like processes that project into the lumen. These processes are called *villi*. Each villus has a surface lining of epithelium and a core formed by an extension of the connective tissue of the lamina propria.

5. The luminal surfaces of the epithelial cells bear numerous microvilli (page 24).

The epithelium of the gut also performs a very important secretory function. The secretory cells are arranged in the form of numerous glands as follows.

(a) Some glands are unicellular, the secretory cells being scattered among the cells of the lining epithelium.

(b) In many situations, the epithelium dips into the lamina propria forming simple tubular glands. (These are the crypts referred to above) .

(c) In other situations (e.g., in the duodenum) there are compound tubulo-alveolar glands (page 51) lying in the submucosa. They open into the lumen of the gut through ducts traversing the mucosa.

(d) Finally, there are the pancreas and the liver, that form distinct organs lying outside the gut wall. They pour their secretions into the lumen of the gut through large ducts. (In this respect, these glands are similar to the salivary glands). The liver and pancreas, and most of the salivary glands, are derivatives of the epithelial lining of the gut. Embryologically, this epithelium is derived from endoderm.

The Lamina Propria

The lamina propria is made up of collagen and reticular fibres embedded in a glycosaminoglycan matrix. Some fibroblasts, blood capillaries, lymph vessels, and nerves are seen in this layer. In the small intestine the lamina propria forms the core of each villus. It surrounds and supports glandular elements.

Prominent aggregations of lymphoid tissue (as well as scattered lymphocytes) are present in the lamina propria. Some of this lymphoid tissue extends into the submucosa. This gut related lymphoid tissue (GALT) has been considered on page 190.

The Muscularis Mucosae

This is a thin layer of smooth muscle that separates the connective tissue of the lamina propria from the submucosa. It consists of an inner layer in which the muscle fibres are arranged circularly (around the lumen) and an outer layer in which the muscle fibres run longitudinally. The muscularis mucosae extends into mucosal folds, but not into villi. Contractions of the muscularis mucosae are important for the local mixing of intestinal contents.

The Submucosa

This layer of loose areolar tissue connects the mucosa to the muscularis externa. Its looseness permits some mobility of the mucosa over the muscle. Numerous blood vessels, lymphatics and nerve fibres traverse the submucosa. Smaller branches arising from them enter the mucous membrane.

The Muscularis Externa

Over the greater part of the gut the muscularis externa consists of smooth muscle. The only exception is the upper part of the oesophagus where this layer contains striated muscle fibres. Some striated muscle fibres are also closely associated with the wall of the anal canal.

The muscle layer consists (typically) of an inner layer of circularly arranged muscle fibres, and an outer longitudinal layer.

> Both layers really consist of spirally arranged fasciculi, the turns of the spiral being compact in the circular layer, and elongated in the longitudinal layer.

The arrangement of muscle fibres shows some variation from region to region. In the stomach an additional oblique layer is present. In the colon the longitudinal fibres are gathered to form prominent bundles called the *taenia coli*.

Localized thickenings of circular muscle fibres form *sphincters* that can occlude the lumen of the gut. For example, the *pyloric sphincter* is present around the pyloric end of the stomach, and the *internal anal sphincter* surround the anal canal. A functional sphincter is seen at the junction of the oesophagus with the stomach. A valvular arrangement at the ileocaecal junction (ileocaecal valve) prevents regurgitation of caecal contents into the ileum.

The Serous and Adventitial Layers

Covering the muscle coat, there is the serous layer. This layer is merely the visceral peritoneum that covers most parts of the gastro-intestinal tract. In some places where a peritoneal covering is absent (e.g., over part of the oesophagus) the muscle coat is covered by an adventitia made up of connective tissue.

Nerve Plexuses

The gut is richly supplied with nerves. A number of nerve plexuses are present as follows.

(a) The *myenteric plexus (of Auerbach)* lies between the circular and longitudinal coats of muscle.

(b) The *submucosal plexus (of Meissner)* lies in the submucosa (near its junction with the circular muscle layer).

(c) A third plexus is present near the muscularis mucosae.

The nerve fibres in these plexuses are both afferent and efferent. The efferent fibres supply smooth muscle and glands. Postganglionic neurons meant for these structures lie amongst the nerve fibres forming these plexuses.

THE OESOPHAGUS

The oesophagus is a tube, the wall of which has the usual four layers described on page 230 viz., mucous membrane, submucosa, muscle layer and an external adventitia. The oesophagus does not have a serous covering except over a short length near its lower end. Other points worth noting about the structure of the oesophagus are as follows (Fig. 15.2).

The Mucosa

1. The mucous membrane of the oesophagus shows several longitudinal folds that disappear when the tube is distended.

2. The mucosa is lined by stratified squamous epithelium, which is normally not keratinized.

> Occasional melanocytes and endocrine cells (page 247) are present. A columnar epithelium, similar to that lining the cardiac end of the stomach, may extend for some distance into the abdominal part of the oesophagus.

3. Finger like processes (or papillae) of the connective tissue of the lamina propria project into the epithelial layer (just like dermal papillae). This helps to prevent separation of epithelium from underlying connective tissue.

4. At the upper and lower ends of the oesophagus some tubulo-alveolar mucous glands are present in the lamina propria.

5. The muscularis mucosae is absent or poorly developed in the upper part of the oesophagus. It is distinct in the lower part of the oesophagus, and is thickest near the eosophagogastric junction. It consists chiefly of longitudinal muscular fibres, but a few circular fibres are also present.

The Submucosa

The only special feature of the submucosa is the presence at some places of compound tubulo-alveolar mucous glands. They are most frequently seen at the level of the bifurcation of the trachea. Small aggregations of lymphoid tissue may be present in the submucosa, specially near the lower end. Some plasma cells and macrophages are also present.

The Muscle Layer

The muscle layer consists of the usual circular and longitudinal layers. However, it is unusual

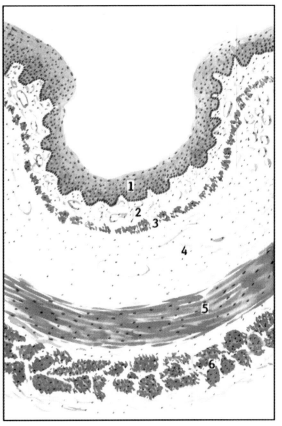

Fig. 15.2. Section through oesophagus. 1-Stratified squamous epithelium. 2-Lamina propria. 3-Muscularis mucosae. 4-Submucosa. 5-Circular muscle. 6- Longitudinal muscle.

in that the muscle fibres are partly striated and partly smooth. In the upper one third (or so) of the oesophagus the muscle fibres are entirely of the striated variety, while in the lower one third all the fibres are of the smooth variety Both types of fibres are present in the middle one third of the oesophagus.

The circular muscle fibres present at the lower end of the oesophagus could possibly act as a sphincter guarding the cardiooesophageal junction. However, the circular muscle is not thicker here than elsewhere in the oesophagus, and its role as a sphincter is not generally accepted. However, a *physiological sphincter* does appear to exist. The anatomical factors that could account for this sphincteric action are not agreed upon.

The muscle layer of the oesophagus is surrounded by a layer of dense fibrous tissue that forms an adventitial coat for the oesophagus. The lowest part of the oesophagus is intra-abdominal and has a covering of peritoneum.

THE STOMACH

The wall of the stomach has the four basic layers described on page 230: a mucous membrane, a submucosa, a muscularis externa, and a serous layer. The mucous membrane and the muscularis externa have some special features that are described below.

The Mucous Membrane

As seen with the naked eye the mucous membrane shows numerous folds (or *rugae*) that disappear when the stomach is distended.

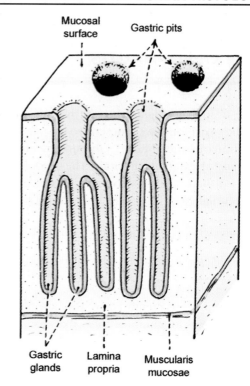

Fig. 15.3. Scheme to show the basic structure of the mucous membrane of the stomach.

Lining Epithelium

The lining epithelium is columnar and mucous secreting. The apical parts of the lining cells are filled by mucin which is usually removed during processing of tissues so that the cells look empty (or vacuolated). Mucous secreted by cells of the lining epithelium protects the gastric mucosa against acid and enzymes produced by the mucosa itself. [The mucous cells lining the surface are also believed to produce blood group factors].

At numerous places the lining epithelium dips into the lamina propria to form the walls of depressions called *gastric pits*. These pits extend for a variable distance into the thickness of the mucosa. Deep to the gastric pits the mucous membrane is packed with numerous *gastric glands*. These glands are of three types: main gastric, cardiac and pyloric.

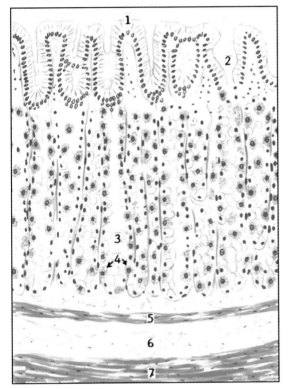

Fig. 15.4. Section through body of the stomach. 1-Lining by columnar epithelium. 2-Gastric pit. 3-Gastric glands. 4-Oxyntic cells. 5-Muscularis mucosae. 6-Submucosa. 7-Circular muscle.

The Main Gastric Glands

The main gastric glands are present over most of the stomach, but not in the pyloric region and in a small area near the cardiac end. In other words they are present in the body of the stomach, and in the fundus (Fig. 15.4). (Note that these glands are often inappropriately called fundic glands in many books of histology: they are not confined to the fundus).

The main gastric glands are simple or branched tubular glands that lie at right angles to the mucosal surface. The glands open into gastric pits, each pit receiving the openings of several glands. Here the gastric pits occupy the superficial one fourth or less of the mucosa, the remaining thickness being closely packed with gastric glands. The following varieties of cells are present in the epithelium lining the glands (Fig. 15.4).

(a) The most numerous cells are called *chief cells*, *peptic cells*, or *zymogen cells*. They are particularly numerous in the basal parts of the glands. The cells are cuboidal or low columnar. Their cytoplasm is basophilic. With special methods the chief cells are seen to contain prominent secretory granules in the apical parts of their cytoplasm. The granules contain pepsinogen which is a precursor of pepsin. With the EM the cytoplasm is seen to contain abundant rough endoplasmic reticulum and a prominent Golgi complex. The luminal surfaces of the cells bear small irregular microvilli.

Chief cells secrete the digestive enzymes of the stomach including pepsin. Pepsin is produced by action of gastric acid on pepsinogen. Pepsin breaks down proteins into small peptides. It is mainly through the action of pepsin that solid food is liquefied.

(b) The *oxyntic* or *parietal cells* are large, ovoid or polyhedral, with a large central nucleus.

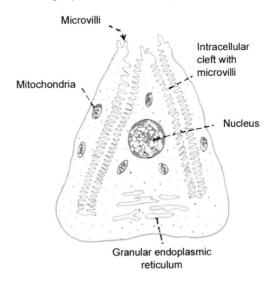

Fig. 15.5. Diagram to show some features of the EM structure of an oxyntic cell.

They are present singly, amongst the peptic cells. They are more numerous in the upper half of the gland than in its lower half. They are called oxyntic cells because they stain strongly with eosin. They are called parietal cells as they lie against the basement membrane, and often bulge outwards (into the lamina propria) creating a beaded appearance. With the light microscope they appear to be buried amongst the chief cells. The EM shows, however, that each parietal cell has a narrow apical part that reaches the lumen of the gland. The cell membrane of this apical region shows several invaginations into the cytoplasm, producing tortuous intracellular canaliculi that communicate with the glandular lumen. The walls of the canaliculi bear microvilli that project into the canaliculi. The cytoplasm (in the intervals between the canaliculi) is packed with mitochondria. The mitochondria are responsible for the granular appearance and eosinophilia of the cytoplasm (seen with the light microscope). Secretory granules are not present.

Oxyntic cells are responsible for the secretion of hydrochloric acid. They also produce an *intrinsic factor* (a glucoprotein) which combines with vitamin B12 (present in ingested food and constituting an *extrinsic factor*) to form a complex necessary for normal formation of erythrocytes.

(c) Near the upper end (or 'neck') of the glands there are mucous secreting cells that are called *mucous neck cells*. These are large cells with a clear cytoplasm. The nucleus is flattened and is pushed to the base of the cell by accumulated mucous. The supranuclear part of the cell contains prominent granules. The chemical structure of the mucous secreted by these cells is different from that secreted by mucous cells lining the surface of the gastric mucosa.

(d) Near the basal parts of the gastric glands there are *endocrine cells* that contain membrane bound neurosecretory granules. As

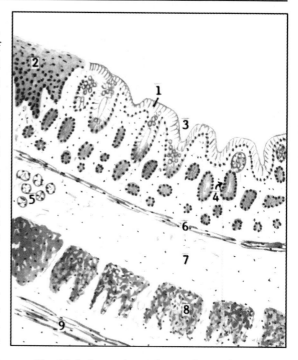

Fig. 15.6. Stomach, cardiac end. 1-Columnar epithelium. 2-Stratified squamus lining of lower end of oesophagus. 3-Gastric pit. 4-Cardiac gland. 5-Oesophageal gland. 6-Muscularis mucosae. 7-Submucosa. 8-Circular muscle. 9-Longitudinal muscle.

the granules stain with silver salts these have, in the past, been called *argentaffin cells.* These cells are flattened. They do not reach the lumen, but lie between the chief cells and the basement membrane. These cells probably secrete the hormone *gastrin*. Some of the cells can be shown to contain serotonin (5HT). For further details see page 236

(e) Some undifferentiated cells (stem cells) that multiply to replace other cells are also present. They increase in number when the gastric epithelium is damaged (for example when there is a gastric ulcer), and play an important role in healing.

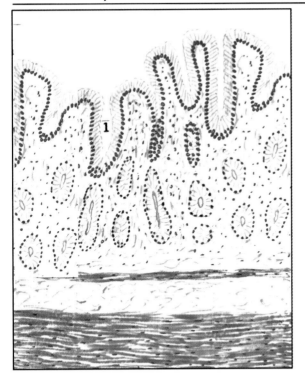

Fig. 15.7. Stomach, pyloric part. 1-Gastric pit. 2-Pyloric gland. 3-Muscularis mucosae. 4-Submucosa. 5. Circular muscle.

The Cardiac Glands

These are confined to a small area near the opening of the oesophagus. In this region the mucosa is relatively thin. Gastric pits are shallow (as in the body of the stomach). The cardiac glands are either simple tubular, or compound tubulo-alveolar (Fig. 15.6). They are mucous secreting. An occasional oxyntic or peptic cell may be present.

The Pyloric Glands

In the pyloric region of the stomach the gastric pits are deep and occupy two thirds of the depth of the mucosa. The pyloric glands which open into these pits are short and occupy the deeper one third of the mucosa. They are simple or branched tubular glands that are coiled. The glands are lined by mucous secreting cells (Fig. 15.7). Occasional oxyntic and argentaffin cells may be present. Some pyloric glands may pass through the muscularis mucosae to enter the submucosa. In addition to other substances, pyloric glands secrete the hormone gastrin.

The Lamina Propria

As seen above the mucous membrane of the stomach is packed with glands. The connective tissue of the lamina propria is, therefore, scanty. It contains the usual connective tissue cells. Occasional aggregations of lymphoid tissue are present in it.

The Muscularis Mucosae

The muscularis mucosae of the stomach is well developed. Apart from the usual circular (inner) and longitudinal (outer) layers an additional circular layer may be present outside the longitudinal layer.

The Muscularis Externa

The muscularis externa of the stomach is well developed. Three layers, oblique, circular and longitudinal (from inside out) are usually described. The appearance of the layers in sections is, however, highly variable depending upon the part of the stomach sectioned. The circular fibres are greatly thickened at the pylorus where they form the pyloric sphincter. There is no corresponding thickening at the cardiac end.

THE SMALL INTESTINE

The small intestine is a tube about five meters long. It is divided into three parts. These are (in craniocaudal sequence) the ***duodenum*** (about 25 cm long); the ***jejunum*** (about 2 meters long); and the ***ileum*** (about 3 meters long). [Gut length is shorter in the living person than in a cadaver, because of muscle tone].

The wall of the small intestine is made up of the four layers described on page 230: serous, muscular, submucous, and mucous. The serous and muscular layers correspond exactly to the description on page 232. The submucosa is also typical except in the duodenum, where it

contains the ***glands of Brunner*** (see page 233). The mucous membrane exhibits several special features that are described below.

The Mucous Membrane

The surface area of the mucous membrane of the small intestine is extensive (to allow adequate absorption of food). This is achieved by virtue of the following.

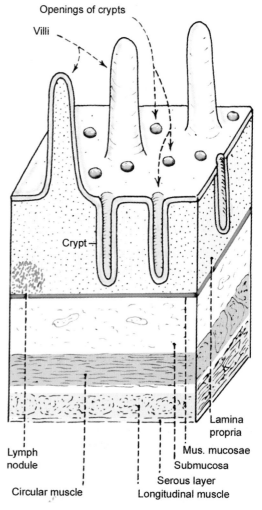

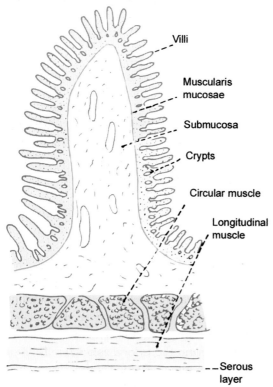

Fig. 15.8. Longitudinal section through a part of the small intestine seen at a very low magnification to show a mucosal fold.

Fig. 15.9. Scheme to show the basic structure of the small intestine.

(a) The considerable length of the intestine.

(b) The presence of numerous circular folds in the mucosa.

(c) The presence of numerous finger-like processes, or *villi*, that project from the surface of the mucosa into the lumen.

(d) The presence of numerous depressions or *crypts* that invade the lamina propria.

(e) The presence of microvilli on the luminal surfaces of the cells lining the mucosa.

Circular Folds

The circular folds are also called the *valves of Kerkring*. Each fold is made up of all layers of the mucosa (lining epithelium, lamina propria and muscularis mucosae). The submucosa also extends into the folds. The folds are large and readily seen with the naked eye. They are absent in the first one or two inches of the duodenum. They are prominent in the rest of the duodenum, and in the whole of the jejunum. The folds gradually become fewer and less marked in the ileum. The terminal parts of the ileum have no such folds.

Apart from adding considerably to the surface area of the mucous membrane, the circular folds tend to slow down the passage of contents through the small intestine thus facilitating absorption.

The Villi

The villi are, typically, finger like projections consisting of a core of reticular tissue covered by a surface epithelium (described below). The connective tissue core contains numerous blood capillaries forming a plexus. The endothelium lining the capillaries is fenestrated thus allowing rapid absorption of nutrients into the blood.

Each villus contains a central lymphatic vessel called a *lacteal*. Distally, the lacteal ends blindly near the tip of the villus; and proximally it ends in a plexus of lymphatic vessels present in the lamina propria. Occasionally, the lacteal may be double. Some muscle fibres derived from the muscularis mucosae extend into the villus core.

In some situations the villi, instead of being finger like, are flattened and leaf like, while in some other situations they are in the form of ridges. The villi are greatest and most numerous (for a given area) in the duodenum. They progressively decrease in size, and in number, in proceeding caudally along the small intestine. It has been estimated that the presence of villi increases the surface area of the epithelial lining of the small intestine about eight times. The cells lining the villi are described below.

The Crypts

The crypts (of Lieberkuhn) are tubular invaginations of the epithelium into the lamina propria. They are really simple tubular *intestinal glands* that are lined by epithelium. The epithelium is supported on the outside by a basement membrane. The cells lining the crypts are considered below.

The Epithelial Lining

The epithelium covering the villi, and areas of the mucosal surface intervening between them, consists predominantly of columnar cells that are specialized for absorption. These are called *enterocytes*. Scattered amongst the columnar cells there are mucous secreting goblet cells. The crypts (intestinal glands) are lined mainly by undifferentiated cells that multiply to give rise to absorptive columnar cells and to goblet cells. Near the bases of the crypts there are *Paneth cells* that secrete enzymes. Endocrine cells

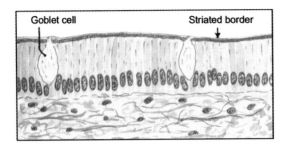

Fig. 15.10. Columnar epithelium lining the small intestine. Note the striated border and some goblet cells.

(bearing membrane bound granules filled with various neuroactive peptides) are also present. The various cells mentioned above are briefly described below.

Absorptive Columnar Cells

The general characteristics of columnar epithelium have been described on page 44. This description applies to the columnar cells lining the mucous membrane of the small intestine. Each cell has an oval nucleus located in its lower part. When seen with the light microscope the luminal surface of the cell appears to be thickened and to have striations in it, perpendicular to the surface (Fig. 15.10). With the EM this *striated border* is seen to be produced by microvilli arranged in a very regular manner (page 24). The presence of microvilli greatly increases the absorptive surface of the cell.

Each microvillus has a wall of plasma membrane within which there are fine filaments. These filaments are continuous with a plexus of similar filaments present in the apical part of the cell and is called the *terminal web*. The surface of each microvillus is covered by a layer of fine fibrils and mucous (*glycocalyx*).

The plasma membrane on the lateral sides of absorptive cells shows folds that interdigitate with those of adjoining cells. Adjacent cells are united by typical junctional complexes (page 13) and by scattered desmosomes. Intercellular canals may

be present between adjacent cells. The cytoplasm of absorptive cells contains the usual organelles, including lysosomes and smooth ER. These cells are responsible for absorption of amino acids, carbohydrates, and lipids present in digested food.

Goblet Cells

[A goblet is literally a drinking glass which is broad above, and has a narrow stem attached to a base. Goblet cells are so named because of a similar shape].

Each goblet cell has an expanded upper part that is distended with mucin granules (Fig. 15.10). The nucleus is flattened and is situated near the base of the cell. Goblet cells are mucous secreting cells. In consonance with their

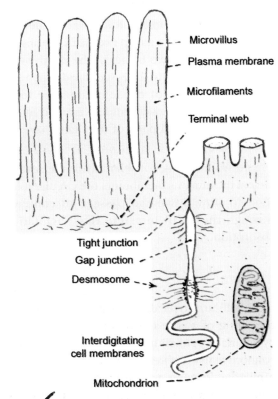

Fig. 15.11. Apical parts of two absorptive cells of the small intestine to show microvilli and the junctional complex uniting the two cells.

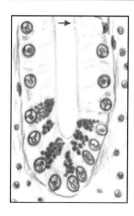

Fig. 15.12. High power view of an intestinal crypt showing Paneth cells with red staining supranuclear granules.

secretory function these cells have a well developed Golgi complex and abundant rough endoplasmic reticulum. The luminal surface of the cell bears some irregular microvilli. In haematoxylin and eosin stained preparations, the mucin content of goblet cells appears to be unstained. It stains brightly with the PAS technique. Mucous cells increase in number as we pass down the small intestine, being few in the duodenum and most numerous in the terminal ileum.

Undifferentiated Cells

These are columnar cells present in the walls of intestinal crypts. They are similar to absorptive cells, but their microvilli and terminal webs are not so well developed. The cytoplasm contains secretory granules.

Undifferentiated cells proliferate actively by mitosis. The newly formed cells migrate upwards from the crypt to reach the walls of villi. Here they differentiate either into typical absorptive cells, or into goblet cells. These cells migrate towards the tips of the villi where they are shed off. In this way, the epithelial lining is being constantly replaced, each cell having a life of only a few days. The term *intermediate cells* has been applied to differentiating stem cells that show features intermediate between those of stem cells and fully differentiated cells.

Zymogen Cells (Paneth Cells)

These cells are found only in the deeper parts of intestinal crypts. They contain prominent eosinophilic secretory granules (Fig. 15.12). With the EM Paneth cells are seen to contain considerable rough endoplasmic reticulum. Other organelles and some irregular microvilli are present. The cells are rich in zinc.

The function of zymogen cells is not well known. They are known to produce lysozyme which destroys bacteria. They may also produce other enzymes.

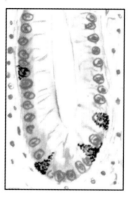

Fig. 15.13. High power view of intestinal crypt showing argentaffin cell with black staining granules that are mostly infranuclear.

Endocrine Cells

Cells containing membrane bound vesicles filled with neuroactive substances are present in the epithelial lining of the small intestine. They are most numerous near the lower ends of crypts. As the granules in them stain with silver salts these cells have, in the past, been termed argentaffin cells (Fig. 15.13). Some of them also give a positive chromaffin reaction. They are, therefore, also called *enterochromaffin cells*. With the introduction of immunohistochemical techniques it has now been demonstrated that these cells are of various functional types, and contain many amines having an endocrine function. These are consider further on page 247.

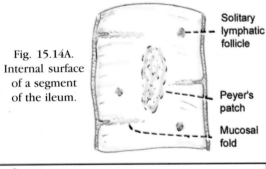

Fig. 15.14A.
Internal surface
of a segment
of the ileum.

Solitary
lymphatic
follicle

Peyer's
patch

Mucosal
fold

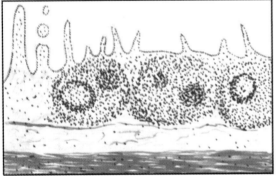

Fig. 15.14B. Terminal ileum showing an aggregated lymphatic follicle (Peyer's patch)
in the submucosa.

Lymphoid Tissue of the Small Intestine

Solitary and aggregated lymphatic follicles
(Peyer's patches) are present in the lamina
propria of the small intestine. They have been
described on page 191. The solitary follicles
become more numerous, and the aggregated
follicles larger, in proceeding caudally along the
small intestine. They are most prominent in the
terminal ileum (Fig. 15.14 A, B). Their lymphoid
tissue may occasionally extend into the
submucosa. Villi are few or missing in the mucosa
overlying aggregated follicles.

The epithelium overlying lymphatic follicles
contains special *follicle-associated epithelial
cells* or *M-cells* (M for 'microfold' or
'membrane'). These cells are columnar. They are
believed to take up antigens present in the lumen
of the intestine and to transport them to
subjacent lymphoid tissue, which can then
produce antibodies against the antigens. The
lateral borders of these cells are deeply indented
by small lymphocytes (lying within the thickness
of the epithelium).

Other Cells in the Lamina Propria

Apart from connective tissue associated
fibroblasts, and lymphocytes (mentioned above)
the lamina propria of the small intestine contains
eosinophil leucocytes, macrophages, and mast
cells. Plasma cells are present in relation to
aggregations of lymphoid tissue.

Distinguishing Features of Duodenum, Jejunum, & Ileum

1. Sections through the small intestine are
readily distinguished from those of other parts
of the gut because of the presence of villi.

2. The duodenum is easily distinguished from
the jejunum or ileum because of the presence in
it of glands in the submucosa. (No glands are
present in the submucosa of the jejunum or
ileum). These *duodenal glands* (of Brunner)
are compound tubulo-alveolar glands (Fig.
15.15). Their ducts pass through the muscularis
mucosae to open into the intestinal crypts (of
Lieberkuhn). The alveoli of the duodenal glands
are lined predominantly by mucous secreting
columnar cells having flattened basal nuclei.
Some endocrine cells are also present. The
duodenal glands are most numerous in the
proximal part of the duodenum. They are few
(or missing) in the distal part. The secretions of
the duodenal glands contain mucous,
bicarbonate ions (to neutralize gastric acid
entering the duodenum) and an enzyme that
activates trypsinogen produced by the pancreas.

3. The proximal part of the jejunum shows
significant differences in structure from the
terminal part of the ileum. The changes take

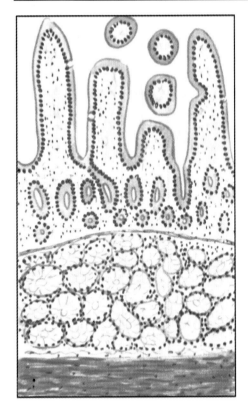

Fig. 15.15. Duodenum. Note that the submucosa is packed with mucous secreting glands (of Brunner).

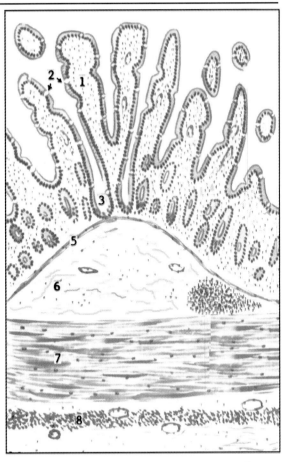

Fig. 15.16. Jejunum. 1-Villus. 2-Goblet cells. 3-Crypt. 5- Muscularis mucosae. 6-Submucosa. Note the solitary lymphatic nodule seen towards the right side. 7-Circular muscle. 8. Longitudinal muscle.

place gradually in proceeding caudally along the small intestine, there being no hard and fast line of distinction between the jejunum and the ileum. As compared to the ileum the jejunum has the following features (Fig. 15.16).

(**a**) A larger diameter.

(**b**) A thicker wall.

(**c**) Larger and more numerous circular folds.

(**d**) Larger villi.

(**e**) Fewer solitary lymphatic follicles. Aggreated lymphatic follicles are absent in the proximal jejunum, and small in the distal jejunum.

(**f**) Greater vascularity.

THE LARGE INTESTINE

The Colon

The structure of the colon conforms to the general description of the structure of the gut given on page 230. The following additional points may be noted (Fig. 15.17B).

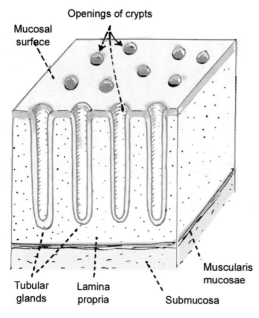

Fig. 15.17A. Scheme to show the basic features of the structure of the mucous membrane of the large intestine.

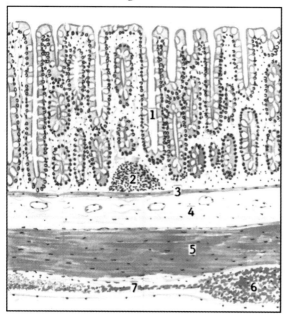

Fig. 15.17B. Section through a part of the large intestine. 1-Crypt. 2-Lymphatic nodule. 3-Muscularis mucosae. 4-Submucosa. 5-Muscle coat. 6-Taenia coli. 7-Longitudinal muscle.

The mucous membrane of the colon shows numerous crescent-shaped folds. There are no villi. The mucosa shows numerous closely arranged tubular glands or crypts similar to those in the small intestine. The mucosal surface, and the glands, are lined by an epithelium made up predominantly of columnar cells with a striated border. Their main function is to absorb excess water and electrolytes from intestinal contents. Many columnar cells secrete mucous and antibodies (IgA). The antibodies provide protection against pathogenic organisms. Numerous goblet cells are present, their number increasing in proceeding caudally. The mucous secreted by them serves as a lubricant that facilitates the passage of semisolid contents through the colon. Paneth cells are not present. Some endocrine cells, and some stem cells, are seen.

The epithelium overlying solitary lymphatic follicles (present in the lamina propria) contains M-cells similar to those described in the small intestine. Scattered cells bearing tufts of long microvilli are also seen. They are probably sensory cells.

The submucosa often contains fat cells. Some cells that contain PAS-positive granules, termed *muciphages*, are also present. These are most numerous in the rectum.

The longitudinal layer of muscle is unusual. Most of the fibres in it are collected to form three thick bands, the *taenia coli*. A thin layer of longitudinal fibres is present in the intervals between the taenia. The taenia are shorter in length than other layers of the wall of the colon. This results in the production of *sacculations* (also called *haustrations*) on the wall of the colon.

The serous layer is missing over the posterior aspect of the ascending and descending colon. In many situations the peritoneum forms small pouch-like processes that are filled with fat. These yellow masses are called the ***appendices epiploicae***.

The Vermiform Appendix

The structure of the vermiform appendix resembles that of the colon (described above) with the following differences (Fig. 15.19).

1. The appendix is the narrowest part of the gut.

2. The crypts are poorly formed.

3. The longitudinal muscle coat is complete and equally thick all round. Taenia coli are not present.

4. The submucosa contains abundant lymphoid tissue which may completely fill the submucosa. The lymphoid tissue is not present at birth. It gradually increases and is best seen in children about 10 year old. Subsequently, there is progressive reduction in quantity of lymphoid tissue.

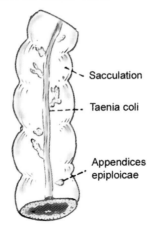

Fig. 15.18. Diagram to show a segment of the colon.

The Rectum

The structure of the rectum is similar to that of the colon except for the following.

1. A continuous coat of longitudinal muscle is present and there are no taenia.

2. Peritoneum covers the front and sides of the upper one-third of the rectum; and only the front of the middle third. The rest of the rectum is devoid of a serous covering.

3. There are no appendices epiploicae.

The Anal Canal

The anal canal is about 4 cm long. The upper 3 cm are lined by mucous membrane, and the lower 1 cm by skin. The area lined by mucous membrane can be further divided into an upper part (15 mm) and a lower part (15 mm).

The mucous membrane of the upper 15 mm of the canal is lined by columnar epithelium. The mucous membrane of this part shows six to twelve longitudinal folds that are called the ***anal***

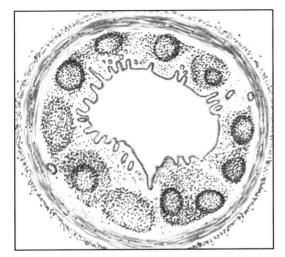

Fig. 15.19. Vermiform appendix. Note the lymphatic nodules filling the submucosa almost completely.

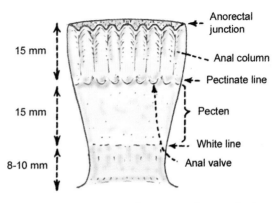

Fig. 15.20. Diagram to show some features in the interior of the anal canal.

		15.21. Different types of endocrine cells in the gut and in the pancreas			
Cell type	Secretory products	Distribution (+ = present)			
		Stomach	Small intestine	Large intestine	Pancreas
D_1	Vasoactive intestinal polypeptide	+	+	+	+
D	Somatostatin	+	+	+	+
EC_1	5HT + Substance P		+	+	
L	Enteroglucagon		+	+	
G	Gastric encephalin	+	+		
EC_2	5HT + Motilin		+		
S	Secretin		+		
I	Cholecystokinin pancreozymin		+		
K	Gastric inhibitory peptide		+		
N	Neurokinin		+		
ECn	5HT + unknown	+			
B	Insulin				+
A	Glucagon	?	?		+
PP	Pancreatic polypeptide		?		+

columns. The lower ends of the anal columns are united to each other by short transverse folds called the *anal valves*. The anal valves together form a transverse line that runs all round the anal canal: this is the *pectinate line*. The mucous membrane of the next 15 mm of the rectum is lined by nonkeratinized stratified squamous epithelium. This region does not have anal columns. The mucosa has a bluish appearance because of the presence of a dense venous plexus between it an the muscle coat. This region is called the *pecten* or *transitional zone*. The lower limit of the pecten forms the *white line* (*of Hilton*).

The lowest 8 to 10 mm of the anal canal are lined by true skin in which hair follicles, sebaceous glands and sweat glands are present.

Above each anal valve there is a depression called the *anal sinus*. Atypical (apocrine) sweat glands open into each sinus. They are called the *anal (or circumanal) glands*.

The anal canal is surrounded by circular and longitudinal layers of muscle continuous with those of the rectum. The circular muscle is thickened to form the *internal anal sphincter*. Outside the layer of smooth muscle, there is the *external anal sphincter* which is made up of striated muscle. For further details of the anal musculature see a book on gross anatomy.

Prominent venous plexuses are present in the submucosa of the anal canal. The internal haemorrhoidal plexus lies above the level of the pectinate line, while the external haemorrhoidal plexus lies near the lower end of the canal.

THE ENDOCRINE CELLS OF THE GUT

The lining epithelium of the stomach, and of the small and large intestines, contains scattered cells that have an endocrine function. These were recognized by early workers because of the presence, in them, of infranuclear granules that blackened with silver salts. They were, therefore, termed *argentaffin* cells. The granules also show a positive chromaffin reaction and have, therefore, also been called *enterochromaffin* cells. More recently, by the use of immunohistochemical methods, several other biologically active substances (amines or polypeptides) have been located in these cells. Many of these substances are also found in the nervous system where they function as neurotransmitters. They also act as hormones. This action is either local on neighbouring cells (paracrine effect); or on cells at distant sites (through the blood stream). Very similar cells are also to be seen in the pancreas. All these cells are now grouped together under the term *gastro-entero-pancreatic endocrine system*. Some of the cell types recognized, and their secretory products are given in the Table 15.11.

Some features of this system are similar to those of amine producing cells in other organs. All these are included under the term APUD cell system which is considered in Chapter 20.

16

The Liver and Pancreas

THE LIVER

Introductory Remarks

The liver may be regarded as a modified exocrine gland that also has other functions. It is made up, predominantly, of liver cells or **hepatocytes**. Each hepatocyte is a large cell with a round open faced nucleus, with prominent nucleoli (Figs. 16.1 to 16.3).

The liver substance is divisible into a large number of large lobes, each of which consists of numerous lobules. The exocrine secretion of the liver cells is called **bile**. Bile is poured out from liver cells into very delicate **bile canaliculi** that are present in intimate relationship to the cells (Fig. 16.3). From the canaliculi bile drains into progressively larger ducts which end in the **bile duct**. This duct conveys bile into the duodenum where bile plays a role in digestion of fat.

All blood draining from the stomach and intestines (and containing absorbed food materials) reaches the liver through the portal vein and its branches. Within the liver this blood passes through sinusoids and comes into very intimate relationship with liver cells. The liver is

thus able to 'screen' all substances entering the body through the gut. Some of them (e.g., amino acids) are used for synthesis of new proteins needed by the body. Others (e.g., glucose, lipids) are stored in liver cells for subsequent use; while harmful substances (e.g., drugs, alcohol) are

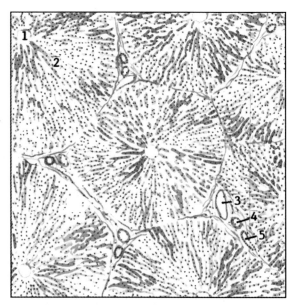

Fig. 16.1. Section through liver (low power view). 1-Central vein. 2-Liver cells arranged as radiating cords or plates that form hexagonal lobules.. 3-Branch of portal vein. 4- Branch of hepatic artery. 5-Interlobular duct. 3, 4 and 5 form a portal triad.

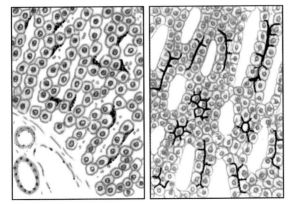

Figs. 16.2   Fig. 16.3

These are high power views of parts of the liver. In Fig. 16.2. note cords of cells separated by sinusoids. Phagocytic cells (of Kupffer) (containing dark injested material) are seen scattered along the walls of sinusoids. In Fig. 16.3. Note the bile capillaries (black) intervening between liver cells.

Basic Histology of the Liver

In sections through the liver, the substance of the organ appears to be made up of hexagonal areas that constitute the **hepatic lobules** (Figs. 16.1 to 16.3). In some species (e.g., the pig) the lobules are distinctly demarcated by connective tissue septa, but in the human liver the connective tissue is scanty and the lobules often appear to merge with one another. In transverse sections each lobule appears to be made up of cords of liver cells that are separated by sinusoids. However, the cells are really arranged in the form of plates (one cell thick) that branch and anastomose with one another to form a network. Spaces within the network are occupied by sinusoids.

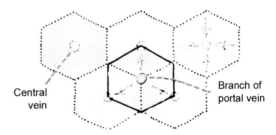

Central vein   Branch of portal vein

Fig. 16.4. Scheme to show the concept of portal lobules (pink). Hepatic lobules are shaded green. Note that the portal lobule is made up of parts of three hepatic lobules.

detoxified. The need for intimate contact between blood in the sinusoids, and liver cells, thus becomes obvious. The portal vein also brings blood from the spleen to the liver. This blood contains high concentrations of products formed by breakdown of erythrocytes in the spleen. Some of these products (e.g., bilirubin) are excreted in bile, while some (e.g., iron) are stored for re-use in new erythrocytes.

In addition to deoxygenated blood reaching the liver through the portal vein, the organ also receives oxygenated blood through the **hepatic artery** and its branches. The blood entering the liver from both these sources passes through the hepatic sinusoids and is collected by tributaries of hepatic veins. One such tributary runs through the centre of each lobule of the liver where it is called the **central vein** (see below).

Branches of the hepatic artery, the portal vein, and the hepatic ducts, travel together through the liver. The tributaries of hepatic veins follow a separate course as described below.

Along the periphery of each lobule there are angular intervals filled by connective tissue. These intervals are called **portal canals**, the 'canals' forming a connective tissue network permeating the entire liver substance. Each 'canal' contains (a) a branch of the portal vein; (b) a branch of the hepatic artery, and (c) an interlobular bile duct. These three structures collectively form a **portal triad**. Blood from the branch of the portal vein, and from the branch of the hepatic artery, enters the sinusoids at the periphery of the lobule and passes towards its centre. Here the sinusoids open into a **central vein** which occupies the centre of the lobule. We have already seen that

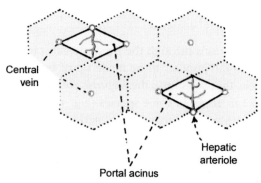

Fig. 16.5. Scheme to show the concept of portal acini (pink). Compare with Fig. 16.4.

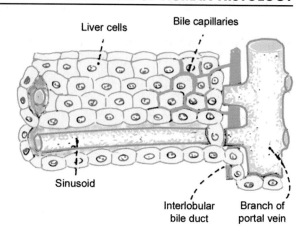

Fig. 16.6. Diagram to show relationship of bile capillaries to liver cells.

the central vein drains into hepatic veins (which leave the liver to end in the inferior vena cava).

The vessels in a portal triad usually give branches to parts of three adjoining lobules. The area of liver tissue (comprising parts of three hepatic lobules) supplied by one branch of the portal vein is regarded by many authorities as the true functional unit of liver tissue, and is referred to as a *portal lobule* (in distinction to a hepatic lobule described above). A still smaller unit, the *portal acinus* has also been described. It consists of the area of liver tissue supplied by one hepatic arteriole (Fig.16.5) running along the line of junction of two hepatic lobules. Two central veins lie at the ends of the acinus.

The liver is covered by a connective tissue *capsule* (Glisson's capsule). This connective tissue extends into the liver substance through the portal canals (mentioned above) where it surrounds the portal triads. Sinusoids are surrounded by reticular fibres. Connective tissue does not intervene between adjoining liver cells.

Bile is secreted by liver cells into *bile canaliculi*. These canaliculi have no walls of their own. They are merely spaces present between plasma membranes of adjacent liver cells. The canaliculi form hexagonal networks around the liver cells. At the periphery of a lobule the canaliculi become continuous with delicate *intralobular ductules*, which in turn become

continuous with larger *interlobular ductules* of portal triads. The interlobular ductules are lined by cuboidal epithelium. Some smooth muscle is present in the walls of larger ducts.

Further Details of Liver Structure

1. The cytoplasm of liver cells contains numerous mitochondria, abundant rough and smooth endoplasmic reticulum, a well developed Golgi complex, lysosomes, and vacuoles containing various enzymes. Numerous free ribosomes are present. These features are to be correlated with the high metabolic activity of liver cells. Stored glycogen, lipids, and iron (as crystals of ferratin and haemosidrin) are usually present. Glycogen is often present in relation to smooth ER. Many hepatocytes show two nuclei; or a single polyploid nucleus.

2. Although the liver performs numerous functions all liver cells look alike. Each cell is probably capable of performing all functions. However, the cells at the periphery of a lobule receive more highly oxygenated blood than those nearer the centre of the lobule. Functional differences exist between hepatocytes in these regions.

3. We have seen that liver cells are arranged

in the form of anastomosing plates, one cell thick; and that the plates form a network in the spaces of which sinusoids lie. In this way each liver cell has a sinusoid on two sides. The sinusoids are lined by an endothelium in which there are numerous pores (fenestrae). A basement membrane is not seen. Interspersed amongst the endothelial cells there are hepatic macrophages (**Kupffer cells**). The surface of the liver cell is separated from the endothelial lining of the sinusoid by a narrow **perisinusoidal space** (of Disse). Microvilli, present on the liver cells, extend into this space. As a result of these factors hepatocytes are brought into a very intimate

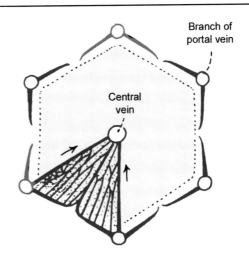

Fig. 16.8. Scheme to show the presence of several branches of the portal vein around a hepatic lobule. The manner in which they open into sinusoids is shown. The intervals between the sinusoids are occupied by liver cells.

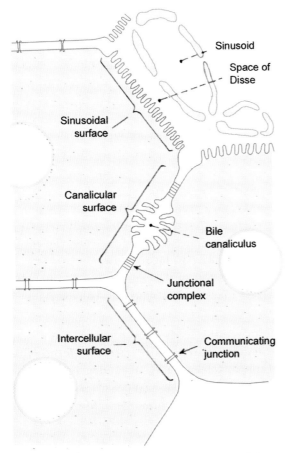

Fig. 16.7. Three functional specializations of the cell surface of a hepatocyte.

relationship with the circulating blood. Some fat cells may also be seen in the space of Disse.

4. Blood vessels and hepatic ducts present in portal canals are surrounded by a narrow interval called the **space of Mall**.

5. The surface of a hepatocyte can show three kinds of specialization.

(a) **Sinusoidal surface**: As mentioned above the cell surface adjoining sinusoids bears microvilli that project into the space of Disse. The cell surface here also shows many coated pits (see page 8) which are concerned with exocytosis. Both these features are to be associated with active transfer of materials from sinusoids to hepatocytes, and **vice versa**. About 70% of the surface of hepatocytes is of this type.

(b) **Canalicular surface**: Such areas of cell membrane bear longitudinal depressions that are apposed to similar depressions on neighbouring hepatocytes, to form the wall of a bile canaliculus. Irregular microvilli project into the canaliculus. On either side of the canaliculus, the two cell membranes are united by junctional complexes (page 13). About 15% of the hepatocyte surface is canalicular.

(c) *Intercellular surface*: These are areas of cell surface where adjacent hepatocytes are united to each other just as in typical cells. Communicating junctions allow exchanges between the cells. About 15% of the hepatocyte surface is intercellular.

Functions of the Liver

The liver performs numerous functions. Some of these are as follows.

1. We have seen that the liver acts as an exocrine gland for the secretion of bile. However, the architecture of the liver has greater resemblance to that of an endocrine gland, the cells being in intimate relationship to blood in sinusoids. This is to be correlated with the fact that liver cells take up numerous substances from the blood, and also pour many substances back into it.

2. The liver plays a prominent role in metabolism of carbohydrates, proteins and fats. Metabolic functions include synthesis of plasma proteins fibrinogen and prothrombin, and the regulation of blood glucose and lipids.

3. The liver acts as a store for various substances including glucose (as glycogen), lipids, vitamins and iron. When necessary the liver can convert lipids and amino acids into glucose (*gluconeogenesis*).

4. The liver plays a protective role by detoxifying substances (including drugs and alcohol). Removal of bile pigments from blood (and their excretion through bile) is part of this process. Amino acids are deaminated to produce urea, which enters the blood stream to be excreted through the kidneys. The macrophage cells (of Kupffer) lining the sinusoids of the liver have a role similar to that of other cells of the mononuclear phagocyte system (page 86). They are of particular importance as they are the first cells of this system that come in contact with materials absorbed through the gut. They also remove damaged erythrocytes from blood.

5. During fetal life the liver is a centre for haemopoiesis.

Some Disorders of the Liver

1. Inflammation in the liver is called hepatitis. It is frequently caused by viruses (*viral hepatitis*), and by a protozoan parasite *entamoeba histolytica* (*amoebic hepatitis*). An abscess may form in the liver as a sequel of amoebic hepatitis.

2. Cirrhosis of the liver is a disease in which many hepatocytes are destroyed, the areas being filled by fibrous tissue. This gradually leads to collapse of the normal architecture of the liver.

3. One effect of cirrhosis of the liver is to disrupt the flow of blood through the liver. As a result of increased resistance to blood flow there is increased blood pressure in the portal circulation (*portal hypertension*). In portal hypertension anastomoses between the portal and systemic veins dilate to form varices (e.g., at the lower end of the oesophagus). Rupture of these varices can result in fatal bleeding.

4. When a large number of hepatocytes are destroyed this leads to liver failure. The various functions (listed above) are interfered with. Hepatic failure may be acute or chronic. Accumulation of waste products in blood (due to lack of detoxification by the liver) ultimately leads to unconsciousness (*hepatic coma*) and death.

EXTRAHEPATIC BILIARY APPARATUS

The extrahepatic biliary apparatus consists of the gall bladder and the extrahepatic bile ducts.

The Gall Bladder

The gall bladder stores and concentrates bile. This bile is discharged into the duodenum when required. The wall of the gall bladder is made up of a mucous membrane, a fibromuscular coat, and a serous layer that covers part of the organ.

The mucous membrane of the gall bladder is lined by a tall columnar epithelium with a striated border. The mucosa is highly folded. The folds are called *rugae*. In sections, the folds may look like villi. [Because of this resemblance to villi students sometimes mistake sections of the gall bladder for those of the intestines. The two are easily distinguished if it is remembered that

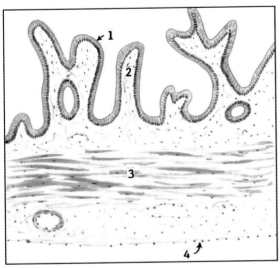

Fig. 16.9. Gall bladder. 1- Mucous membrane lined by columnar epithelium. 2-Mucosal fold. 3-Muscle coat. 4-Serous layer (peritoneum) lined by flattened mesothelium.

there are no goblet cells in the epithelium of the gall bladder]. The folds may branch and anastomose with one another to give a reticular appearance.

The fibromuscular coat is made up mainly of connective tissue containing the usual elements. Smooth muscle fibres are present and run in various directions.

The serous layer has a lining of mesothelium resting on connective tissue.

With the EM the lining cells of the gall bladder are seen to have irregular microvilli on their luminal surfaces. Near the lumen the lateral margins of the cells are united by well developed junctional complexes. More basally the lateral margins are separated by enlarged intercellular spaces into which complex folds of plasma membrane extend. Numerous blood capillaries are present near the bases of the cells. These features indicate that bile is concentrated by absorption of water at the luminal surface of the cell. This water is poured out of the cell into basal intercellular spaces from where it passes into blood. Absorption of salt and water from bile into blood is facilitated by presence of Na^+ and K^+ ATPases in cell membranes of cells lining the gall bladder.

Inflammation of the gall bladder is called *cholecystitis*. Stones may form in the gall bladder (*gall stones*; *cholelithiasis*). In such cases surgical removal of the gall bladder may be necessary (*cholecystectomy*).

The Extrahepatic Ducts

These are the right, left and common hepatic ducts; the cystic duct; and the bile duct. All of them have a common structure. They have a mucosa surrounded by a wall made up of connective tissue, in which some smooth muscle may be present.

The mucosa is lined by a tall columnar epithelium with a striated border.

At its lower end the bile duct is joined by the main pancreatic duct, the two usually forming a common **hepato-pancreatic duct** (or **ampulla**) which opens into the duodenum at the summit of the major duodenal papilla. The mucosa of the hepato-pancreatic duct is highly folded. These folds are believed to constitute a valvular mechanism that prevents duodenal contents from entering the bile and pancreatic ducts.

Well developed smooth muscle is present in the region of the lower end of the bile duct. This muscle forms the **sphincter of Oddi**. From a functional point of view this sphincter consists of three separate parts. The **sphincter choledochus** surrounds the lower end of the bile duct. It is always present, and its contraction is responsible for filling of the gall bladder. A less developed **sphincter pancreaticus** surrounds the terminal part of the main pancreatic duct. A third sphincter surrounds the

hepato-pancreatic duct (or ampulla) and often forms a ring round the lower ends of both the bile and pancreatic ducts. This is the **sphincter ampullae**. The sphincter ampullae and the sphincter pancreaticus are often missing.

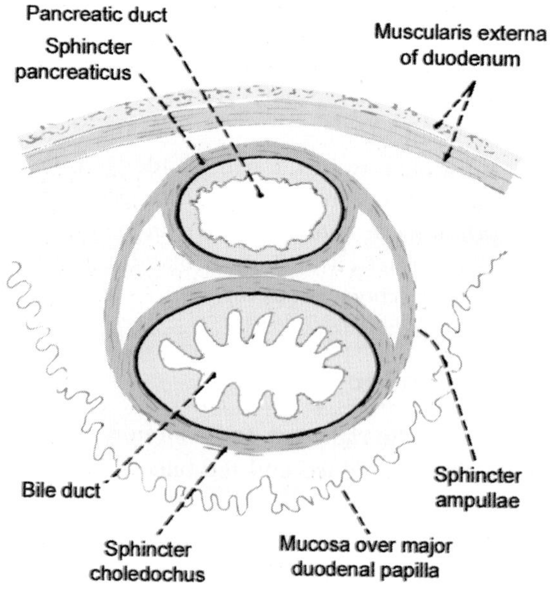

Blockage of the bile duct (by inflammation, by a gall stone, or by carcinoma) leads to accumulation of bile in the biliary duct system, and within the bile capillaries. As pressure in the passages increases bile passes into blood leading to **jaundice**. The sclera, the skin, and the nails appear to be yellow in colour, and bile salts and pigments are excreted in urine. Jaundice occurring as a result of such obstruction is called **obstructive jaundice**. Jaundice is seen in the absence of obstruction in cases of hepatitis.

A gall stone passing through the bile duct can cause severe pain. This pain is **biliary colic**.

THE PANCREAS

Introductory Remarks

The pancreas is a gland that is partly exocrine, and partly endocrine, the main bulk of the gland being constituted by its exocrine part (Fig. 16.11). The exocrine pancreas secretes enzymes that play a very important role in the digestion of carbohydrates, proteins and fats. We have seen that after digestion, and absorption through the gut, these products are carried to the liver through the portal vein. The endocrine part of the pancreas produces two very important hormones, **insulin** and **glucagon**. These two hormones are also carried through the portal vein to the liver where they have a profound influence on the metabolism of carbohydrates, proteins and fats. The functions of the exocrine and endocrine parts of the pancreas are thus linked. The linkage

Fig. 16.10. Section through the major duodenal papilla to show the components of the sphincter of Oddi.

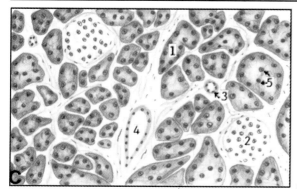

Fig. 16.11. Pancreas. 1-Serous acini. 2-Pancreatic islet. 3-Intralobular duct. 4-Interlobular duct.

between the two parts is also seen in their common embryonic derivation from the endodermal lining of the gut.

The Exocrine Part

The exocrine part of the pancreas is in the form of a serous, compound tubulo-alveolar gland. [Its general structure is very similar to that of the parotid gland, but the two are easily distinguished because of the presence in the pancreas of endocrine elements described below].

The pancreas is surrounded by a delicate capsule. Septa extend from the capsule into the gland and divide it into lobules.

The secretory elements of the exocrine pancreas are long and tubular (but they are usually described as alveoli as they appear rounded or oval in sections). Their lumen is small. The lining cells appear triangular in section, and have spherical nuclei located basally. In sections stained with haematoxylin and eosin the cytoplasm is highly basophilic (blue) specially in the basal part. With suitable fixation and staining numerous secretory (or zymogen) granules can be demonstrated in the cytoplasm, specially in the apical part of the cell. These granules are eosinophilic. They decrease considerably after the cell has poured out its secretion.

With the EM the cells lining the alveoli show features that are typical of secretory cells. Their basal cytoplasm is packed with rough endoplasmic reticulum (this being responsible for the basophilia of this region). A well developed Golgi complex is present in the supranuclear part of the cell. Numerous secretory granules (membrane bound, and filled with enzymes) occupy the greater part of the cytoplasm (except the most basal part).

The secretory cells produce two types of secretion.

(1) One of these is watery and rich in bicarbonate. Bicarbonate is probably added to pancreatic secretion by cells lining the ducts. It helps to neutralise the acid contents entering the duodenum from the stomach. Production of this secretion is stimulated mainly by the hormone *secretin* liberated by the duodenal mucosa.

(2) The other secretion is thicker and contains numerous enzymes (including trypsinogen, chymotrypsinogen, amylase, lipases etc.). The production of this secretion is stimulated mainly by the hormone cholecystokinin (pancreozymin) liberated by endocrine cells in the duodenal mucosa.

Secretion by cells of the exocrine pancreas, and the composition of the secretion, is influenced by several other amines produced either in the gastrointestinal mucosa or in pancreatic islets. (These include gastrin, vasoactive intestinal polypeptide, and pancreatic polypeptide). Secretion is also influenced by autonomic nerves, mainly parasympathetic.

The enzymes are synthesized in the rough endoplasmic reticulum. From here they pass to the Golgi complex where they are surrounded by membranes, and are released into the cytoplasm as secretory granules. The granules move to the luminal surface of the cell where the secretions are poured out by exocytosis. Within the cell the enzymes are in an inactive form. They become active only after mixing with duodenal contents. Activation is influenced by enzymes present in the epithelium lining the duodenum.

In addition to secretory cells, the alveoli of the exocrine pancreas contain *centroacinar cells* that are so called because they appear to be located near the centre of the acinus (or alveolus). These cells really belong to the intercalated ducts (see below) which are invaginated into the secretory elements. Some cell bodies of autonomic neurons, and undifferentiated cells are also present in relation to the secretory elements.

Secretions produced in the alveoli are poured into *intercalated ducts* (also called *intralobular ducts*). These ducts are invaginated deeply into the secretory elements. As a result of this invagination the ducts are not conspicuous in sections. (Contrast this with the parotid in which the intralobular ducts are easily seen: compare Figs.16.11 with 14.8). From the intercalated ducts the secretions pass into larger, *interlobular ducts*. They finally pass into the duodenum through the *main pancreatic duct* and the *accessory pancreatic duct.* The cells lining the pancreatic ducts control the bicarbonate and water content of pancreatic secretion. These actions are under hormonal and neural control. The walls of the larger ducts are formed mainly of fibrous tissue. They are lined by a columnar epithelium.

The terminal part of the main pancreatic duct is surrounded by a sphincter (Fig. 16.10). A similar sphincter may also be present around the terminal part of the accessory pancreatic duct.

The Endocrine Part

The endocrine part of the pancreas is in the form of numerous rounded collections of cells that are embedded within the exocrine part. These collections of cells are called the *pancreatic islets*, or the *islets of Langerhans* (Fig. 16.12). The human pancreas has about one million islets. They are most numerous in the

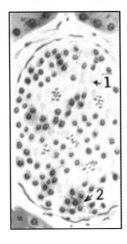

Fig. 16.12. Pancreatic islet. 1-Alpha cells. 2-Beta cells. 3-Capillary.

tail of the pancreas.

Each islet is separated from the surrounding alveoli by a thin layer of reticular tissue. The islets are very richly supplied with blood through a dense capillary plexus. The intervals between the capillaries are occupied by cells arranged in groups or as cords. In ordinary preparations stained with haematoxylin and eosin, all the cells appear similar, but with the use of special procedures three main types of cells can be distinguished as follows.

(a) The *alpha cells* (or *A-cells*) secrete the hormone *glucagon*. They form about 20% of the islet cells.

(b) The *beta cells* (or *B-cells*) secrete the hormone *insulin*. About 70% of the cells are of this type.

(c) The *delta cells* (or *D-cells*) probably produce the hormones *gastrin* and *somatostatin*. Somatostatin inhibits the secretion of glucagon by alpha cells, and (to a lesser extent) that of insulin by beta cells.

In islets of the human pancreas the alpha cells tend to be arranged towards the periphery (or *cortex*) of the islets. In contrast the beta cells tend to lie near the centre (or *medulla*) of the islet. Delta cells are also peripherally placed.

The beta cells contain granules that can be stained with aldehyde fuchsin. The alpha cells contain smaller granules that stain brightly with acid fuchsin. They do not stain with aldehyde fuchsin.

The delta cells (also called type III cells) stain black with silver salts (i.e., they are argyrophile). They resemble alpha cells in having granules that stain with acid fuchsin; and are, therefore, sometimes called A1 cells in distinction to the glucagon producing cells that are designated A2. The two can be distinguished by the fact that A2 cells are not argyrophile.

With the EM the granules of islet cells are seen to be membrane bound. The granules of alpha cells (A2) are round or ovoid with high electron density, while those of delta cells (A1) are of low electron density. The granules of beta cells are fewer, larger, and of less electron density than those of alpha cells.

Apart from the three main types of cells described above some other types are also present. These are the PP cells containing pancreatic polypeptide (and located mainly in the head and neck of the pancreas), and D1 cells (or type IV cells) probably containing vasoactive intestinal polypeptide (or a similar amine). A few cells secreting serotonin, motilin and substance P are also present (page 246). As described on page 247 the cells of pancreatic islets belong to the gastro-entero-pancreatic endocrine system. Pancreatic islets are richly innervated by autonomic nerves.

Noradrenalin and acetyl choline released at nerve endings influence secretion by islet cells.

Some islet cell tumours secrete gastrin, but this substance has not been demonstrated in the normal pancreas.

Connective Tissue Basis, Blood Vessels, and Nerves of the Pancreas

The pancreas is covered by connective tissue that forms a capsule for it. Septa arising from the capsule extend into the gland dividing it into lobules. Each pancreatic islet is surrounded by a network of reticular fibres.

The gland is richly supplied with blood vessels that run through the connective tissue. The capillary network is most dense in the islets. Here the endothelial lining is fenestrated providing intimate contact of islet cells and circulating blood.

The connective tissue also serves as a pathway for nerve fibres, both myelinated and unmyelinated. Groups of neurons are also present.

Lymphatics are present in the pancreas.

The urinary organs are the right and left kidneys and ureters, the urinary bladder and the urethra. These organs are responsible for the production, storage, and passing of urine, Many harmful waste products (that result from metabolism) are removed from blood through urine. These include urea and creatinine which are end products of protein metabolism.

Many drugs, or their breakdown products, are also excreted in urine. In diseased conditions urine can contain glucose (as in diabetes mellitus), or proteins (in kidney disease), the excretion of which is normally prevented. Considerable amount of water is excreted through urine. The quantity is strictly controlled being greatest when there is heavy intake of water, and least when intake is low or when there is substantial water loss in some other way (for example by perspiration in hot weather). This enables the water content of plasma and tissues to remain fairly constant.

Urine production, and the control of its composition, is done exclusively by the kidneys. The urinary bladder is responsible for storage of urine until it is voided. The ureter and urethra are simple passages for transport of urine.

THE KIDNEYS : BASIC STRUCTURE

Some features of the kidney that can be seen by naked eye

Each kidney has a characteristic bean-like shape. It has a convex lateral margin; and a concavity on the medial side which is called the *hilum*. The hilum leads into a space called the *renal sinus*. The renal sinus is occupied by the upper expanded part of the ureter which is miscalled the *renal pelvis*. Within the renal sinus the pelvis divides into two (or three) parts called *major calyces*. Each major calyx divides into a number of *minor calyces*. The end of each minor calyx is shaped like a cup. A projection of kidney tissue, called a *papilla* fits into the cup.

Some features of the internal structure of the kidney can be seen when we examine a coronal section through the organ (Fig.17.1). Kidney tissue consists of an outer part called the *cortex*, and an inner part called the *medulla*.

The medulla is made up of triangular areas of

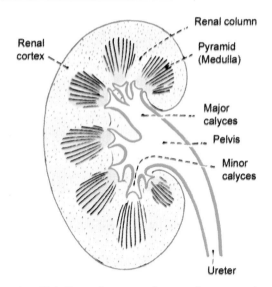

Fig. 17.1. Some features to be seen in a coronal section through the kidney.

The Uriniferous Tubules

From a functional point of view the kidney may be regarded as a collection of numerous *uriniferous tubules* that are specialized for the excretion of urine. Each uriniferous tubule consists of an excretory part called the *nephron*, and of a *collecting tubule*. The collecting tubules draining different nephrons join to form larger tubules called the *papillary ducts* (of Bellini), each of which opens into a minor calyx at the apex of a renal papilla. Each kidney contains one to two million nephrons.

Urinary tubules are held together by scanty connective tissue. Blood vessels, lymphatics and nerves lie in this connective tissue.

Parts of the Nephron

The nephron consists of a *renal corpuscle* (or *Malpighian corpuscle*), and a long complicated *renal tubule*. The renal corpuscle is a rounded structure consisting of (a) a rounded tuft of blood capillaries called the *glomerulus*; and (b) a cup-like, double layered covering for the glomerulus called the *glomerular capsule* (or *Bowman's capsule*). The glomerular capsule represents the cup-shaped blind beginning of the renal tubule. Between the two layers of the capsule there is a *urinary space* which is continuous with the lumen of the renal tubule.

The renal tubule is divisible into several parts that are shown in Fig. 17.3. Starting from the glomerular capsule there are: (a) the *proximal convoluted tubule*; (b) the *loop of Henle* consisting of a *descending limb*, a *loop*, and an *ascending limb*; and (c) the *distal convoluted tubule*, which ends by joining a collecting tubule.

Renal corpuscles, and (the greater parts of) the proximal and distal convoluted tubules are located in the cortex of the kidney. The loops of

renal tissue that are called the *renal pyramids*. Each pyramid has a base directed towards the cortex; and an apex (or papilla) which is directed towards the renal pelvis, and fits into a minor calyx. Pyramids show striations that pass radially towards the apex.

The renal cortex consists of the following:

(a) Tissue lying between the bases of the pyramids and the surface of the kidney, forming the *cortical arches* or *cortical lobules*. This part of the cortex shows light and dark striations. The light lines are called *medullary rays*.

(b) Tissue lying between adjacent pyramids is also a part of the cortex. This part constitutes the *renal columns*.

(c) In this way each pyramid is surrounded by a 'shell' of cortex. The pyramid and the cortex around it constitutes a lobe of the kidney. This lobulation is obvious in the fetal kidney.

Kidney tissue is intimately covered by a thin layer of fibrous tissue which is called the *capsule*. The capsule of a healthy kidney can be easily stripped off, but it becomes adherent in some diseases.

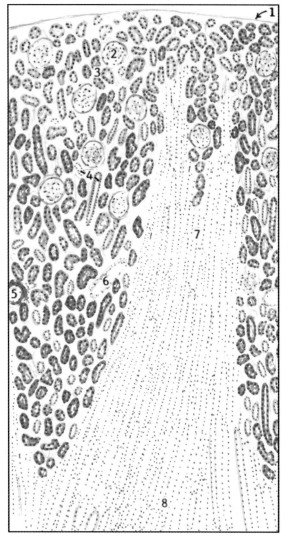

Fig. 17.2. Kidney (low power view). 1-Capsule,
2-Renal corpuscle. 3-Proximal convoluted tubule.
4-Distal convoluted tubule. 5-Artery. 6-Vein.
7-Medullary ray. 8-Collecting duct.

Henle and the collecting ducts lie in the
medullary rays and in the substance of the
pyramids.

The Renal Corpuscle

We have seen that the glomerulus is a rounded
tuft of anastomosing capillaries (Figs. 17.2,

17.4)). Blood enters the tuft through an afferent
arteriole and leaves it through an efferent
arteriole. (Note that the efferent vessel is an
arteriole, and not a venule. It again breaks up
into capillaries as described on page 263). The
afferent and efferent arterioles lie close together
at a point that is referred to as the ***vascular pole***
of the renal corpuscle.

We have seen that the glomerular capsule is a
double layered cup, the two layers of which are
separated by the urinary space. The outer layer
is lined by squamous cells. With the light
microscope the inner wall also appears to be
lined by squamous cells, but the EM shows that
these cells, called ***podocytes***, have a highly
specialized structure (page 265). The urinary
space becomes continuous with the lumen of the

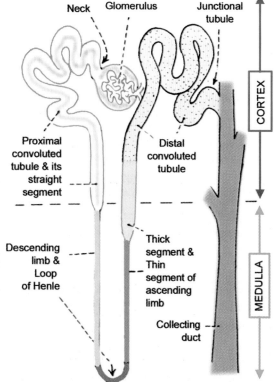

Fig. 17.3. Parts of a nephron. A collecting duct
is also shown.

renal tubule at the **urinary pole** of the renal corpuscle. This pole lies diametrically opposite the vascular pole.

The Renal Tubule

We have seen that the renal tubule is made up (in proximo-distal sequence) of the proximal convoluted tubule, the loop of Henle, and the distal convoluted tubule. The distal convoluted tubule ends by opening into a collecting tubule.

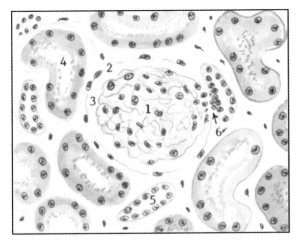

Fig. 17.4. Renal cortex (high power view).
1-Glomerulus. 2-Urinary space. 3-Proximal convoluted tubule. 5-Distal convoluted tubule. 6-Macula densa.

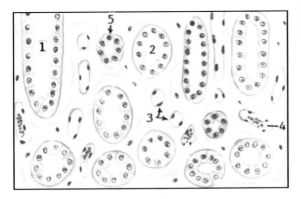

Fig. 17.5. Renal medulla (high power view).
1, 2-Collecting duct (L.S & T.S). 3, 5-Loop of Henle (thin and thick segments). 4-Capillary.

The following additional details may be noted.

(**a**) The junction of the proximal convoluted tubule with the glomerular capsule is narrow and is referred to as the **neck**.

(**b**) The proximal convoluted tubule is made up of an initial part having many convolutions (lying in the cortex), and of a terminal straight part that descends into the medulla to become continuous with the descending limb of the loop of Henle.

(**c**) The descending limb, the loop itself, and part of the ascending limb of the loop of Henle are narrow and thin walled. They constitute the **thin segment** of the loop. The upper part of the ascending limb has a larger diameter and thicker wall and is called the **thick segment**. (See below for some departures from this terminology).

(**d**) The distal convoluted tubule has a straight part continuous with the ascending limb of the loop of Henle, and a convoluted part lying in the cortex. At the junction between the two parts, the distal tubule lies very close to the renal corpuscle of the nephron to which it belongs. The terminal part of the distal convoluted tubule is again straight. This part is called the **junctional tubule** or **connecting tubule**, and ends by joining a collecting duct.

Students may be confused by somewhat different terminology used in some books. The straight part of the proximal convoluted tubule is sometimes described as part of the loop of Henle, and is termed the **descending thick segment**, in distinction to the (ascending) thick segment. Some workers regard the thin segment alone to be the loop of Henle. They include the descending and ascending thick segments with the proximal and distal convoluted tubules respectively.

A short **zigzag tubule** (or **irregular tubule**) may lie between the distal convoluted tubule and the junctional tubule. The glomerular capsule (described here as part of the renal corpuscle) is sometimes described as part of the renal tubule.

Epithelium Lining the Renal Tubule

Along its entire length the renal tubule is lined by a single layer of epithelial cells that are supported on a basal lamina. The features of the lining cells, as seen with the light microscope in different parts of the renal tubule, are described below.

The **neck** is lined by simple squamous epithelium continuous with that of the glomerular capsule. (Some texts refer to the neck as part of the glomerulus).

The **proximal convoluted tubules** are 40-60 µm in diameter. They have a relatively small lumen. They are lined by cuboidal (or columnar) cells having a prominent brush border. The nuclei are central and euchromatic. The cytoplasm stains pink (with haematoxylin and eosin). The basal part of the cell shows a vertical striation. (For EM structure see page 255).

The thin segment of the loop of Henle is about 15-30 µm in diameter. It is lined by low cuboidal or squamous cells. The thick segment of the loop is lined by cuboidal cells.

The distal convoluted tubules are 20-50 µm in diameter. They can be distinguished (in sections) from the proximal tubules as (a) they have a much larger lumen; (b) the cuboidal cells lining them do not have a brush border; and (c) they stain less intensely pink (with eosin).

The smallest collecting tubules are 40-50 µm in diameter, and the largest as much as 200 µm. They are lined by a simple cuboidal or columnar epithelium. Collecting tubules can be easily distinguished from convoluted tubules as follows.

(a) Collecting tubules have larger lumina. In transverse sections their profiles are circular in contrast to the irregular shapes of convoluted tubules.

(b) The lining cells have clear, lightly staining

cytoplasm, and the cell outlines are usually distinct. They do not have a brush border.

Renal Blood Vessels

A knowledge of some features of the arrangement of blood vessels within the kidney is essential to the understanding of renal function.

At the hilum of the kidney each renal artery

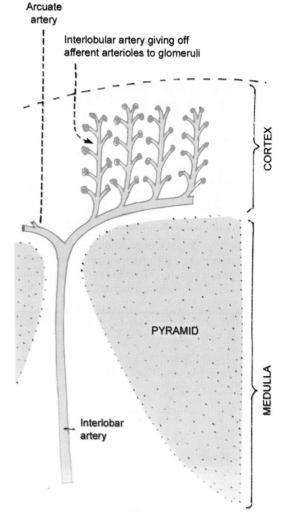

Fig. 17.6. Scheme to show the arrangement of arteries within the kidney.

divides into a number of *lobar arteries* (one for each pyramid). Each lobar artery divides into two (or more) *interlobar arteries* that enter the tissue of the renal columns and run towards the surface of the kidney. Reaching the level of the bases of the pyramids, the interlobar arteries divide into *arcuate arteries*. The arcuate arteries run at right angles to the parent interlobar arteries.

They lie parallel to the renal surface at the junction of the pyramid and the cortex. They give off a series of *interlobular arteries* that run through the cortex at right angles to the renal surface to end in a subcapsular plexus. Each

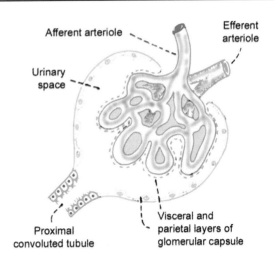

Fig. 17.8. Scheme to show the basic structure of a renal corpuscle.

interlobular artery gives off a series of arterioles that enter glomeruli as *afferent arterioles*.

Blood from these arterioles circulates through gomerular capillaries which join to form *efferent arterioles* that emerge from glomeruli.

The behaviour of efferent arterioles leaving the glomeruli differs in the case of glomeruli located more superficially in the cortex, and those lying near the pyramids. Efferent arterioles arising from the majority of glomeruli (superficial) divide into capillaries that surround the proximal and distal convoluted tubules. These capillaries drain into *interlobular veins*, and through them into *arcuate veins* and *interlobar veins*. Efferent arterioles arising from glomeruli nearer the medulla (*juxtamedullary glomeruli*) divide into 12 to 25 straight vessels that descend into the medulla. These are the *descending vasa recta*. Side branches arising from the vasa recta join a capillary plexus that surrounds the descending and ascending limbs of the loop of Henle (and also the collecting tubules). The capillary plexus consists predominantly of vessels running longitudinally along the tubules. It is drained by *ascending vasa recta* that run upwards parallel to the descending vasa recta to

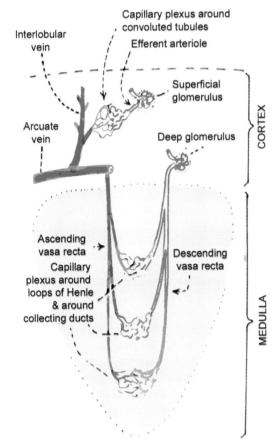

Fig. 17.7. Scheme to show behaviour of efferent arterioles of glomeruli in the superficial and deeper parts of the renal cortex.

reach the cortex. Here they drain into interlobular or arcuate veins. The parallel orientation of the ascending and descending vasa recta and their close relationship to the ascending and descending limbs of the loops of Henle is of considerable physiological importance (page 257).

From this account of the renal blood vessels it will be clear that two sets of arterioles and capillaries intervene between the renal artery and vein. The first capillary system, present in glomeruli, is concerned exclusively with the removal of waste products from blood. It does not supply oxygen to renal tissues. Exchanges of gases (oxygen, carbon dioxide) between blood and renal tissue is entirely through the second capillary system (present around tubules).

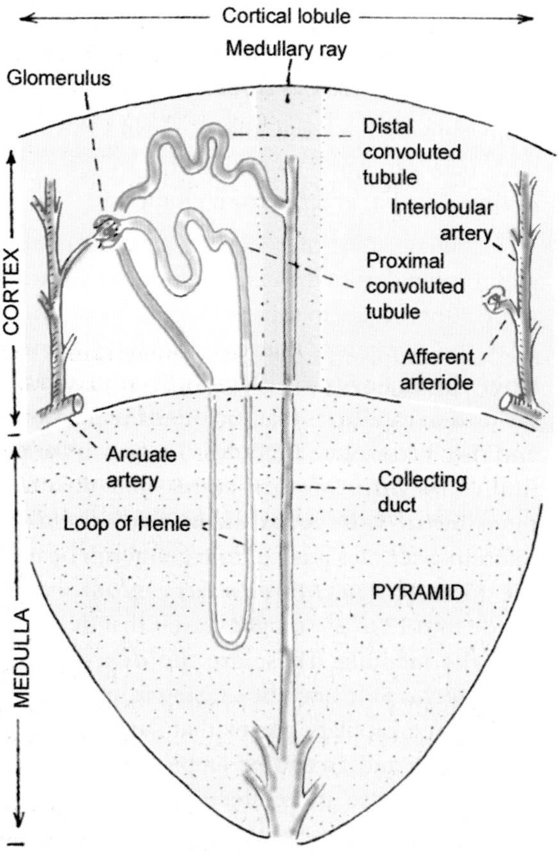

It has been said that in most tissues the blood supply exists to provide service to the parenchyma (in the form of the supply of oxygen and nutrients, and the removal of carbon dioxide and other waste products). In the kidney, on the other hand, the parenchyma exists to provide service to blood (by removal of waste products in it).

It has also been held that interlobular arteries divide the renal cortex into small lobules. Each lobule is defined as the region of cortex lying between two adjacent interlobular arteries. A medullary ray, containing a collecting duct, runs vertically through the middle of the lobule (midway between the two arteries) (Fig. 17.9). Glomeruli lie in a zone adjacent to the arteries while other parts of the nephron lie nearer the centre of the lobule.

Fig. 17.9. Scheme to illustrate the concept of cortical lobules.

FURTHER DETAILS OF RENAL STRUCTURE

Further details about the Renal Corpuscle

Glomerular Filtration Barrier

A preliminary description of the renal corpuscle has been given on page 260. In the renal corpuscle water and various small molecules pass, by filtration, from blood (in the glomerular capillaries) to the urinary space of the glomerular capsule. Theoretically the barrier across which the filtration would have to occur is constituted by (a) the capillary endothelium, (b) by the cells (podocytes) forming the glomerular (or visceral) layer of the glomerular capsule, and (c) by a *glomerular basement membrane* which intervenes between the two layers of cells named above, and represents the fused basal laminae of

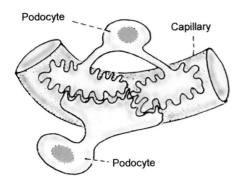

Fig. 17.10. Diagram showing relationship of podocytes to a glomerular capillary. Note that the entire surface of the capillary is covered by processes of podocytes, the bare areas being shown only for sake of clarity.

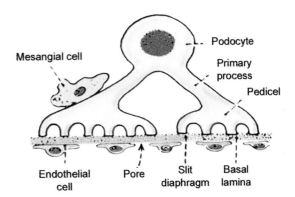

Fig. 17.11. Scheme to show filtration slits.

the two layers. In fact, however, the barrier is modified as follows.

(1) Firstly, the endothelial cells show numerous fenestrae or pores that are larger than pores in many other situations. The fenestrae are not closed by membrane. As a result filtrate passes easily through the pores, and the endothelial cells do not form an effective barrier.

(2) The *podocytes* are so called because they possess foot-like processes. Each podocyte has a few *primary processes* that give the cell a star shaped appearance. These processes are wrapped around glomerular capillaries and interdigitate with those of neighbouring podocytes. Each primary process terminates in numerous *secondary processes* also called *pedicels* (or end feet) which rest on the basal lamina. The cell body of the podocyte comes in contact with the basal lamina only through the pedicels. Between the areas of attachment of individual pedicels there are gaps in which the basal lamina is not covered by podocyte cytoplasm. Filtration takes place through the basal lamina at these gaps which are, therefore, called *filtration slits* or *slit pores*. These slits are covered by a layer of fine filaments that constitute the *glomerular slit diaphragm*. From what has been said above it will be clear that the filtrate does not have to pass through podocyte cytoplasm.

It follows, therefore, that the only real barrier across which filtration occurs is the basal lamina (or the glomerular basement membrane) which is thickened at the filtration slits by the glomerular slit diaphragm. The efficacy of the barrier is greatly enhanced by the presence of a high negative charge in the basement membrane and in podocyte processes. [Loss of this charge, in some diseases, leads to excessive leakage of protein through the barrier].

Glomerular Basement Membrane

As compared to typical membranes the glomerular basement membrane is very thick (about 300 nm). It is made up of three layers. There is a central electron dense layer (*lamina densa*), and inner and outer electron lucent layers (*lamina rara interna* and *externa*). The lamina densa contains a network of collagen (type IV) fibrils, and thus acts as a physical barrier. The electron lucent layers contain the glycosaminoglycan heparan sulphate. This bears the negative charges referred to above. The glomerular basement membrane is, therefore, both a physical barrier and an electrical barrier to the passage of large molecules.

As shown in Fig. 17.12 the glomerular basement membrane (and overlying podocyte cytoplasm) does not go all round a glomerular capillary. The gap is filled in by mesangium described below. A thin membrane continuous with the lamina rara

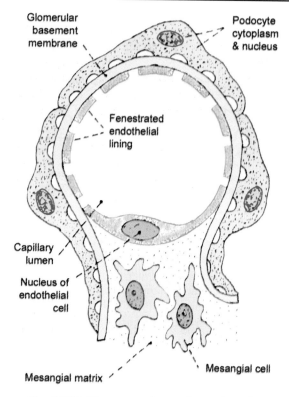

Fig. 17.12. Diagram to show relationship of a glomerular capillary to podocytes, basement membrane and mesangium.

interna may separate endothelial cytoplasm from mesangium. Also note that in the interval between capillaries the basement membrane is in contact with mesangium.

Defects in the glomerular basement membrane are responsible for the nephrotic syndrome in which large amounts of protein are lost through urine. The regular arrangement of podocyte processes is also disorganized in this condition.

The Mesangium

On entering the glomerulus the afferent arteriole divides (usually) into five branches, each branch leading into an independent capillary network. The glomerular circulation can, therefore, be divided into a number of lobules or segments.

Glomerular capillaries are supported by the *mesangium* which is made up of mesangial cells surrounded by a non-cellular mesangial matrix. The mesangium forms a mesentery like fold over the capillary loop. (In Fig. 17.12. note the similarity of mesangium to the mesentery of the small intestine). Mesangial cells give off processes that run through the matrix. Mesangium intervenes between the capillaries of the glomerular segments (mentioned above).

Mesangial cells contain filaments similar to myosin. They bear angiotensin II receptors. It is believed that stimulation by angiotensin causes the fibrils to contract. In this way mesangial cells may play a role in controlling blood flow through the glomerulus. Other functions attributed to mesangial cells include phagocytosis, and maintenance of glomerular basement membrane. The mesangium becomes prominent in a disease called glomerulonephritis.

Further details about the Renal Tubule

With the EM the lining cells of the proximal convoluted tubules show microvilli on their luminal surfaces. The striae, seen with the light microscope near the base of each cell, are shown by EM to be produced by infoldings of the basal plasma membrane, and by numerous mitochondria that lie longitudinally in the cytoplasm intervening between the folds. The presence of microvilli, and of the basal infoldings greatly increases the surface area available for transport. Adjacent cells show some lateral interdigitations. Numerous enzymes associated with ionic transport are present in the cytoplasm.

The loop of Henle is also called the *ansa nephroni*. With the EM the flat cells lining the thin segment of the loop of Henle show very few organelles indicating that the cells play only a passive role in ionic movements across them. In some areas the lining epithelium may show short microvilli, and some basal and lateral infoldings.

The length of the thin segment of the loop of Henle is variable. The loops of nephrons having

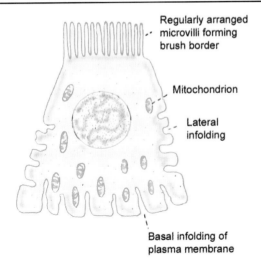

Regularly arranged microvilli forming brush border

Mitochondrion

Lateral infolding

Basal infolding of plasma membrane

Fig. 17.13. Some features of the ultrastructure of a cell lining a proximal convoluted tubule.

glomeruli lying deep in the cortex (juxtamedullary glomeruli) pass deep into the medulla. Those associated with glomeruli lying in the middle of the cortical thickness extend into the medulla to a lesser degree, so that part of the loop of Henle lies in the cortex. Some loops (associated with glomeruli placed in the superficial part of the cortex) may lie entirely within the cortex.

The structure of the (ascending) thick segment of the loop of Henle is similar to that of distal convoluted tubules. The cells of the distal convoluted tubules resemble those of the proximal convoluted tubules with the following differences.

(a) They have only a few small microvilli.

(b) The basal infoldings of plasma membrane are very prominent and reach almost to the luminal surface of the cell. This feature is characteristic of cells involved in the active transport of ions. Enzymes concerned with active transport of ions are present in the cells. At the junction of the straight and convoluted parts of the distal convoluted tubules, the cells show specializations that are described below in connection with the juxta-glomerular apparatus.

The walls of collecting tubules (in the proximal part of the collecting system) are lined by two types

of cells. The majority of cells (called *clear cells*) have very few organelles, a few microvilli and some basal infoldings. The lining epithelium also contains some *dark cells* (or *intercalated cells*). These bear microvilli, but no basal infoldings are seen. They contain numerous mitochondria.

The cells of the collecting ducts do not have microvilli, or lateral infoldings of plasma membrane. Very few organelles are present in the cytoplasm.

Correlation of Structure and Function of the Nephron

We have seen that water and various other molecules pass from blood into the urinary space of the glomerular capsule by a process of filtration. It has been emphasized that the process is greatly facilitated by the presence of fenestrae in the endothelial cells, and by the presence of filtration slits between the pedicels of podocytes.

As the filtrate passes through the renal tubule it undergoes considerable modification by selective absorption of substances that the body needs to retain. Some cells of the tubules also secrete certain substances into the tubules. The

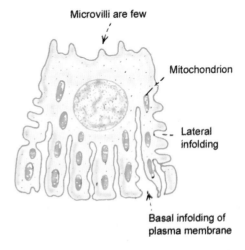

Microvilli are few

Mitochondrion

Lateral infolding

Basal infolding of plasma membrane

Fig. 17.14. Some features of ultrastructure of a cell lining a distal convoluted tubule.

ultimate composition of urine leaving the kidneys depends upon these three processes of filtration, reabsorption, and secretion.

Role of Proximal Convoluted Tubules

These tubules play a vital role in selective reabsorption of many substances from the glomerular filtrate. The substances reabsorbed include water, glucose, amino acids, proteins of small molecular size, and various ions including sodium, chloride, phosphate, bicarbonate and calcium. Reabsorption is facilitated by the presence of microvilli and foldings of the lateral and basal plasma membranes. Energy for the process is provided by the numerous mitochondria present.

Role of Loop of Henle (thin segment)

The main role of the loop of Henle is to create a hypertonic environment in the medulla. This environment plays a very important part in reabsorption of large quantities of water by collecting ducts. The hypertonic environment is created as follows.

(a) The spaces surrounding the descending and ascending limbs of the loops of Henle are surrounded by a fluid which is hypertonic. The hypertonicity is achieved by active transport of chloride and sodium ions out of the ascending limbs of the loops, into the surrounding space, but flow of water is not allowed. (This is the *countercurrent multiplier system*. For details consult a book on Physiology). The result is that filtrate leaving the loop of Henle is hypotonic.

(b) Normally, blood flowing through the medulla of the kidney would remove the ions, present in excess, from the intertubular space, to neutralise hypertonicity. However, this does not happen because of the fact that ions taken up by blood into ascending vasa recta diffuse into the descending vasa recta. This diffusion occurs because the former vessels contain a higher concentration of ions. (This is the *counter-current exchange* system). This diffusion is facilitated by the close approximation of the ascending and descending vasa recta.

Role of Distal Convoluted Tubules

(a) Like the proximal convoluted tubules, the distal tubules are involved in selective reabsorption of ions (chiefly sodium and bicarbonate).

(b) The tubules secrete hydrogen ions into the filtrate. This, combined with the reabsorption of bicarbonate, makes the urine acidic. This process is controlled by aldosterone (produced in the adrenal cortex).

(c) We have seen that filtrate entering the distal convoluted tubules (from the loop of Henle) is hypotonic. Selective absorption of sodium ions makes it even more hypotonic. This hypotonicity creates an osmotic gradient that forces water out of tubules into interstitial tissue, and from there into blood. This is possible as the distal tubules are permeable to water. Permeability is controlled by the antidiuretic hormone (ADH) (produced by the pars posterior of the hypophysis cerebri).

The absorption of water from the filtrate as described above, would be expected to make the filtrate hypertonic. However, this does not happen as absorption of water is accompanied by selective absorption of sodium and chloride by cells of the ascending limb of the loop of Henle and the distal convoluted tubule. As a result the filtrate entering the collecting ducts is in fact hypotonic.

The proximal and distal convoluted tubules add various substances to the glomerular filtrate. These include hydrogen ions (that make the urine acid), ammonia, creatinine and para-amino-hippuric acid. Various drugs, or their breakdown products, are also excreted in this way.

Role of Collecting Ducts

The collecting tubules and ducts play a very important role is final concentration of urine. As the filtrate passes through the collecting ducts, it once more enters the hypertonic environment of the medulla. This hypertonic environment, combined with the high permeability of the collecting ducts to water, forces water out of the ducts (into the interstitial space, and from there into blood). This renders the urine hypertonic by the time it is poured into the renal pelvis. However, the permeability of the collecting ducts is variable and is controlled by antidiuretic hormone (ADH). This hormone can thus regulate the dilution of urine depending upon functional requirements. Absence or deficiency of ADH is marked by excretion of very large volumes of dilute urine (*diabetes insipidus*).

The efficacy of the mechanism for resorption of water from the glomerular filtrate is shown by the fact that the filtrate is reduced from an original volume of about 200 litres a day to an average urine output of 1.5 litres per day.

Juxtaglomerular Apparatus

We have seen that a part of the distal convoluted tubule (at the junction of its straight and convoluted parts) lies close to the vascular pole of the renal corpuscle, between the afferent and efferent arterioles. In this region the muscle cells in the wall of the afferent arteriole are modified. They are large and rounded (epitheloid) and have spherical nuclei. Their cytoplasm contains granules that can be stained with special methods. These are *juxtaglomerular cells*. They are innervated by unmyelinated adrenergic nerve fibres. Juxta medullary cells are regarded, by some, as highly modified myoepithelial cells as they contain contractile filaments in the cytoplasm.

The wall of the distal convoluted tubule is also modified at the site of contact with the arteriole. Here the cells lining it are densely packed together, and are columnar (rather than cuboidal as in the rest of the tubule). These cells form the *macula densa* (Fig. 17.4). The cells of the

macula densa lie in close contact with the juxtaglomerular cells, the two together forming the *juxtaglomerular apparatus* or complex.

The granules of the juxtaglomerular cells are seen by EM to be membrane bound secretory granules. They contain an enzyme called *renin*. Renin acts on a substance called *angiotensinogen* present in blood and converts it into *angiotensin I*. Another enzyme (present mainly in the lungs) converts angiotensin I into *angiotensin II*. Angiotensin II increases blood pressure. It also stimulates the secretion of aldosterone by the adrenal cortex, thus influencing the reabsorption of sodium ions by the distal convoluted tubules, and that of water through the collecting ducts.

In addition to the renin producing cells, and the macula densa, the juxtaglomerular apparatus has a third component: these are *lacis cells*. These cells are so called as they bear processes that form a lace like network. They are located in the interval between the macula densa and the afferent and efferent arterioles. The function of lacis cells is unknown.

The juxtaglomerular apparatus is a mechanism that controls the degree of resorption of ions by the renal tubule. It appears likely that cells of the macula densa monitor the ionic constitution of the fluid passing across them (within the tubule). The cells of the macula densa appear to influence the release of renin by the juxtaglomerular cells. As described above renin influences aldosterone production (through angiotensin II) and hence controls tubular resorption. In this way it helps to regulate plasma volume and blood pressure.

The juxtaglomerular cells also probably act as baroreceptors reacting to a fall in blood pressure by release of renin. Secretion of renin is also stimulated by low sodium blood levels and by sympathetic stimulation.

In addition to renin the kidney produces the hormone erythropoietin (which stimulates erythrocyte production). Some workers have claimed that erythropoietin is produced by juxtaglomerular cells, but the site of production of the hormone is uncertain.

Interstitial Tissue of the Kidney

Most of the interstitial space in the renal cortex is occupied by blood vessels and lymphatics. In the medulla the interstitium is composed mainly of a matrix containing proteins and glycosaminoglycans. Collagen fibres and interstitial cells are present.

It has been held that interstitial cells produce prostaglandins, but it now appears that prostaglandins are produced by epithelial cells of collecting ducts.

THE URETERS

The wall of the ureter has three layers: an outer fibrous coat, a middle layer of smooth muscle, and an inner lining of mucous membrane (Fig. 17.15).

The mucous membrane has a lining of transitional epithelium which is 4 to 5 cell thick. The epithelium does not have a distinct basal lamina. It rests on a layer of fibrous tissue containing many elastic fibres.

(As mentioned on page 48 some observers hold that all cells of transitional epithelium reach the base, and that the epithelium should, therefore, be classified as pseudostratified).

The mucosa (consisting of epithelium and the underlying connective tissue) shows a number of longitudinal folds that give the lumen a star-

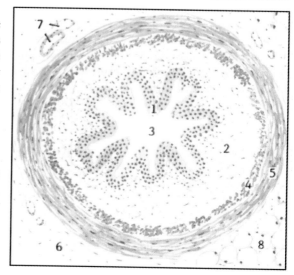

Fig. 17.15. Ureter. 1-Mucosa lined by transitional epithelium. 2-Connective tissue. 3-Lumen (star shaped). 4, 5-Muscle coat (inner longitudinal, and outer circular). 6-Connective tissue. 7-Blood vessel.

shaped appearance in transverse section. The folds disappear when the ureter is distended.

The muscle coat is usually described as having an inner longitudinal layer and an outer circular layer of smooth muscle. A third layer of longitudinal fibres is present outside the circular coat in the middle and lower parts of the ureter. The layers are not distinctly marked off from each other. Some workers have reported that the musculature of the ureter is really in the form of a meshwork formed by branching and anastomosing bundles of muscle fibres.

The outer fibrous coat consists of loose connective tissue. It contains numerous blood vessels, nerves, lymphatics and some fat cells.

Reflux of urine from the urinary bladder into the ureters is prevented by the oblique path followed by the terminal part of the ureter, through the bladder wall. When the musculature of the bladder contracts this part of the ureter is compressed. This mechanism constitutes a physiological sphincter.

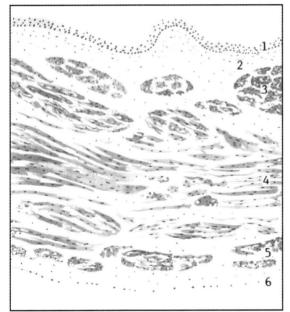

Fig. 17.16. Urinary bladder. 1-Transitional epithelium. 2-Connective tissue. 3, 4, 5-Muscle layers.

In the empty bladder the mucous membrane is thrown into numerous folds (or rugae) that disappear when the bladder is distended. Some mucous glands may be present in the mucosa specially near the internal urethral orifice.

The muscle layer is thick. The smooth muscle in it forms a meshwork. Internally and externally the fibres tend to be longitudinal. In between them there is a thicker layer of circular (or oblique) fibres. Contraction of this muscle coat is responsible for emptying of the bladder. That is why it is called the ***detrusor muscle***. Just above the junction of the bladder with the urethra the circular fibres are thickened to form the ***sphincter vesicae***.

The serous coat lines part of the bladder and has the usual structure.

THE URINARY BLADDER

The wall of the urinary bladder consists of an outer serous layer, a thick coat of smooth muscle, and a mucous membrane.

The mucous membrane is lined by transitional epithelium (page 48). The epithelium rests on a layer of loose fibrous tissue. There is no muscularis mucosae.

When the bladder is distended (with urine) the lining epithelium becomes thinner. This results from the ability of the epithelial cells to change shape and shift over one another.

The transitional epithelium lining the urinary bladder (and the rest of the urinary passages) is capable of withstanding osmotic changes caused by variations in concentrations of urine. It is also resistant to toxic substances present in urine.

THE URETHRA

Although the male urethra is much longer than the female urethra the structure of the two is the same. The wall of the urethra is composed of mucous, submucous and muscular layers. In the case of the male, the prostatic urethra is surrounded by prostatic tissue; and the penile urethra by erectile tissue of the corpus spongiosum (Figs. A90, A91).

The mucous membrane consists of a lining epithelium that rests on connective tissue. The epithelium varies in different parts of the urethra. Both in the male and female the greater part of the urethra is lined by pseudostratified columnar epithelium. A short part adjoining the urinary bladder is lined by transitional epithelium, while the part near the external orifice is lined by stratified squamous epithelium.

The mucosa shows invaginations or recesses

into which mucous glands open.

The submucosa consists of loose connective tissue. The muscle coat consists of an inner longitudinal layer and an outer circular layer of smooth muscle. This coat is better defined in the female urethra. In the male urethra it is well defined only in the membranous and prostatic parts, the penile part being surrounded by occasional fibres only.

In addition to this smooth muscle the membranous part of the male urethra, and the corresponding part of the female urethra are surrounded by striated muscle that forms the *external urethral sphincter*.

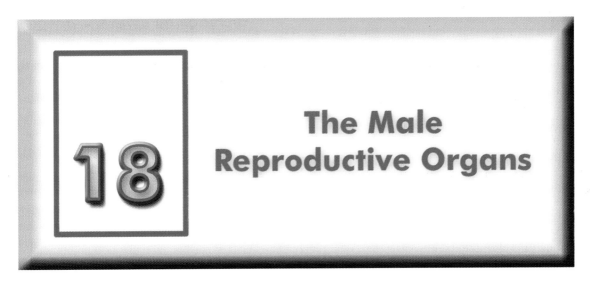

The Male Reproductive Organs

The male reproductive organs are the testis, the epididymis, the ductus deferens, and the seminal vesicle which are paired; and the prostate, the male urethra, and the penis which are unpaired.

THE TESTIS

Some features of Gross Structure

The right and left testes produce the male gametes or **spermatozoa**. Each testis is an oval structure about 4 cm long. The outermost layer of the organ is formed by a dense fibrous membrane called the **tunica albuginea**. The tunica albuginea consists of closely packed collagen fibres amongst which there are many elastic fibres. In the posterior part of the testis the connective tissue of the tunica albuginea expands into a thick mass that projects into the substance of the testis. This projection is called the **mediastinum testis**. Numerous septa pass from the mediastinum testis to the tunica albuginea, and divide the substance of the testis into a large number of lobules. Each lobule is roughly conical, the apex of the cone being directed towards the mediastinum testis. Each lobule contains one or more highly convoluted **seminiferous tubules**.

When stretched out each tubule is 70-80 cm in length. It has a diameter of about $150\,\mu$m. These tubules are lined by cells which are concerned with the production of spermatozoa. It has been estimated that each testis has about 200 lobules, and that each lobule has one to three seminiferous tubules. The total number of

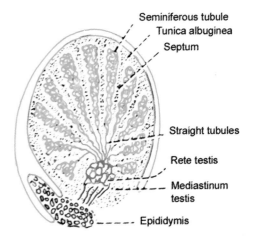

Fig. 18.1. Scheme to show the basic structure of the testis.

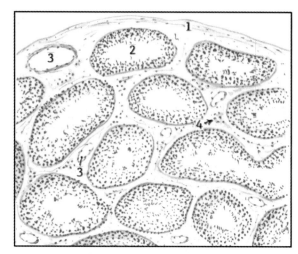

Fig. 18.2.Testis, low power view. 1-Tunica albuginea.
2-Seminiferous tubule. 3-Blood vessel.
4-Interstitial cells.

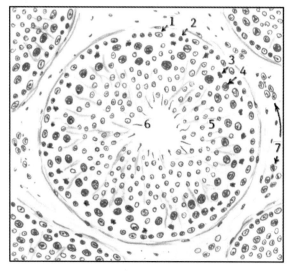

Fig. 18.3. Testis, high power view. 1-Sustentacular
cells. 2-Spermatogonia. 3-Dividing spermatogonia.
4-Spermatocyte. 5-Spermatid. 6-Spermatozoa.
7-Interstitial cells.

tubules is between 400 and 600. The combined length of all seminiferous tubules in one testis is between 300 and 900 metres. It is believed that each seminiferous tubule is in the form of a loop, both ends of the loop becoming continuous with a straight tubule (See below). Within a lobule, the spaces between seminiferous tubules are filled by very loose connective tissue, containing blood vessels and lymphatics. Lying in this connective tissue there are groups of *interstitial cells* (of Leydig). These cells have an endocrine function and secrete the male sex hormone (Fig. 18.3). Their cytoplasm contains yellow pigment.

Near the apex of the lobule the seminiferous tubules lose their convolutions and join one another to form about 20 to 30 larger, *straight tubules* (or *tubuli recti*). These straight tubules enter the fibrous tissue of the mediastinum testis and unite to form a network called the *retetestis*. At its upper end the retetestis gives off 12 to 20 *efferent ductules*. These ductules pass from the upper part of the testis into the *epididymis*. The epididymis has a head, a body and a tail. The head of the epididymis is made up of highly convoluted continuations of the efferent ductules. At the lower end of the head of the epididymis these tubules join to form a single tube called the *duct of the epididymis*. This duct is highly coiled on itself and forms the body and tail of the epididymis. At the lower end of the tail of the epididymis the duct becomes continuous with the *ductus deferens*.

The testis lies within a double layered serous sac called the *tunica vaginalis*. The visceral layer of this sac covers the tunica albuginea, except in the region of the mediastinum testis.

General Structure of Seminiferous Tubules

As seminiferous tubules are highly convoluted, each tube is cut up several times in any section through the testis. For the same reason the profiles of the tubules assume various shapes. The wall of each tubule is made up of an outer layer of fibrous tissue which also contains muscle-like (myoid) cells. Contractions of these cells probably help to move spermatozoa along the tubule. Between this connective tissue and the lumen of the tubule there are several layers of cells. The cells rest on a basal lamina. They are of various shapes and sizes. Most of the cells represent stages in the formation of spermatozoa: they are referred to as *germ cells*. Other cells that have a supporting function are called *sustentacular cells* or the *cells of Sertoli*.

The appearance of the cellular lining of the seminiferous tubules is characteristic, and a student who has studied sections through them carefully (even at low magnification) is not likely to mistake the seminiferous tubules for anything else. The points to note are (a) the many layers of cells; (b) the great variety in size and shape of the cells and of their nuclei; (c) the lack of a well defined margin of the lumen; and (d) inconspicuous cell boundaries. Some features of the cells lining the tubules are considered below.

Cells Representing Stages in Spermatogenesis

The process of the formation of spermatozoa is called *spermatogenesis*. It consists of several stages. Although it may not be possible to distinguish individual stages in class room slides a knowledge of these stages is essential.

1. The stem cells from which all stages described below are derived are called *spermatogonia*. These cells lie near the basal lamina. Spermatogonia undergo several mitotic divisions and, because of this, spermatogonia of varied structure are seen in the wall of a seminiferous tubule. These mitoses give rise to more spermatogonia, and to primary spermatocytes (see below). (For further details see page 279).

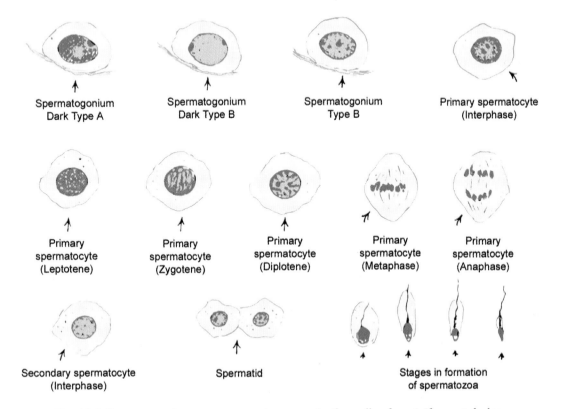

Spermatogonium
Dark Type A

Spermatogonium
Dark Type B

Spermatogonium
Type B

Primary spermatocyte
(Interphase)

Primary
spermatocyte
(Leptotene)

Primary
spermatocyte
(Zygotene)

Primary
spermatocyte
(Diplotene)

Primary
spermatocyte
(Metaphase)

Primary
spermatocyte
(Anaphase)

Secondary spermatocyte
(Interphase)

Spermatid

Stages in formation
of spermatozoa

Fig. 18.4. Some stages in spermatogenesis as seen in the walls of seminiferous tubules.

2. *Primary spermatocytes* are formed by mitotic division of spermatogonia. These are large cells with large spherical nuclei. Each primary spermatocyte undergoes meiosis (described in detail on page 39) to give rise to two secondary spermatocytes (see below). This is the first meiotic division in which the number of chromosomes is reduced to half. (Each primary spermatocyte has 46 chromosomes, whereas each secondary spermatocyte has only 23).

3. *Secondary spermatocytes* are smaller than primary spermatocytes, and so are their nuclei. We have seen that each secondary spermatocyte has the haploid number of chromosomes (i.e., 23). It divides to form two spermatids (see below). This is the second meiotic division (page 41) and this time there is no further reduction in chromosome number.

4. Each *spermatid* is a rounded cell with a spherical nucleus. Both cell and nucleus are much smaller than in the case of spermatogonia or spermatocytes. The spermatid undergoes changes in shape, and in the orientation of its organelles, to form a spermatozoon. This process is called *spermiogenesis*.

For further details of the various stages in spermatogenesis see page 279.

Diploid and Haploid Chromosome Number and DNA content

We have seen that a typical cell contains 46 chromosomes, this being referred to as the diploid number. Spermatozoa (or ova) have only half this number i.e., 23 which is the haploid number. At fertilization, the diploid number is restored, the zygote receiving 23 chromosomes from the ovum, and 23 from the sperm.

A primary spermatocyte contains the diploid number of chromosomes (46). During the first meiotic division the number is halved so that secondary spermatocytes have the haploid number (23).

Now let us look at these facts in relation to DNA content, rather than chromosome number. Let us designate the DNA content of a gamete (sperm or ovum) as n. The DNA content of a zygote formed as a result of fertilization is, therefore, $n + n = 2n$. Before the zygote can undergo division its DNA has to be replicated. In other words it has to become $4n$, of which $2n$ goes to each daughter cell.

When first formed primary spermatocytes (or oocytes) have $2n$ DNA. After replication this becomes $4n$. At the first meiotic division $2n$ goes to each secondary spermatocyte. The point to note is that although the chromosome number in a secondary spermatocyte is haploid, DNA is $2n$. There is no replication of DNA in secondary spermatocytes. As a result the DNA content of spermatids formed as a result of the second meiotic division is n. Therefore, note that although there is no reduction in chromosome number during the second meiotic division, DNA content is reduced from $2n$ to n.

Sustentacular Cells or Cells of Sertoli

These are tall, slender cells having an irregularly pyramidal or columnar shape. The nucleus lies near the base of the cell. It is light staining and is of irregular shape. There is a prominent nucleolus. The base of each sustentacular cell rests on the basement membrane, spermatogonia being interposed amongst the sustentacular cells. The apex of the sustentacular cell reaches the lumen of the seminiferous tubule. Numerous spermatids, at various stages of differentiation into spermatozoa, appear to be embedded in the apical part of the cytoplasm. Nearer the basement membrane spermatocytes and spermatogonia indent the sustentacular cell cytoplasm.

Sustentacular cells support developing germ cells and provide them with nutrition. They

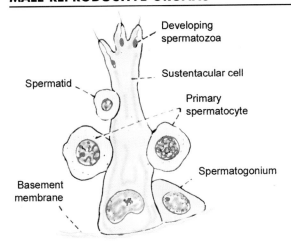

Fig. 18.5. Scheme to show a sustentacular cell and some related germ cells.

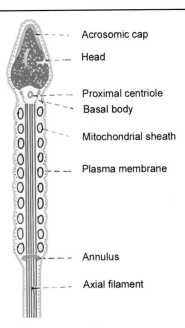

Fig. 18.6. Structure of a spermatozoon as seen by EM.

probably secrete fluid that helps to move spermatozoa along the seminiferous tubules. This fluid is rich in testosterone, which may stimulate activity of cells lining the epididymis. Sustentacular cells may also act as macrophages. In the adult testis sustentacular cells are less prominent than germ cells. They are more prominent than germ cells before puberty, and in old age. (For further details see page 280).

Structure of a Mature Spermatozoon

The spermatozoon has a *head*, a *neck*, a *middle piece* and a *principal piece* or *tail*. The head is covered by a cap called the *acrosomic cap*, *anterior nuclear cap*, or *galea capitis*.

> The acrosome is made up of glycoprotein. It can be regarded as a large lysosome containing numerous enzymes (proteases, acid phosphatase, neuraminidase, hyaluronidase).

The neck of the spermatozoon is narrow. It contains a funnel-shaped *basal body* and a spherical *centriole*. An *axial filament* (or *axoneme*) begins just behind this centriole. It passes through the middle piece and extends into the tail. At the point where the middle piece

joins the tail, this axial filament passes through a ring-like *annulus*. That part of the axial filament which lies in the middle piece is surrounded by a *spiral sheath* made up of mitochondria.

The *head* of the human spermatozoon is flattened from before backwards so that it is oval when seen from the front, but appears to be pointed (somewhat like a spear-head) when seen from one side, or in section. It consists of chromatin (mostly DNA) that is extremely condensed and, therefore, appears to have a homogeneous structure even when examined by EM. This condensation makes it highly resistant to various physical stresses.

The chief structure to be seen in the neck is the *basal body*. It is also called the *connecting piece* because it helps to establish an intimate union between the head and the remainder of the spermatozoon. The basal body is made up of nine segmented rod-like structures each of which is continuous distally with one coarse fibre of the axial filament (see below). On its proximal side (i.e., towards the head of the spermatozoon)

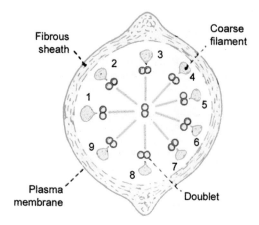

Fig. 18.7. Transverse section across the tail of a spermatozoon to show the arrangement of fibrils.

the basal body has a convex *articular surface* which fits into a depression (called the *implantation fossa*) present in the head.

The *axial filament*, that passes through the middle piece and most of the tail, is really composed of several fibrils arranged as illustrated in Fig. 18.7. There is a pair of central fibrils, surrounded by nine pairs (or *doublets*) arranged in a circle around the central pair. (This arrangement of one central pair of fibrils surrounded by nine doublets is similar to that seen in cilia. Compare also with the structure of the centriole, page 21).

In addition to these doublets there are nine coarser petal-shaped fibrils of unequal size, one such fibril lying just outside each doublet. These coarse fibrils are present in the middle piece and most of the tail, but do not extend into the terminal part of the tail. The whole system of fibrils is kept in position by a series of coverings. Immediately outside the fibrils there is a fibrous sheath. In the region of the middle piece the fibrous sheath is surrounded by spirally arranged mitochondria. Finally, the entire sperm is enclosed in a plasma membrane.

From Fig. 18.7 it will be seen that one of the coarse fibrils is larger than the others. This is

called fibril 1, the others being numbered in a clockwise direction from it. The fibrous sheath is adherent to fibrils 3 and 8. The line joining fibrils 3 and 8 divides the tail into a major compartment containing 4 fibrils and a minor compartment containing 3 fibrils. This line also passes through both the central fibrils and provides an axis in reference to which sperm movements can be analysed.

Spermiogenesis

The process by which a spermatid becomes a spermatozoon is called *spermiogenesis* (or *spermateleosis*). The spermatid is a more or less circular cell containing a nucleus, Golgi complex, centriole and mitochondria. All these components take part in forming the spermatozoon. The nucleus undergoes condensation and changes shape to form the head. The Golgi complex is transformed into the acrosomic cap which comes to lie over one side of the nucleus. The acrosome marks the future anterior pole of the spermatozoon. The centriole divides into two parts which are at first close together. They migrate to the pole of the cell that is away from the acrosome. The axial filament grows out of the distal centriole. The region occupied by the two centrioles later becomes the neck of the spermatozoon. The proximal centriole probably forms the basal body. The part of the axial filament between the head and the annulus becomes surrounded by mitochondria, and together with them forms the middle piece. Most of the cytoplasm of the spermatid is shed, and is phagocytosed by Sertoli cells. The cell membrane persists as a covering for the spermatozoon.

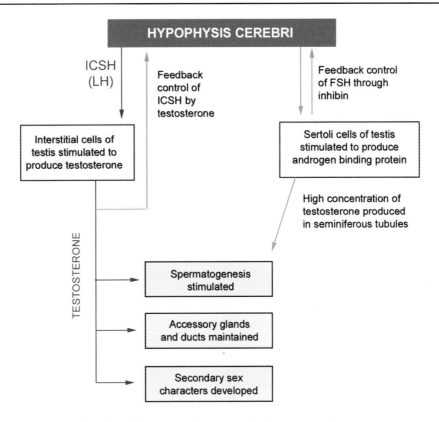

Fig. 18.8. Scheme to show control of male genital system.

Some Further Details of Cells Lining the Seminiferous Tubules

1. Three main types of spermatogonia are described: *dark type-A (AD)*, *light* (or *pale*) *type-A (AP)*, and *type-B*. In type A spermatogonia (dark and light) the nuclei are oval and possess nucleoli that are eccentric, and are attached to the nuclear membrane. The terms dark and light, applied to these cells, refer to the intensity of staining of the nuclei. In type B spermatogonia the nuclei are spherical. Each nucleus has a spherical nucleolus.

Dark type A spermatogonia (also called type A_1) represent a reserve of resting stem cells. They divide to form more dark type A cells and also some light type A cells (or A_2 cells). Light type A spermatogonia divide to form more light type A spermatogonia, and also some spermatogonia of type B. Each type B spermatogonium divides several times (probably four times in man). The resulting cells are designated B_1, B_2, B_3 etc. Each of the resulting cells divides to form two primary spermatocytes.

2. We have seen (page 39) that the prophase of the first meiotic division is prolonged and passes through several stages (leptotene, zygotene, pachytene, diplotene) in which the appearance of the nucleus shows considerable alterations. As a result, primary spermatocytes at various stages of prophase (and subsequent stages of division) can be recognized in the wall of a seminiferous tubule (Fig.18.4).

3. **Spermatogenic Cycle:** We have noted that many types of cells are to be seen in the walls of the seminiferous tubules, as there are several types of spermatogonia and several stages in maturation of spermatocytes and of spermatids (Fig.18.4).

However, all types of cells are not seen in any one part of the seminiferous tubule at a given time. Detailed studies have brought to light the following.

(a) In a given segment of the tubule there is a gradual change in the type of cells encountered (with passage of time). Six phases have been recognized.

(b) At a given point of time different segments of a seminiferous tubule show cell patterns corresponding to the six phases.

It has, therefore, been suggested that over a period of time waves of maturation (of germ cells) pass along the length of a seminiferous tubule. Details of the various phases will not be considered here.

4. **Sustentacular Cells:** The basic structure of these cells has been described on page 276. With the EM it is seen that the sides and apices of these cells are marked by recesses which are occupied by spermatogonia, spermatocytes, and spermatids. However, there is no cytoplasmic continuity between these cells and the sustentacular cell. On the basis of light microscopic studies some workers were of the view that the sustentacular cells formed a syncytium. However, EM studies have shown that the cells are distinct. The plasma membranes of adjoining sustentacular cells are connected by tight junctions (page 12) which divide the wall of the seminiferous tubule into two compartments, **superficial** (or **adluminal**) and **deep** (**abluminal**). The deep compartment contains spermatogonia (and preleptotene spermatocytes) and the superficial compartment contains other stages of spermatogenesis. The two compartments are believed to be separated by a **blood-testis barrier**. Sustentacular cells contain abundant mitochondria, endoplasmic reticulum, and other organelles. Microfilaments and microtubules form a cytoskeleton that appears to be important in cohesive functions of these cells.

Several functions have been attributed to Sertoli cells.

(a) They provide physical support to germ cells, and provide them with nutrients. Waste products from germ cells are transferred to blood or lymph through them.

(b) They phagocytose residual cytoplasm that remains after conversion of spermatids to spermatozoa.

(c) Sertoli cells produce a number of hormones. In the eighth month of fetal life they secrete a hormone (**Mullerian inhibitory substance** or **MIS**) that suppresses development of the paramesonephric (Mullerian) ducts (in male fetuses). They are also believed to produce a substance that inhibits spermatogenesis before puberty.

(d) In the male adult, Sertoli cells produce **androgen binding protein (ABP)** which binds to testosterone (and hydroxytestosterone) making these available in high concentration to germ cells within seminiferous tubules. Secretion of ABP is influenced by FSH. A hormone **inhibin** produced by Sertoli cells inhibits production of FSH (Fig. 18.8).

Maturation and capacitation of spermatozoa

As fully formed spermatozoa pass through the male genital passages they undergo a process of **maturation**. Spermatozoa acquire some motility only after passing through the epididymis. The secretions of the epididymis, seminal vesicles and the prostate have a stimulating effect on sperm motility, but spermatozoa become fully motile only after ejaculation. When introduced into the vagina, spermatozoa reach the uterine tubes much sooner than their own motility would allow, suggesting that contractions of uterine and tubal musculature exert a sucking effect.

Spermatozoa acquire the ability to fertilize the ovum only after they have been in the female genital tract for some time. This final step in their maturation is called **capacitation**. During capacitation some proteins and glycoproteins are removed from the plasma membrane overlying the acrosome. When the sperm reaches near the ovum, changes take place in membranes over the acrosome and enable release of lysosomal enzymes present within the acrosome. This is called the *acrosome reaction*. The substances released include hyaluronidase which helps in separating corona radiata cells present over the ovum. *Trypsin like substances* and a substance called *acrosin*, help in digesting the zona pellucida and penetration of the sperm through it. Changes in the properties of the zona pellucida constitute the *zona reaction*.

Interstitial Cells

The interstitial cells (of Leydig) are large, round or polyhedral cells lying in the connective tissue that intervenes between the coils of seminiferous tubules (Fig. 18.3). Their nuclei are eccentric. The cytoplasm stains lightly and often has a foamy appearance (because of the removal of lipids during processing of tissues). It contains yellow granules which are seen by EM to be vacuoles containing various enzymes. Rod shaped crystalloids (Reinke's crystalloids) are also present in the cytoplasm. Much agranular endoplasmic reticulum is present. Yellow-brown pigment (lipofuscin) is seen in some cells.

Interstitial cells secrete male sex hormone (testicular androgens). Secretion is stimulated by the interstitial cell stimulating hormone of the hypophysis cerebri (Chapter 20). (This hormone is identical with the luteinising hormone present in the female).

Some interstitial cells may be present in the mediastinum testis, in the epididymis, or even in the spermatic cord.

Apart from interstitial cells, the interstitial tissue contains collagen fibres, fibroblasts, macrophages, mast cells, blood vessels and lymphatics.

Structure of Rete Testis & Efferent Ductules

The rete testis consists of anastomosing tubules that are lined by flattened or cuboidal cells. They bear microvilli. The epithelium is surrounded by connective tissue of the mediastinum testis.

The efferent ductules are lined by ciliated columnar epithelium. Some non-ciliated cells bearing microvilli are also present. The tubules have some smooth muscle in their walls. Movement of spermatozoa through the tubules is facilitated by ciliary action, and by peristaltic contraction of smooth muscle.

ACCESSORY UROGENITAL ORGANS

The Epididymis

Structurally, the epididymis consists of two parts. The head is formed by highly convoluted continuations of the efferent ductules (Fig. 18.9). These are lined by ciliated columnar epithelium. The body and tail of the epididymis are made up of the duct of the epididymis, which is greatly coiled on itself. The duct is lined by pseudostratified columnar epithelium in which there are tall columnar cells, and shorter basal cells that do not reach the lumen. The luminal surface of each columnar cell bears non-motile projections that resemble cilia. These stereocilia are seen by EM to be thick microvilli. They do not have the structure of true cilia. The EM also shows the presence in these cells of agranular endoplasmic reticulum, lysosomes and a prominent Golgi complex. The basal cells are precursors of the tall cells. The tubules of the epididymis are surrounded by smooth muscle

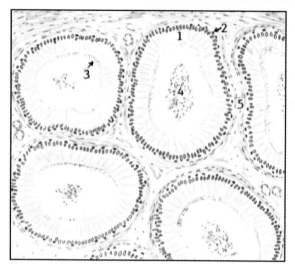

Fig. 18.9. Epidydimis. 1-Lining of tall columnar cells. 2-Basal cell. 3-Stereocilia. 4-Clump of spermatozoa.

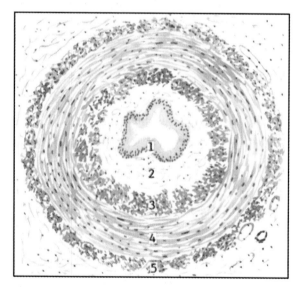

Fig. 18.10. Ductus deferens. 1-Pseudostratified columnar epithelium. 2-Lamina propria. 3, 4, 5-Muscle layers (inner longitudinal, middle circular, outer longitudinal).

and by a rich network of capillaries.

Some functions attributed to epithelial cells of the epididymis are as follows.

(a) Phagocytosis of defective spermatozoa.

(b) Absorption of excess fluid.

(c) Secretion of substances (sialic acid, glyceryl-phosphoryl-choline) that play a role in maturation of spermatozoa.

The Ductus Deferens

The wall of the ductus deferens (deferent duct or vas deferens) consists (from inside out) of mucous membrane, muscle and connective tissue (Fig. 18.10).

The mucous membrane shows a number of longitudinal folds so that the lumen appears to be stellate in section. The lining epithelium is simple columnar, but becomes pseudostratified columnar in the distal part of the duct. The cells are ciliated in the extra-abdominal part of the duct. The epithelium is supported by a lamina propria in which there are many elastic fibres.

The muscle coat is very thick and consists of smooth muscle. It is arranged in the form of an inner circular layer and an outer longitudinal layer. An inner longitudinal layer is present in the proximal part of the duct.

The terminal dilated part of the ductus deferens is called the *ampulla*. It has the same structure as that of the seminal vesicle (see below).

The Seminal Vesicle

The seminal vesicle is a sac-like mass that is really a convoluted tube. The tube is cut several times in any section (Figs. 18.11, 18.12). The tube has an outer covering of connective tissue, a thin intermediate layer made up of smooth muscle , and an inner mucosal lining. The mucosal lining is thrown into numerous thin folds that branch and anastomose thus forming a network. The lining epithelium is simple columnar, or pseudostratified. Goblet cells are present in the epithelium. The muscle layer contains outer longitudinal and inner circular

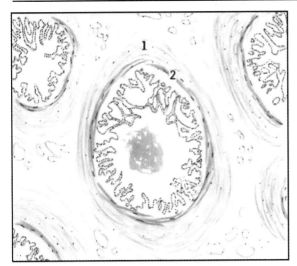

Fig. 18.11.Seminal vesicle (low power). It is made up of a convoluted tubule that is cut up several times. 1-Connective tissue. 2-Smooth muscle.

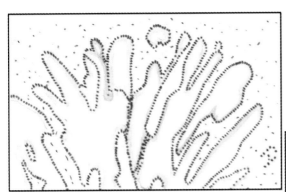

Fig. 18.12. Seminal vesicle (high power). Note that the tubule is lined by columnar epithelium.

fibres.

The seminal vesicles do not function as stores for spermatozoa. They produce a thick secretion which forms the bulk of semen. The secretion contains fructose (which provides nutrition to spermatozoa). It also contains amino acids, proteins, prostaglandins, ascorbic acid and citric acid. This secretion is expelled during ejaculation by contraction of the smooth muscle of the vesicle.

The Prostate

The prostate is made up of 30 to 50 compound tubulo-alveolar glands that are embedded in a framework of fibromuscular tissue. In sections, the glandular tissue is seen in the form of numerous follicles that are lined by columnar epithelium (Figs. 18.13, 18.14). The epithelium is thrown into numerous folds (along with some underlying connective tissue). The follicles drain into 12 to 20 excretory ducts which open into the prostatic urethra. The ducts are lined by a double layered epithelium. The superficial (luminal) layer is columnar, and the deeper layer is cuboidal.

Small rounded masses of uniform or lamellated structure are found within the lumen of the follicles. They are called *amyloid bodies* or *corpora amylacea*. These are more abundant in older individuals. These consist of condensed glycoprotein. They are often calcified.

The fibromuscular tissue forms a conspicuous feature of sections of the prostate. It contains

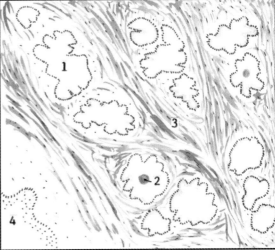

Fig. 18.13. Prostate (low power view). 1-Follicle of irregular shape. 2-Amyloid body. 3-Fibromuscular tissue. 4-Prostatic urethra lined by transitional epithelium.

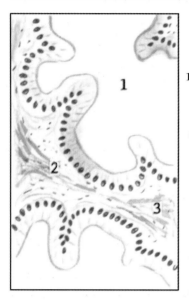

Fig. 18.14. Prostate (high power view). 1-Follicle lined by columnar epithelium. 2,3- Fibro-muscular tissue.

collagen fibres and smooth muscle. Within the gland the fibromuscular tissue forms septa that separate the glandular elements. These septa are continuous with a fibrous capsule that surrounds the prostate. The capsule contains numerous veins and parasympathetic ganglion cells.

The prostate produces a secretion which forms a considerable part of semen. The secretion is rich in enzymes (acid phosphatase, amylase, protease) and in citric acid. The prostate also produces substances called ***prostaglandins*** which have numerous actions.

The glandular part of the prostate is poorly developed at birth. It undergoes considerable proliferation at puberty, and degenerates in old age.

The prostate is traversed by the prostatic urethra which has been described on page 259. The gland is also traversed by the ejaculatory ducts. The gland is divided into lobes for details of which see a book on gross anatomy.

On the basis of differences in the size and nature of the glands the prostate can be divided into an ***outer*** (or ***peripheral***) ***zone***, and an ***internal zone***. An innermost zone lying immediately around the prostatic urethra is also described.

The glands in the outer zone are the main prostatic glands. They open into long ducts that join the urethra. The internal (or submucous) glands have short ducts. The innermost (or mucous) glands open directly into the urethra. The internal and innermost zones together form the central zone. The peripheral zone is often the site of carcinoma. The central zone commonly undergoes benign hypertrophy in old persons. Enlargement of the prostate can compress the urethra leading to problems in passing urine.

The Penis

The penis consists of a ***root*** that is fixed to the perineum, and of a free part which is called the ***body*** or ***corpus***. A transverse section through the free part of the penis is shown in Fig. 18.15. The penis is covered all round by thin skin that is attached loosely to underlying tissue. The substance of the penis is made up of three masses of erectile tissue, two dorsal and one ventral. The

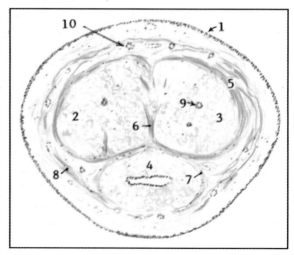

Fig. 18.15. Penis. 1-Skin. 2, 3, 5-Corpora cavernosa and sheaths for them. 6-Median septum. 4,7-Corpus spongiosum and its sheath. 8-Common sheath. 10-Dorsal artery.

dorsal masses are the right and left *corpora cavernosa*, while the ventral mass is the *corpus spongiosum*. The corpora cavernosa lie side by side and are separated only by a median fibrous septum. The corpus spongiosum is placed in the midline ventral to the corpora cavernosa. It is traversed by the penile urethra.

Each corpus cavernosum is surrounded by a dense sheath containing collagen fibres, elastic fibres and some smooth muscle. In the midline the sheaths of the right and left corpora cavernosa fuse to form a median septum. The corpus spongiosum is also surrounded by a sheath, but this sheath is much thinner than that around the corpora cavernosa. An additional sheath surrounds both the corpora cavernosa and the corpus spongiosum.

Erectile Tissue

Numerous septa arising from the connective tissue sheath extend into the corpora cavernosa and into the corpus spongiosum, and form a network (Fig. 18.16). The spaces of the network are lined by endothelium. The spaces are in communication with arteries and veins. They are normally empty. During erection of the penis they are filled with blood under pressure. This results in enlargement and rigidity of the organ. The process of erection involves the corpora cavernosa more than the corpus spongiosum, rigidity of the former being made possible by the presence of a dense fibrous sheath. The corpus spongiosum does not become so rigid as its sheath is elastic, and the vascular spaces within it are smaller. As a result, the penile urethra remains patent during erection, and semen can flow through it.

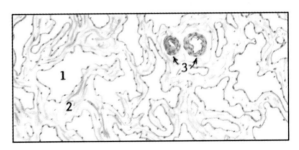

Fig. 18.16. Erectile tissue (from part of penis). 1-space lined by endothelium. 2-Connective tissue. 3-Artery with thick muscular wall.

Blood to the corpora cavernosa is supplied mainly by the deep arteries of the penis. These arteries give off branches that follow a spiral course before opening into the cavernous spaces. They are called *helicrine arteries* and have an unusual structure. The circular muscle in their media is very thick so that the vessels can be completely occluded. The tunica intima shows longitudinal thickenings. Erection is produced by complete relaxation of smooth muscle both in the walls of arteries and in the septa. Helicrine arteries are connected to veins by arteriovenous anastomoses. Normally, the anastomoses are patent. Their closure (caused by parasympathetic nerves) causes cavernous spaces to fill leading to erection. As the cavernous spaces fill with blood, increasing pressure in them compresses the veins which lie just deep to the fibrous sheath. In this way blood is prevented from draining out of the spaces. At the end of erection smooth muscle in the walls of arteries contracts stopping inflow of blood. Contraction of muscle in the trabeculae gradually forces blood out of the spaces.

Many sensory nerve endings are present in the penis, particularly on the glans.

The female reproductive organs are the right and left ovaries and uterine tubes, the uterus, the vagina, the external genitalia, and the mammary glands.

THE OVARIES

General Structure

The ovaries are the female gonads, responsible for the formation of ova. They also produce hormones that are responsible for the development of the female secondary sex characters, and produce marked cyclical changes in the uterine endometrium.

Each ovary is an oval structure about 3 cm in long diameter. Its free surface is covered by a single layer of cubical cells that constitute the *germinal epithelium*. This epithelium is continuous with the mesothelium lining the peritoneum, and represents a modification of the latter.

> The term germinal epithelium is a misnomer. The epithelium does not produce germ cells. The cells of this epithelium bear microvilli, and contain numerous mitochondria. They become larger in pregnancy.

The substance of the ovary is divisible into a thick cortex and a much smaller medulla (Fig. 19.1).

Immediately deep to the germinal epithelium the *cortex* is covered by a condensation of connective tissue called the *tunica albuginea*. The tunica albuginea of the ovary is much thinner, and less dense, than that of the testis. Deep to the tunica albuginea the cortex has a stroma made up of reticular fibres and numerous fusiform cells that resemble mesenchymal cells. Scattered in this stroma there are *ovarian follicles* at various stages of development. Each follicle contains a developing ovum. The formation of ova, and the development and fate of ovarian follicles are described below.

The *medulla* consists of connective tissue in which numerous blood vessels (mostly veins) are seen. Elastic fibres and smooth muscle are also present. The hilum of the ovary is the site for entry of blood vessels and lymphatics. It is continuous with the medulla. The hilum also contains some remnants of the mesonephric ducts; and *hilus cells* that are similar to interstitial cells of the testis.

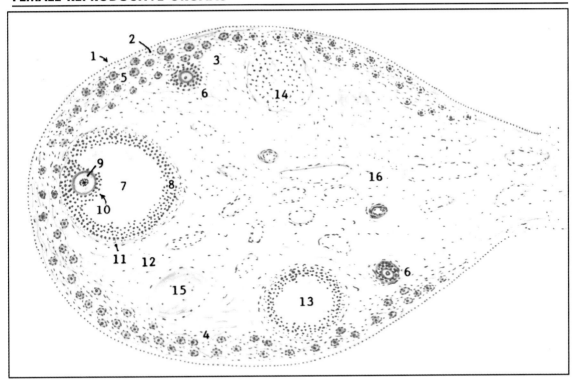

Fig. 19.1. Ovary, panoramic view. 1-Cuboidal epithelium over surface. 2-Tunica albuginea.
3, 4-Cortex. 5-Primordial follicle. 6-Secondary follicle. 7-Follicular cavity. 8-Granulosa cells.
9-Ovum. 10-Cumulus oophoricus. 11-Capsule of follicle. 12-Stroma. 14-Corpus luteum.

Oogenesis

The stem cells from which ova are derived are called **oogonia**. These are large round cells present in the cortex of the ovary. Oogonia are derived (in fetal life) from **primordial germ cells** that are formed in the region of the yolk sac, and migrate into the developing ovary. They increase in number by mitosis.

All oogonia to be used throughout the life of a woman are produced at a very early stage (before birth) and do not multiply thereafter. At birth the number of oogonia in an ovary is about one million. Many oogonia formed in this way degenerate, the process starting before birth and progressing throughout life, so that the number of oogonia becomes less and less with increasing age.

An oogonium enlarges to form a **primary oocyte**. The primary oocyte contains the diploid number of chromosomes i.e., 46. It undergoes the first meiotic division (page 39) to form two daughter cells each of which has 23 chromosomes. However, the cytoplasm of the primary oocyte is not equally divided. Most of it goes to one daughter cell which is large and is called the **secondary oocyte**. The second daughter cell has hardly any cytoplasm, and forms the **first polar body**. The secondary oocyte now undergoes the second meiotic division (page 41), the daughter cells being again unequal in size. The larger daughter cell produced as a result of this division is the **mature ovum**. The smaller daughter cell (which has hardly any cytoplasm) is the **second polar body**. From the above it will be seen that one primary oocyte ultimately gives rise to only one ovum.

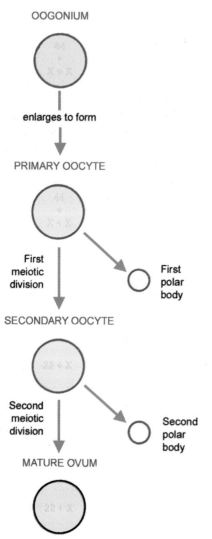

Fig. 19.2 Scheme to show the stages in oogenesis.

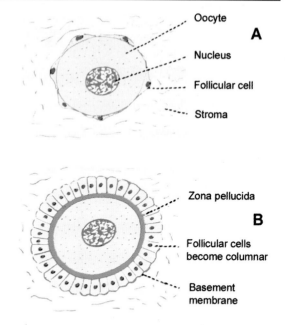

Fig. 19.3. Diagrammatic presentation of: A. Primordial follicle. B. Primary follicle.

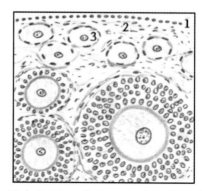

Fig. 19.4. Section of ovary (high power) showing early stages in formation of follicles. 1-Germinal epithelium. 2-Tunica albuginea. 3-Primordial follicle. One primary follicle and two secondary follicles are also seen.

Formation of Ovarian Follicles

Ovarian follicles (or *Graafian follicles*) are derived from stromal cells that surround developing ova as follows.

1. Some cells of the stroma become flattened and surround an oocyte (Fig. 19.3A). These stromal cells are now called *follicular cells*.

The ovum and the flat surrounding cells form a *primordial follicle*. Numerous primordial follicles are present in the ovary at birth. They undergo further development only at puberty.

2. The first indication that a primordial follicle is beginning to undergo further development is that the flattened follicular cells become columnar (Fig. 19.3B). Follicles at this stage of development are called *primary follicles*.

3. A homogeneous membrane, the *zona*

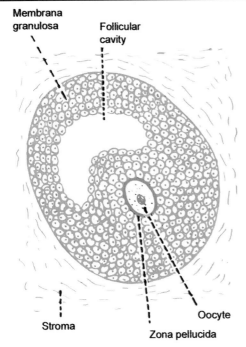

Fig. 19.5. Developing ovarian follicle after establishment of a follicular cavity.

pellucida, appears between the follicular cells and the oocyte (Fig.19.3B). With the appearance of the zona pellucida the follicle is now referred to as a *multilaminar primary follicle*

> The origin of the zona pellucida is controversial. It consists of glycoprotein which is eosinophilic and PAS positive. It is traversed by microvilli projecting outwards from the oocyte. Thin cytoplasmic processes from follicular cells also enter it.

4. The follicular cells proliferate to form several layers of cells which constitute the *membrana granulosa*. The cells are now called *granulosa cells*. This is a *secondary follicle*.

5. So far the granulosa cells are in the form of a compact mass. However, the cells to one side of the ovum soon partially separate from one another so that a *follicular cavity* (or *antrum folliculi*) appears between them. It is with the appearance of this cavity that a true follicle (= small sac) can be said to have been formed. The

follicular cavity is filled by a fluid, the *liquor folliculi* (Fig. 19.5).

6. The follicular cavity rapidly increases in size. As a result, the wall of the follicle (formed by the granulosa cells) becomes relatively thin (Fig. 19.6). The oocyte now lies eccentrically in the follicle surrounded by some granulosa cells that are given the name of *cumulus oophoricus* (or *cumulus oophorus*, or *cumulus ovaricus*). The granulosa cells that attach the oocyte to the wall of the follicle constitute the *discus proligerus*.

7. As the follicle expands the stromal cells surrounding the membrana granulosa become condensed to form a covering called the *theca interna* (theca = cover). The cells of the theca interna later secrete a hormone called *oestrogen*, and they are then called the cells of the *thecal gland*.

8. Outside the theca interna some fibrous tissue becomes condensed to form another covering

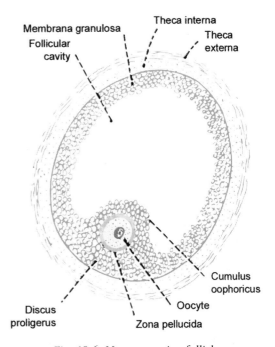

Fig. 19.6. Mature ovarian follicle.

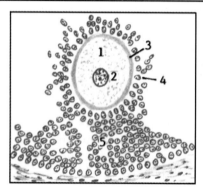

Fig. 19.7. Part of ovarian follicle seen at high power.
1-Ovum. 2-Nucleus of ovum. 3-Zona pellucida.
4-Cumulus oophoricus. 5-Discus proligerus.

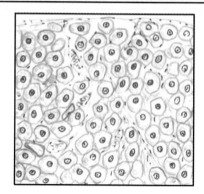

Fig. 19.9. Corpus luteum as seen in a section after
haemataoxylin and eosin staining (high power
view). Note large polyhedral cells and capillaries
present amongst them.

for the follicle. This is the ***theca externa***. The theca interna and externa are collectively called the ***theca folliculi***, the two layers being described as the ***tunica interna*** and the ***tunica externa*** respectively.

9. The ovarian follicle is at first very small compared to the thickness of the ovarian cortex. As the follicle enlarges it becomes so big that it not only reaches the surface of the ovary, but forms a bulging in this situation. As a result the stroma and the theca on this side of the follicle are stretched and become very thin. An avascular area (***stigma***) appears over the most convex point of the follicle. At the same time the cells of the cumulus oophoricus become loosened by accumulation of fluid between them. The follicle ultimately ruptures and the ovum is shed from the ovary. The shedding of the ovum is called ***ovulation***. The 'ovum' that is shed from the ovary is not fully mature. It is really a secondary oocyte.

10. After ovulation, the remaining part of the follicle undergoes changes that convert it into an important structure called the ***corpus luteum***.

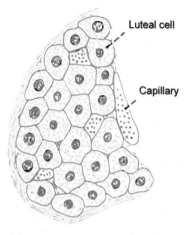

Luteal cell

Capillary

Fig. 19.8. Corpus luteum (diagrammatic). Note the large hexagonal cells filled with yellow granules.

Corpus Luteum

The corpus luteum is an important structure. It secretes a hormone, ***progesterone***. The corpus luteum is derived from the ovarian follicle, after the latter has ruptured to shed the ovum, as follows (Fig. 19.10).

(a) When the follicle ruptures its wall collapses and becomes folded. Sudden reduction in pressure caused by rupture of the follicle results in bleeding into the follicle. The follicle filled with blood is called the ***corpus haemorrhagicum***.

(b) At this stage, the follicular cells are small

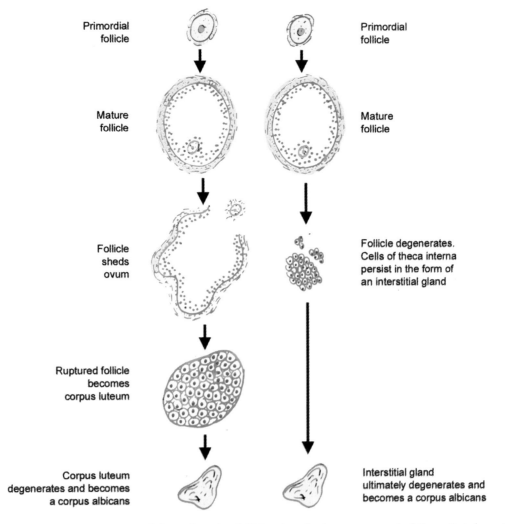

Primordial follicle

Mature follicle

Follicle sheds ovum

Ruptured follicle becomes corpus luteum

Corpus luteum degenerates and becomes a corpus albicans

Primordial follicle

Mature follicle

Follicle degenerates. Cells of theca interna persist in the form of an interstitial gland

Interstitial gland ultimately degenerates and becomes a corpus albicans

Fig. 19.10. Comparison of fate of ovarian follicles that shed an ovum, and of those that do not.

and rounded. They now enlarge rapidly. As they increase in size their walls press against those of neighbouring cells so that the cells acquire a polyhedral shape (Fig.19.8). Their cytoplasm becomes filled with a yellow pigment called *lutein*. They are now called *luteal cells*. The presence of this yellow pigment gives the structure a yellow colour, and that is why it is called the corpus luteum (= yellow body). Some cells of the theca interna also enlarge and contribute to the corpus luteum. The cells of the corpus luteum contain abundant smooth ER and

considerable amount of lipids.

(c) We have seen that the corpus luteum secretes progesterone. This secretion has to be poured into blood like secretions of endocrine glands. All endocrine glands are richly supplied with blood vessels for this purpose. The ovarian follicle itself has no blood vessels, but the surrounding theca interna is full of them. When the corpus luteum is forming, blood vessels from the theca interna invade it and provide it with a rich blood supply.

The subsequent fate of the corpus luteum depends on whether the ovum is fertilized or not.

(a) If the ovum is not fertilized, the corpus luteum persists for about 14 days. During this period it secretes progesterone. It remains relatively small and is called the *corpus luteum of menstruation*. At the end of its functional life, it degenerates and becomes converted into a mass of fibrous tissue called the *corpus albicans* (= white body) (Fig. 19.10).

(b) If the ovum is fertilized and pregnancy results, the corpus luteum persists for three to four months. It is larger than the corpus luteum of menstruation, and is called the *corpus luteum of pregnancy*. The progesterone secreted by it is essential for the maintenance of pregnancy in the first few months. After the fourth month, the corpus luteum is no longer needed, as the placenta begins to secrete progesterone.

The series of changes that begin with the formation of an ovarian follicle, and end with the degeneration of the corpus luteum constitute what is called an *ovarian cycle*.

Fate of Ovarian Follicles

We have seen that in each ovarian cycle one follicle reaches maturity, sheds an ovum, and becomes a corpus luteum. At the same time, several other follicles also begin to develop, but do not reach maturity. It is interesting to note that, contrary to what one might expect, these follicles do not persist into the next ovarian cycle, but undergo degeneration. The ovum and granulosa cells of each follicle disappear. The cells of the theca interna, however, proliferate to form the *interstitial glands*, also called the *corpora atretica*. These glands are believed to secrete oestrogens. After a period of activity, each gland becomes a mass of scar tissue indistinguishable from the corpus albicans formed from the corpus luteum.

From the above it will be clear that the cortex of an ovary (taken from a woman in the reproductive period) can show ovarian follicles (at various stages of maturation), corpora lutea, corpora albicantes, and corpora atretica.

The changes taking place during the ovarian cycle are greatly influenced by certain hormones produced by the hypophysis cerebri. The hormones produced by the theca interna and by the corpus luteum in turn influence other parts of the female reproductive system, notably the uterus, resulting in a cycle of changes referred to as the *uterine cycle* or *menstrual cycle*.

THE UTERINE TUBES

Each uterine tube has a medial or uterine end, attached to (and opening into) the uterus, and a lateral end that opens into the peritoneal cavity near the ovary. The tube has (from medial to lateral side) a *uterine part* that passes through the thick uterine wall; a relatively narrow, thick walled part called the *isthmus*; and a thin walled dilated part called the *ampulla*. The lateral end of the tube is funnel shaped and is called the *infundibulum*. It is prolonged into a number of finger like processes or *fimbria*.

The uterine tube conveys ova, shed by the ovary, to the uterus. Ova enter the tube at its fimbriated end. Spermatozoa enter the uterine tube through the vagina and uterus. Fertilization normally takes place in the ampulla. When fertilization occurs, the fertilized ovum travels towards the uterus through the tube. Secretions present in the tubes provide nutrition, oxygen and other requirements for ova and spermatozoa passing through the tube.

The wall of the uterine tube is made up of

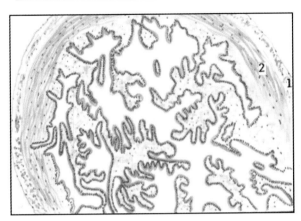

Fig. 19.11. Uterine tube. 1,2-Muscle layer (longitudinal and circular). Mucous membrane shows branching folds covered by ciliated columnar epithelium.

mucous membrane, surrounded by a muscle coat (Fig. 19.11). It is covered externally by peritoneum.

The mucous membrane shows numerous branching folds which almost fill the lumen of the tube. These folds are most conspicuous in the ampulla. Each fold has a highly cellular core of connective tissue. It is lined by columnar epithelium that rests on a basement membrane. Some of the lining cells are ciliated: ciliary action helps to move ova towards the uterus. Other cells are secretory. They contain secretory granules and are not ciliated. Their surface shows microvilli. A third variety of *intercalary cells* is also described.

The muscle coat has an inner circular layer and an outer longitudinal layer of smooth muscle. An additional inner longitudinal layer may also be present. The circular layer is thickest in the uterine part of the tube. Some authorities claim that there is some kind of sphincteric mechanism here that can cut off the uterus from the uterine tube (and through it) from the peritoneal cavity. However, there is no anatomical evidence of the presence of a sphincter. The circular muscle is thickest in the isthmus. The pattern of mucosal

folds is also different in this region. There is some evidence that the isthmus may have some control on the passage of a fertilized ovum through it.

THE UTERUS

The uterus consists of an upper larger part called the body, and a lower smaller part called the cervix. The description that follows applies to the body of the uterus. The cervix is described on page 295.

The uterus has a very thick wall made up mainly of muscle. The lumen is small and is lined by mucous membrane. (Figs. 19.12, 19.14). Part of the uterus is covered on the outside by peritoneum.

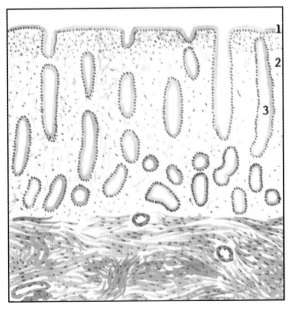

Fig. 19.12. Uterus (Proliferative phase). 1-Lining of columnar epithelium. 2-Stroma. 3-Uterine gland. Also observe the muscular coat.

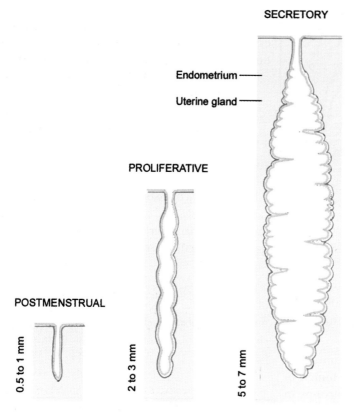

Fig. 19.13. Uterine glands at various stages of the menstrual cycle. The thickness of the endometrium is also indicated.

The Myometrium

The muscle layer of the uterus is also called the *myometrium*. It consists of bundles of smooth muscle amongst which there is connective tissue. Numerous blood vessels, nerves and lymphatics are also present in it.

The muscle fibres run in various directions and distinct layers are difficult to define. However, three layers, external, middle and internal are usually described. The fibres in the external layer are predominantly longitudinal. In the internal layer some bundles are longitudinal and others are circular. In the middle layer there is a mixture of bundles running in various directions.

The muscle cells of the uterus are capable of undergoing great elongation in association with the great enlargement of the organ in pregnancy. New muscle fibres are also formed. Contractions of the myometrium are responsible for expulsion of the fetus at the time of child birth.

The Endometrium

The mucous membrane of the uterus is called the *endometrium*. The endometrium consists of a lining epithelium that rests on a stroma. Numerous uterine glands are present in the stroma.

The lining epithelium is columnar. Before menarche (i,e., the age of onset of menstruation) the cells are ciliated, but thereafter most of the cells may not have cilia. The epithelium rests on a stroma which is highly cellular and contains numerous blood vessels. It also contains numerous simple tubular uterine glands. The glands are lined by columnar epithelium.

The endometrium undergoes marked cyclical changes that constitute the *menstrual cycle*. The most prominent feature of this cycle is the monthly flow of blood from the uterus. This is called *menstruation*. The menstrual cycle is divided (for descriptive convenience) into the following phases: *postmenstrual*, *proliferative*, *secretory* and *menstrual*. The cyclical changes in the endometrium take place under the influence of hormones (oestrogen, progesterone) produced by the ovary. They are summarized below. (For details see the author's HUMAN EMBRYOLOGY).

1. In the postmenstrual phase the endometrium is thin. It progressively increases in thickness being thickest at the end of the secretory phase.

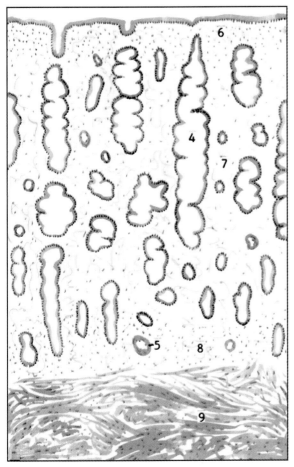

Fig. 19.14. Uterus (secretory phase). 4-Enlarged uterine gland. 5-Artery. 6-Stratum compactum. 7-Stratum spongiosum. 8-Stratum basale. 9-Muscle layer.

At the time of the next menstruation the greater part of its thickness (called the *pars functionalis*) is shed off and flows out along with the menstrual blood. The part that remains is called the *pars basalis*.

2. The uterine glands are straight in the postmenstrual phase. As the endometrium increases in thickness the glands elongate, increase in diameter, and become twisted on themselves. Because of this twisting, they acquire a saw-toothed appearance in sections (Fig. 19.13). At the time of menstruation the greater parts of the uterine glands are lost (along with the entire lining epithelium) leaving behind only their most basal parts. The lining epithelium is reformed (just after the cessation of menstruation) by proliferation of epithelial cells in the basal parts of the glands.

The stroma and blood vessels of the endometrium also undergo cyclical changes.

The Cervix

The structure of the cervix of the uterus is somewhat different from that of the body. Here the mucous membrane (or ***endocervix***) has a number of obliquely placed ***palmate folds***. It contains deep branching glands which secrete mucous. The mucosa also shows small cysts which probably represent glandular elements that are distended with secretion. These cysts are called the ***ovula Nabothi***. The mucous membrane of the upper two thirds of the cervical canal is lined by ciliated columnar epithelium, but over its lower one third the epithelium is non-ciliated columnar. Near the external os the canal is lined by stratified squamous epithelium. Part of the cervix projects into the upper part of the vagina. As a result, this part of the cervix has an external surface which is covered by stratified squamous epithelium. The stroma underlying the epithelium of the cervix is less cellular than that of the body of the uterus, and the muscle coat is not so thick.

The lumen of the cervix is normally a narrow canal. It has tremendous capacity for dilation and, at the time of child birth, it becomes large enough for the fetal head to pass through.

Hormones influencing Ovulation and Menstruation

We have seen that the changes taking place in the uterine endometrium during the menstrual cycle occur under the influence of:

(a) oestrogens produced by the thecal gland (theca interna) and by the interstitial gland cells), and possibly by granulosa cells.

(**b**) progesterone produced by the corpus luteum.

The development of the ovarian follicle, and of the corpus luteum, is in turn dependent on hormones produced by the anterior lobe of the hypophysis cerebri. These are:

(**a**) the *follicle stimulating hormone* (FSH) which stimulates the formation of follicles and the secretion of oestrogens by them; and

(**b**) the *luteinising hormone* (LH) which helps to convert the ovarian follicle into the corpus luteum, and stimulates the secretion of progesterone. Secretion of FSH and LH is controlled by a *gonadotropin releasing hormone* (GnRH) produced by the hypothalamus. Production of LH is also stimulated by feed back of oestrogens secreted by follicular cells of the ovary. A sudden increase (surge) in the level of LH takes place near the middle of the menstrual cycle, and stimulates ovulation which takes place about 36 hours after the surge. Apart from hormones, nervous and emotional influences may affect the ovarian and menstrual cycles. An emotional disturbance may delay or even prevent menstruation.

THE VAGINA

The wall of the vagina consists of a mucous membrane, a muscle coat, and an outer fibrous coat or adventitia.

The mucous membrane shows numerous longitudinal folds, and is firmly fixed to the underlying muscle layer. It is lined by stratified squamous epithelium (nonkeratinized). The epithelial cells are rich in glycogen. (The glycogen content shows cyclical variation during the menstrual cycle). The epithelium rests on dense

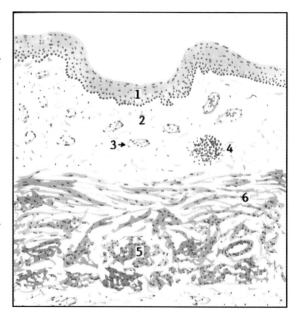

Fig. 19.15. Vagina. 1-Lining of stratified squamous epithelium. 2-Connective tissue. 3-Blood vessels. 4-Lymphoid follicle. 5,6-Muscle coat (longitudinal and circular).

connective tissue (lamina propria) that is highly vascular, many veins being present. The tissue is rich in elastic fibres. No glands are seen in the mucosa, the vaginal surface being kept moist by secretions of glands in the cervix of the uterus.

The muscle coat is made up of an outer layer of longitudinal fibres, and a much thinner inner layer of circular fibres. Many elastic fibres are present among the muscle fibres. The lower end of the vagina is surrounded by striated muscle fibres (of the bulbospongiosus muscle) that form a sphincter for it. The muscle wall is surrounded by an adventitia made up of fibrous tissue containing many elastic fibres.

The vagina is about 8 cm long. It is capable of considerable elongation and distension, this being helped by the rich network of elastic fibres in its wall.

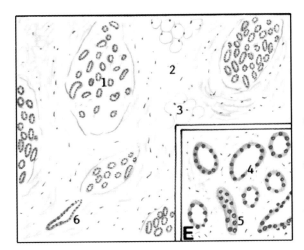

Fig. 19.16. Mammary gland (resting phase).
1, 4-Glandular tissue lined by cuboidal epithelium.
2-Connective tissue. 3-Fat. 5-Duct.

THE FEMALE EXTERNAL GENITALIA

The Labia Minora

These are folds of mucous membrane, made up of a core of connective tissue which is covered by stratified squamous epithelium over. Modified sebaceous glands (not associated with hair follicles) are present.

The Labia Majora

These are folds of skin containing hair, sebaceous glands, and sweat glands. The skin is supported on a core of connective tissue which contains abundant fat.

The Clitoris

The clitoris may be regarded as a miniature penis, with the important difference that the urethra does not pass through it. Two *corpora cavernosa* and a *glans* are present. They contain erectile tissue. The surface of the clitoris is covered by mucous membrane (not skin) which is lined by stratified squamous epithelium. The mucosa is richly supplied with nerves.

THE MAMMARY GLANDS

Although the mammary glands are present in both sexes they remain rudimentary in the male. In the female, they are well developed after puberty. Each breast is a soft rounded elevation present over the pectoral region. The skin over the centre of the elevation shows a darkly pigmented circular area called the *areola*. Overlying the central part of the areola there is a projection called the *nipple*.

Each mammary gland has an outer covering of skin deep to which there are several discrete masses of glandular tissue. These masses are separated (and covered) by considerable quantities of connective tissue and of adipose tissue. The fascia covering the gland is connected to overlying skin by fibrous processes called the *suspensory ligaments* (of Cooper). (In cancer of the breast these processes contract causing pitting of the overlying skin).

The glandular tissue (or mammary gland proper) is made up of 15 to 20 lobes. Each lobe consists of a number of lobules. Each lobe drains into a *lactiferous duct* which opens at the summit of the nipple. Some distance from its termination each lactiferous duct shows a dilation called the *lactiferous sinus*. The smaller ducts are lined by columnar epithelium. In the larger ducts the epithelium has two or three layers of cells. Near their openings on the nipple the lining becomes stratified squamous.

The structure of the glandular elements of the mammary gland varies considerably at different periods of life as follows.

(a) Before the onset of puberty the glandular tissue consists entirely of ducts. Between puberty and the first pregnancy the duct system proliferates. At the end of each duct solid masses of polyhedral cells are formed, but proper alveoli are few or absent. The bulk of the breast consists of connective tissue and fat which widely separate the glandular elements.

(b) During pregnancy the ducts undergo marked proliferation and branching. Their terminal parts develop into proper alveoli. Each lobe is now a compound tubulo-alveolar gland. The ducts and alveoli are surrounded by very cellular periductal tissue. Towards the end of pregnancy the cells of the alveoli start secreting milk and the alveoli become distended.

The development of breast tissue during pregnancy takes place under the influence of hormones produced by the hypophysis cerebri. Cells lining glandular tissue bear receptors for these hormones.

(c) During lactation the glandular tissue is much more prominent than before, and there is a corresponding reduction in the volume of the connective tissue and fat.

(d) When lactation ceases the glandular tissue returns to the resting state. It undergoes atrophy after menopause (i.e., the age after which menstruation ceases).

The cells lining the alveoli vary in appearance in accordance with functional activity. In the 'resting' phase they are cuboidal. When actively producing secretion the cells become columnar. When the secretion begins to be poured into the lumen, distending them, the cells again become cuboidal, but are now much larger. The cells are filled with secretory vacuoles.

With the EM the secretory cells are seen to contain both rough and smooth endoplasmic reticulum, numerous mitochondria, a prominent Golgi complex and lysosomes.

Light microscopic observations suggest that in discharging stored secretion the apical parts of the alveolar cells are shed off. In other words the glands are apocrine (page 53). EM studies have shown that this view is only partly correct. Proteins are present in the cytoplasm in form of membrane bound vesicles. These proteins (which form part of the secretion) are thrown out of the cell by exocytosis (as in merocrine glands). However, fat is stored in the cytoplasm in the form of large globules. As this fat passes out of the cell it carries with it a covering of plasma membrane and a thin layer of cytoplasm. Hence the discharge of fat by the cell is an apocrine process.

Milk secreted for a couple of days following parturition (= childbirth) is called *colostrum*. It is particularly rich in fat globules and in *colostral corpuscles* (the origin of which is controversial). Colostrum is rich in immunoglobulins and provides immunity to the infant against several diseases.

In the resting mammary gland, glandular epithelium is surrounded by an avascular zone containing fibroblasts. It has been claimed that this zone constitutes an *epithelio-stromal junction* which controls passage of materials to glandular cells.

Circular smooth muscle is present in the dermis of the areola. Contraction of this muscle causes erection of the nipple. Many sebaceous glands and apocrine sweat glands are also present in the areola. At the periphery of the areola there are large sebaceous glands that are responsible for the formation of surface elevations called the *tubercles of Montgomery*.

In the male, the mammary gland is rudimentary and consists of ducts that may be represented by solid cords of cells. The ducts do not extend beyond the areola.

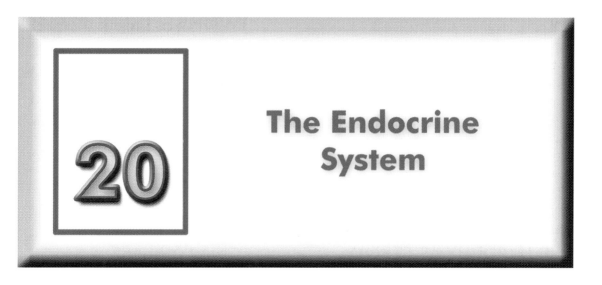

The Endocrine System

Endocrine tissue is made up essentially of cells that produce secretions which are poured directly into blood. The secretions of endocrine cells are called **hormones**. Hormones travel through blood to target cells whose functioning they may influence profoundly. A hormone acts on cells that bear specific receptors for it. Some hormones act only on one organ or on one type of cell, while other hormones may have widespread effects. Along with the autonomic nervous system, the endocrine organs co-ordinate and control the metabolic activities and the internal environment of the body.

Endocrine tissues are highly vascular. The secretory pole of an endocrine cell is towards the wall of a capillary (or sinusoid). [In exocrine glands, the secretory pole is towards the surface over which secretions are discharged].

Endocrine cells are distributed in three different ways.

Some organs are entirely endocrine in function. They are referred to as **endocrine glands** (or **ductless glands**). Those traditionally included under this heading are the hypophysis cerebri (or pituitary), the pineal gland, the thyroid gland, the parathyroid glands, and the suprarenal (or adrenal) glands.

Groups of endocrine cells may be present in organs that have other functions. Several examples of such tissue have been described in previous chapters. They include the islets of the pancreas (page 256), the interstitial cells of the testes (page 281), and the follicles and corpora lutea of the ovaries (page 290). Hormones are also produced by some cells in the kidneys, the thymus, and the placenta. Some authors describe the liver as being partly an endocrine gland (page 252).

Isolated endocrine cells may be distributed in the epithelial lining of an organ. Such cells are seen most typically in the gut. These endocrine cells of the gut have been briefly described on page 247. Similar cells are also present in the epithelium of the respiratory passages. Recent studies have shown that cells in many other locations in the body produce amines that have endocrine functions. Many of these amines also act as neurotransmitters or as neuromodulators. These widely distributed cells are grouped together as the **neuroendocrine system** or the **APUD cell system**.

On the basis of their chemical structure, hormones belong to four main types.

a) **Amino acid derivatives**, for example adrenalin, noradrenalin, and thyroxine.

b) **Small peptides**, for example, encephalin,

vasopressin and thyroid releasing hormone.

c) *Proteins*, for example insulin, parathormone and thyroid stimulating hormone.

d) *Steroids*, for examples progesterone, oestrogens, testosterone and cortisol.

We will come across the various hormones mentioned in subsequent sections.

THE HYPOPHYSIS CEREBRI

The hypophysis cerebri is also called the *pituitary gland*. It is suspended from the floor of the third ventricle (of the brain) by a narrow funnel shaped stalk called the *infundibulum*, and lies in a depression on the upper surface of the sphenoid bone.

The hypophysis cerebri is one of the most important endocrine glands. It produces several hormones some of which profoundly influence the activities of other endocrine tissues. Its own activity is influenced by the hypothalamus, and by the pineal body.

Subdivisions of the Hypophysis Cerebri

The hypophysis cerebri has, in the past, been divided into an anterior part, the *pars anterior*; an intermediate part, the *pars intermedia*; and a posterior part the *pars posterior* (or *pars nervosa*). The pars posterior contains numerous nerve fibres. It is directly continuous with the central core of the infundibular stalk which is made up of nervous tissue. These two parts (pars posterior and infundibular stalk) are together referred to as the *neurohypophysis*. The area in the floor of the third ventricle (tuber cinereum) immediately adjoining the attachment to it of the infundibulum is called the *median eminence*.

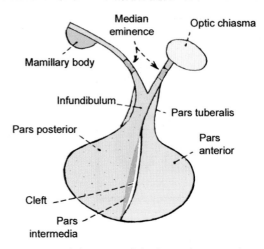

Fig. 20.1. Subdivisions of the hypophysis cerebri.

Some authorities include the median eminence in the neurohypophysis.

The pars anterior (which is also called the *pars distalis*), and the pars intermedia, are both made up of cells having a direct secretory function. They are collectively referred to as the *adenohypophysis*. An extension of the pars anterior surrounds the central nervous core of the infundibulum. Because of its tubular shape this extension is called the *pars tuberalis*. The pars tuberalis is part of the adenohypophysis.

ADENOHYPOPHYSIS

Pars Anterior

The pars anterior consists of cords of cells separated by fenestrated sinusoids. Several types of cells, responsible for the production of different hormones, are present.

Using routine staining procedures the cells of the pars anterior can be divided into *chromophil cells* that have brightly staining granules in their cytoplasm; and *chromophobe cells* in which granules are not prominent. Chromophil cells are further classified as *acidophil* when their granules stain with acid dyes (like eosin or orange

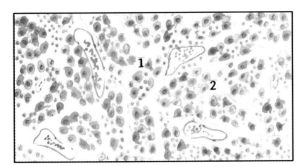

Fig. 20.2. Hypophysis cerebri. Pars anterior.
1-Acidophil. 2-Basophil. Cells in which cytoplasm is
not conspicuous are chromophobes.

G); or *basophil* when the granules stain with basic dyes (like haematoxylin). Basophil granules are also PAS positive. The acidophil cells are often called *alpha cells*, and the basophils are called *beta cells*.

EM examination shows that both acidophil and basophil cells contain abundant dense cored vesicles in the cytoplasm.

Both acidophils and basophils can be divided into sub-types on the basis of the size and shape of the granules in them. These findings have been correlated with those obtained by immunochemical methods: these methods allow cells responsible for production of individual hormones to be recognized. The following functional types of cells have been described.

Types of Acidophil Cells

(1) *Somatotrophs* produce the *somatropic hormone* (also called *somatotropin [STH]*, or *growth hormone [GH]*). This hormone controls body growth, specially before puberty.

(2) *Mammotrophs* (or *lactotrophs*) produce the *mammotropic hormone* (also called *mammotropin*, *prolactin (PRL)*, *lactogenic hormone*, or LTH) which stimulates the growth and activity of the female mammary gland during pregnancy and lactation.

Types of Basophil Cells

(1) The *corticotrophs* (or *corticotropes*) produce the *corticotropic hormone* (also called *adreno-corticotropin* or ACTH). This hormone stimulates the secretion of some hormones of the adrenal cortex (page 311). The staining characters of these cells are intermediate between those of acidophils and basophils. The cells are, therefore, frequently considered to be a variety of acidophils. In the human hypophysis their cytoplasm is weakly basophilic and PAS positive. The granules in the cells contain a complex molecule *of pro-opio-melano-corticotropin*. This is broken down into ACTH and other substances.

> Other corticotropic hormones that have been identified are β-lipotropin (β-LPH), α-melanocyte stimulating hormone (α-MSH)and β-endorphin.

(2) *Thyrotrophs* (or *thyrotropes*) produce the *thyrotropic hormone* (*thyrotropin* or TSH) which stimulates the activity of the thyroid gland.

(3) *Gonadotrophs* (*gonadotropes*, or *delta basophils*) produce two types of hormones each type having a different action in the male and female.

(a) In the female, the first of these hormones stimulates the growth of ovarian follicles. It is, therefore, called the *follicle stimulating hormone* (FSH). It also stimulates the secretion of oestrogens by the ovaries. In the male the same hormone stimulates spermatogenesis.

(b) In the female, the second hormone stimulates the maturation of the corpus luteum, and the secretion by it of progesterone. It is called the *luteinizing hormone* (LH). In the male the same hormone stimulates the production of androgens by the interstitial cells of the testes, and is called the *interstitial cell stimulating hormone* (ICSH).

According to some investigators the two classes of gonadotropic hormones are produced by different cells, but other workers hold that the same cells can produce both the hormones.

Chromophobe Cells

These cells do not stain darkly as they contain very few granules in their cytoplasm. Immunocytochemistry shows that they represent cells similar to the various types of chromophils mentioned above (including mammotrophs, somatotrophs, thyrotrophs, gonadotrophs or corticotrophs).

Some Further Details about cells of the Pars Anterior

1. Somatotrophs constitute about 50%, mammotrophs about 25%, corticotrophs 15-20%, and gonadotrophs about 10% of the cell population of the pars anterior.

2. Somatotrophs are located mainly in the lateral parts of the anterior lobe. Thyrotrophs are concentrated in the anterior, median part; and corticotrophs in the posterior, median part. Gonadotrophs and mammotrophs are scattered throughout the anterior lobe.

3. The size of dense cored vesicles (seen by EM) is highly variable. It is about 400 nm in

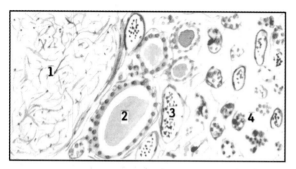

Fig. 20.3. Hypophysis cerebri. Pars posterior (left) and pars intermedia (right). 1-Pars posterior. 2-Vesicle. 3-Capillary. 4-Clumps of cells (including some acidophils and basophils).

somatotrophs, about 300 nm in mammotrophs, 250-700 nm in corticotrophs and 150-400 nm in gonadotrophs.

Pars Tuberalis

The pars tuberalis consists mainly of undifferentiated cells. Some acidophil and basophil cells are also present.

Pars Intermedia

This is poorly developed in the human hypophysis. In ordinary preparations the most conspicuous feature is the presence of colloid filled vesicles (Atlas: 35B). These vesicles are remnants of the pouch of Rathke. Beta cells, other secretory cells, and chromophobe cells are present. Some cells of the pars intermedia produce the ***melanocyte stimulating hormone*** (MSH) which causes increased pigmentation of the skin. Other cells produce ACTH. ***Endorphins*** are present in the cytoplasm of secretory cells.

The secretion of hormones from the adenohypophysis is under control of the hypothalamus as described on page 289.

NEUROHYPOPHYSIS

Pars Posterior

The pars posterior consists of numerous unmyelinated nerve fibres which are the axons of neurons located in the hypothalamus (Atlas: 35B). Most of the nerve fibres arise in the supraoptic and paraventricular nuclei. Situated between these axons there are supporting cells of a special type called ***pituicytes***. These cells have long dendritic processes many of which lie parallel to the nerve fibres. The axons descending into the pars posterior from the hypothalamus end in terminals closely related to capillaries.

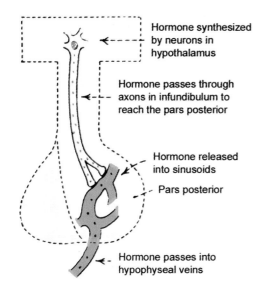

Fig. 20.4. Scheme to show the relationship of the hypothalamus and the pars posterior of the hypophysis cerebri.

The pars posterior of the hypophysis is associated with the release into the blood of two hormones. One of these is ***vasopressin*** (also called the ***antidiuretic hormone*** or ADH). This hormone controls reabsorption of water by kidney tubules. The second hormone is oxytocin. It controls the contraction of smooth muscle of the uterus and also of the mammary gland.

It is now known that these two hormones are not produced in the hypophysis cerebri at all. They are synthesized in neurons located mainly in the supraoptic and paraventricular nuclei of the hypothalamus. Vasopressin is produced mainly in the supraoptic nucleus, and oxytocin in the paraventricular nucleus. These secretions (which are bound with a glycoprotein called ***neurophysin***) pass down the axons of the neurons concerned, through the infundibulum into the pars posterior. Here they are released into the capillaries of the region and enter the general circulation.

Blood Supply of the Hypophysis Cerebri

The hypophysis cerebri is supplied by superior and inferior branches arising from the internal carotid arteries. Some branches also arise from the anterior and posterior cerebral arteries. The inferior hypophyseal arteries are distributed mainly to the pars posterior. Branches from the superior set of arteries supply the median eminence and infundibulum. Here they end in capillary plexuses from which portal vessels arise. These portal vessels descend through the infundibular stalk and end in the sinusoids of the pars anterior. The sinusoids are drained by veins that end in neighbouring venous sinuses.

It will be noticed that the above arrangement is unusual in that two sets of capillaries intervene between the arteries and veins. One of these is in the median eminence and the upper part of the infundibulum. The second set of capillaries

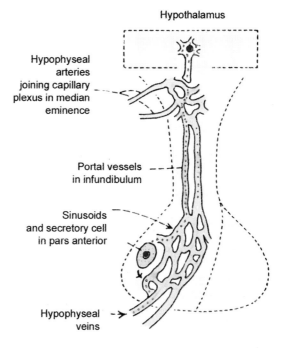

Fig. 20.5. Scheme to show the hypothalamo-hypophyseal portal circulation.

is represented by the sinusoids of the pars anterior. This arrangement is referred to as the ***hypothalamo-hypophyseal portal system***. (Compare with *the* portal system). The functional significance of this system is described below.

> The vessels descending through the infundibular stalk are easily damaged in severe head injuries. This leads to loss of function in the anterior lobe of the hypophysis cerebri.

Control of Secretion of Hormones of the Adenohypophysis

The secretion of hormones by the adenohypophysis takes place under higher control of neurons in the hypothalamus, notably those in the median eminence and in the infundibular nucleus. The axons of these neurons end in relation to capillaries in the median eminence and in the upper part of the infundibulum.

Different neurons produce specific ***releasing factors*** (or releasing hormones) for each hormone of the adenohypophysis. [For details of hypothalamic nuclei and the releasing factors produced by them see the author's TEXTBOOK OF HUMAN NEUROANATOMY]. These factors are released into the capillaries mentioned above. Portal vessels arising from the capillaries carry these factors to the pars anterior of the hypophysis. Here they stimulate the release of appropriate hormones. Some factors inhibit the release of hormones. The synthesis and discharge of releasing factors by the neurons concerned is under nervous control. As these neurons serve as intermediaries between nervous impulses and hormone secretion they have been referred to as ***neuroendocrine transducers***. Some cells called ***tanycytes***, present in ependyma, may transport releasing factors from neurons into the CSF, or from CSF to blood capillaries. They may thus play a role in control of the adenohypophysis.

Recent studies indicate that circulation in relation to the hypophysis cerebri may be more complex than presumed earlier. Some points of interest are as follows.

(**a**) The entire neurohypophysis (from the median eminence to the pars posterior) is permeated by a continuous network of capillaries in which blood may flow ***in either direction***. The capillaries provide a route through which hormones released in the pars posterior can travel back to the hypothalamus, and into CSF.

(**b**) Some veins draining the pars posterior pass into the adenohypophysis. Secretions by the adenohypophysis may thus be controlled not only from the median eminence, but by the entire neurohypophysis.

(**c**) Blood flow in veins connecting the pars anterior and pars posterior may be reversible providing a feed back from adenohypophysis to the neurohypophysis.

THE PINEAL GLAND

The pineal gland (or pineal body) is a small piriform structure present in relation to the posterior wall of the third ventricle of the brain. It is also called the ***epiphysis cerebri***. The pineal has for long been regarded as a vestigial organ of no functional importance. (Hence the name pineal body). However, it is now known to be an endocrine gland of great importance.

Sections of the pineal gland stained with haematoxylin and eosin reveal very little detail. The organ appears to be a mass of cells amongst which there are blood capillaries and nerve fibres. A distinctive feature of the pineal in such sections is the presence of irregular masses made up mainly of calcium salts. These masses constitute

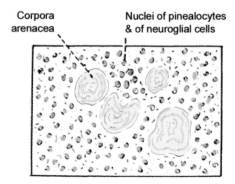

Fig. 20.6. Drawing of a section of the pineal body as seen with a light microscope.

the *corpora arenacea* or *brain sand*. The organ is covered by connective tissue (representing the piamater) from which septa pass into its interior.

With the use of special methods (including silver impregnation, EM, histochemical techniques) the following facts are now known about the pineal gland.

1. The organ is made up mainly of cells called *pinealocytes*. Each cell has a polyhedral body containing a spherical oval or irregular nucleus. The cell body gives off long processes with expanded *terminal buds* that end in relation to the wall of capillaries, or in relation to the ependyma of the third ventricle. The cell bodies of pinealocytes contain both granular and agranular endoplasmic reticulum, a well developed Golgi complex, and many mitochondria. An organelle of unusual structure made up of groups of microfibrils and perforated lamellae may be present (*canaliculate lamellar bodies*). The processes of pinealocytes contain numerous mitochondria. Apart from other organelles the terminal buds contain vesicles in which there are monamines and polypeptide hormones. The neurotransmitter gamma-amino-butyric acid is also present.

2. The pinealocytes are separated from one another by neuroglial cells that resemble astrocytes in structure (page 165).

3. The nerve fibres present in the pineal are sympathetic (adrenergic, unmyelinated). Release of pineal secretions appears to require sympathetic stimulation.

4. The pinealocytes produce a number of hormones (chemically indolamines or polypeptides). These hormones have an important regulating influence (chiefly inhibitory) on many other endocrine organs. The organs influenced include the adenohypophysis, the neurohypophysis, the thyroid, the parathyroids, the adrenal cortex and medulla, the gonads, and the pancreatic islets. The hormones of the pineal body reach the hypophysis both through the blood and through the CSF. Pineal hormones may also influence the adenohypophysis by inhibiting production of releasing factors.

The best known hormone of the pineal gland is the amino acid *melatonin* (so called because it causes changes in skin colour in amphibia). Large concentrations of melatonin are present in the pineal gland. Considerable amounts of 5-

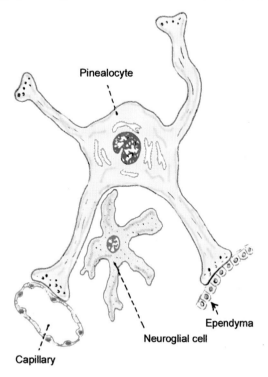

Fig. 20.7. Scheme to show some features of a pinealocyte.

hydroxytryptamine (serotonin), which is a precursor of melatonin, are also present. The presence of related enzymes has been demonstrated.

5. The synthesis and discharge of melatonin is remarkably influenced by exposure of the animal to light, the pineal gland being most active in darkness. The neurological pathways concerned involve the hypothalamus and the sympathetic nerves. Because of this light mediated response, the pineal gland may act as a kind of biological clock which may produce circadian rhythms (variations following a 24 hour cycle) in various parameters.

It has been suggested that the suprachiasmatic nucleus of the hypothalamus plays an important role in the cyclic activity of the pineal gland. This nucleus receives fibres from the retina. In turn it projects to the tegmental reticular nuclei (located in the brainstem). Reticulospinal fibres arising in these nuclei influence the sympathetic preganglionic neurons located in the first thoracic segment of the spinal cord. Axons of these neurons reach the superior cervical ganglion from where the **nervus conarii** arises and supplies the pineal gland.

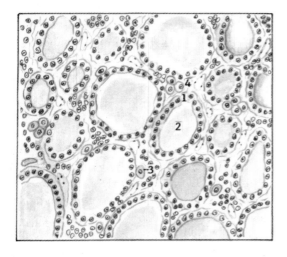

Fig. 20.8. Thyroid gland. 1-Follicle lined by cuboidal epithelium. 2-Colloid. 3-Parafollicular cells. 4-Connective tissue.

6. It has often been stated in the past that the pineal gland degenerates with age. The corpora arenacea were considered to be signs of degeneration. Recent studies show that the organ does not degenerate with age. The corpora arenacea are now regarded as by-products of active secretory activity. It has been postulated that polypeptide hormones first exist in the form of complexes with a carrier protein called **neuroepiphysin**. When hormones are released from the complex the carrier protein combines with calcium ions and is deposited as brain sand.

THE THYROID GLAND

Elementary Histology

The thyroid gland is covered by a fibrous capsule. Septa extending into the gland from the capsule divide it into lobules. On microscopic examination each lobule is seen to be made up of an aggregation of **follicles**. Each follicle is lined by **follicular cells**, that rest on a basement membrane. The follicle has a cavity which is filled by a homogeneous material called **colloid** (which appears pink in haematoxylin and eosin stained sections). The spaces between the follicles are filled by a stroma made up of delicate connective tissue in which there are numerous capillaries and lymphatics. The capillaries lie in close contact with the walls of follicles.

Apart from follicular cells the thyroid gland contains C-cells (or **parafollicular cells**) which intervene (here and there) between the follicular cells and the basement membrane. They may also lie in the intervals between the follicles. Connective tissue stroma surrounding the follicles contain a dense capillary plexus, lymphatic capillaries and sympathetic nerves.

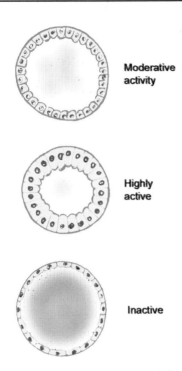

Fig. 20.9. Variations in appearance of thyroid follicles at different levels of activity.

The Follicular Cells

1. The follicular cells vary in shape depending on the level of their activity. Normally (at an average level of activity) the cells are cuboidal, and the colloid in the follicles is moderate in amount. When inactive (or resting) the cells are flat (squamous) and the follicles are distended with abundant colloid. Lastly, when the cells are highly active they become columnar and colloid is scanty. Different follicles may show differing levels of activity.

2. The follicular cells secrete two hormones that influence the rate of metabolism. Iodine is an essential constituent of these hormones. One hormone containing three atoms of iodine in each molecule is called *triiodothyronine* or T3. The second hormone containing four atoms of iodine in each molecule is called tetraiodothyronine, T4, or thyroxine. T3 is much

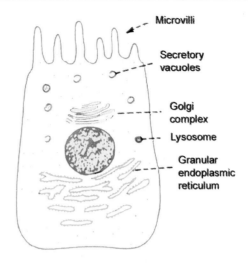

Fig. 20.10. Ultrastructure of a follicular cell of the thyroid gland.

more active than T4.

3. The activity of follicular cells is influenced by the thyroid stimulating hormone (TSH or thyrotropin) produced by the hypophysis cerebri (page 287). There is some evidence to indicate that their activity may also be increased by sympathetic stimulation.

4. With the EM a follicular cell shows the presence of apical microvilli, abundant granular endoplasmic reticulum, and a prominent supranuclear Golgi complex. Lysosomes, microtubules and microfilaments are also present. The apical part of the cell contains many secretory vacuoles.

5. The synthesis and release of thyroid hormone takes place in two phases. In the first phase thyroglobulin (a glycoprotein) is synthesized by granular endoplasmic reticulum and is packed into secretory vacuoles in the Golgi complex. The vacuoles travel to the luminal surface where they release thyroglobulin into the follicular cavity by exocytosis. Here the thyroglobulin combines with iodine to form colloid. Colloid is iodinated thyroglobulin.

In the second phase particles of colloid are

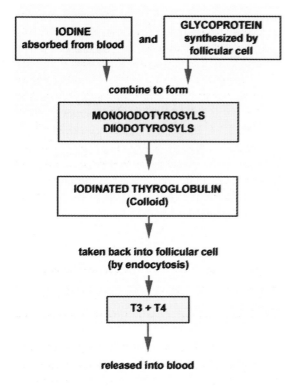

Fig. 20.11. Some steps in the formation of hormones by the thyroid gland.

taken back into the cell by endocytosis. Within the cell the iodinated thyroglobulin is acted upon by enzymes (present in lysosomes) releasing hormones T3 and T4 which pass basally through the cell and are released into blood.

Hormone produced in the thyroid gland is mainly T4 (output of T3 being less than 10%). In the liver, the kidneys (and some other tissues) T4 is converted to T3 by removal of one iodine molecule. T3 and T4 circulating in blood are bound to a protein (thyroxine binding globulin, TBG). The bound form of hormone is not active.

The C-Cells (Parafollicular Cells)

They are also called *clear cells*, or *light cells*. The cells are polyhedral, with oval eccentric nuclei. Typically, they lie between the follicular cells and their basement membrane. They may, however, lie between adjoining follicular cells; but they do not reach the lumen. In some species many parafollicular cells may lie in the connective tissue between the follicles and may be arranged in groups. With the EM the cells show well developed granular endoplasmic reticulum, Golgi complexes, numerous mitochondria, and membrane bound secretory granules.

C-cells secrete the hormone *thyro-calcitonin*. This hormone has an action opposite to that of the parathyroid hormone on calcium metabolism. This hormone comes into play when serum calcium level is high. It tends to lower the calcium level by suppressing release of calcium ions from bone. This is achieved by suppressing bone resorption by osteoclasts.

C-cells share features of the APUD cell system and are included in this system (page 313).

For development and anomalies of the thyroid gland see the author's HUMAN EMBRYOLOGY.

THE PARATHYROID GLANDS

The parathyroid glands are so called because they lie in close relationship to the thyroid gland. Normally, there are two parathyroid glands, one superior and one inferior, on either side; there being four glands in all. Sometimes there may be as many as eight parathyroids.

Each gland has a connective tissue capsule from which some septa extend into the gland substance. Within the gland a network of reticular fibres supports the cells. Many fat cells (adipocytes) are present in the stroma.

The parenchyma of the gland is made up of cells that are arranged in cords. Numerous sinusoids

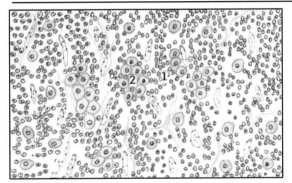

Fig. 20.12. Parathyroid gland. 1-Chief cells (only nuclei seen). 2-Oxyphil cells with pink cytoplasm. Note numerous capillaries.

lie in close relationship to the cells.

The cells of the parathyroid glands are of two main types: *chief cells* (or *principal cells*), and *oxyphil cells* (or *eosinophil cells*). The chief cells are much more numerous than the oxyphil cells. The latter are absent in the young and appear a little before the age of puberty.

With the light microscope the chief cells are seen to be small round cells with vesicular nuclei. Their cytoplasm is clear and either mildly eosinophil or basophil. Sometimes the cell accumulates glycogen and lipids and looks 'clear', In contrast the oxyphil cells are much larger and contain granules that stain strongly with acid dyes. Their nuclei are smaller and stain more intensely than those of chief cells. Three types of chief cells (light, dark, and clear) have been described. Cells intermediate between the chief cells and the oxyphil cells are also described.

The chief cells produce the parathyroid hormone (or parathormone). This hormone tends to increase the level of serum calcium by:

(a) increasing bone resorption through stimulation of osteoclastic activity;

(b) increasing calcium resorption from renal tubules (and inhibiting phosphate resorption);

(c) enhancing calcium absorption from the gut.

With the EM active chief cells are seen to have abundant granular endoplasmic reticulum and well developed Golgi complexes. Small secretory granules are seen, specially in parts of the cytoplasm near adjacent blood sinusoids. These features become much less prominent in inactive cells. Both active and inactive cells contain glycogen, the amount of which is greater in inactive cells. In the normal parathyroid the number of inactive cells is greater than that of active cells.

With the EM it is seen that the granules of oxyphil cells are really mitochondria, large numbers of which are present in the cytoplasm. True secretory granules are not present. The functions of oxyphil cells are unknown.

THE SUPRARENAL GLANDS

As implied by their name the right and left suprarenal glands lie in the abdomen, close to the upper poles of the corresponding kidneys. In many animals they do not occupy a 'supra' renal position, but lie near the kidneys. They are, therefore, commonly called the *adrenal glands*.

Each suprarenal gland is covered by a connective tissue capsule from which septa extend into the gland substance. The gland is made up of two functionally distinct parts: a superficial part called the *cortex*, and a deeper part called the *medulla*. The volume of the cortex is about ten times that of the medulla.

The Suprarenal Cortex

Layers of the Cortex

The suprarenal cortex is made up of cells arranged in cords. Sinusoids intervene between the cords. On the basis of the arrangement of its cells the cortex can be divided into three layers as follows.

(a) The outermost layer is called the *zona*

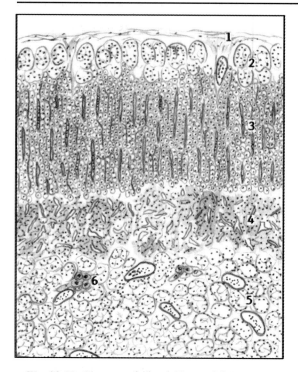

Fig. 20.13. Suprarenal gland. Upper 2/3 is cortex, lower 1/3 is medulla. 1-Capsule. 2-Zona glomerulosa. 3-Zona fasciculata. 4-Zona reticularis. 5-Medulla. 6-Sympathetic neurons.

glomerulosa. Here the cells are arranged as inverted U-shaped formations, or acinus-like groups. The zona glomerulosa constitutes the outer one-fifth of the cortex.

(**b**) The next zone is called the *zona fasciculata*. Here the cells are arranged in straight columns, two cell thick. Sinusoids intervene between the columns. This layer forms the middle three fifths of the cortex.

(**c**) The innermost layer of the cortex (inner one fifth) is called the *zona reticularis*. It is so called because it is made up of cords that branch and anastomose with each other to form a kind of reticulum.

Light Microscopic Structure of

Cells of the Cortex

With the light microscope the cells of the zona glomerulosa are seen to be small, polyhedral or columnar, with basophilic cytoplasm and deeply staining nuclei.

The cells of the zona fasciculata are large, polyhedral, with basophilic cytoplasm and vesicular nuclei. The cells of the zona fasciculata are very rich in lipids which can be demonstrated by suitable stains. With routine methods the lipids are dissolved out during the processing of tissue, giving the cells an 'empty' or vacuolated appearance. These cells also contain considerable amounts of vitamin C.

The cells of the zona reticularis are similar to those of the zona fasciculata, but the lipid content is less. Their cytoplasm is often eosinophilic. The cells often contain brown pigment.

C. EM Structure of Cells of the Cortex

With the EM the cells in all layers of the cortex are characterized by the presence of abundant agranular (or smooth) endoplasmic reticulum. The Golgi complex is best developed in cells of the zona fasciculata. Mitochondria are elongated in the glomerulosa, spherical in the fasciculata, and

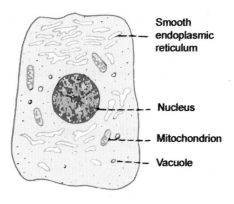

Fig. 20.14. Some features of ultrastructure of a cell from the adrenal cortex.

unusual with tubular cisternae (instead of the usual plates) in the reticularis.

D. Hormones produced by the Suprarenal Cortex

(**a**) The cells of the zona glomerulosa produce the mineralocorticoid hormones **aldosterone** and **deoxycorticosterone**. These hormones influence the electrolyte and water balance of the body. The secretion of aldosterone is influenced by renin secreted by juxta-glomerular cells of the kidney (page 258). The secretion of hormones by the zona glomerulosa appears to be largely independent of the hypophysis cerebri.

(**b**) The cells of the zona fasciculata produce the glucocorticoids **cortisone** and **cortisol** (**dihydrocortisone**). These hormones have widespread effects including those on carbohydrate metabolism and protein metabolism. They appear to decrease antibody responses and have an anti-inflammatory effect.

The zona fascicularis also produces small amounts of **dehydroepiandrosterone** (DHA) which is an androgen.

(**c**) The cells of the zona reticularis also produce some glucocorticoids; and sex hormones, both oestrogens and androgens.

The suprarenal cortex is essential for life. Removal or destruction leads to death unless the hormones produced by it are supplied artificially. Increase in secretion of corticosteroids causes dramatic reduction in number of lymphocytes.

The Suprarenal Medulla

Both functionally and embryologically the medulla of the suprarenal gland is distinct from the cortex. When a suprarenal gland is fixed in a solution containing a salt of chromium (e.g., potassium dichromate) the cells of the medulla

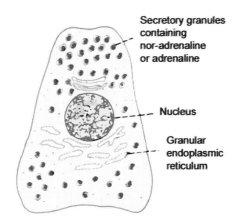

Fig. 20.15. Some features of ultrastructure of a cell from the adrenal medulla.

show yellow granules in their cytoplasm. This is called the **chromaffin reaction**, and the cells that give a positive reaction are called **chromaffin cells**. The cells of the suprarenal cortex do not give this reaction.

The medulla is made up of groups or columns of cells. The cell groups or columns are separated by wide sinusoids. The cells are columnar or polyhedral and have a basophilic cytoplasm. Functionally, the cells of the suprarenal medulla are considered to be modified postganglionic sympathetic neurons. Like typical postganglionic sympathetic neurons they secrete noradrenalin (norepinephrine) and adrenalin (epinephrine) into the blood. This secretion takes place mainly at times of stress (fear, anger) and results in widespread effects similar to those of stimulation of the sympathetic nervous system (e.g., increase in heart rate and blood pressure).

With the EM the cells of the adrenal medulla are seen to contain abundant granular endoplasmic reticulum (in contrast to the agranular endoplasmic reticulum of cortical cells), and a prominent Golgi complex. The cells also contain membrane bound secretory vesicles. In some cells these vesicles are small and electron dense while in others they are large and not so dense. The former are contain noradrenalin and the latter adrenalin.

The suprarenal medulla is now included in the APUD cell system (page 313). In contrast to the suprarenal cortex the medulla is not essential for life as its functions can be performed by other chromaffin tissues (see below).

SOME OTHER ORGANS HAVING ENDOCRINE FUNCTIONS

Paraganglia

Aggregations of cells similar to those of the adrenal medulla are to be found at various sites. They are collectively referred to as paraganglia because most of them are present in close relation to autonomic ganglia. The cells of paraganglia give a positive chromaffin reaction, receive a preganglionic sympathetic innervation, and have secretory granules containing catecholamines in their cytoplasm.

Like the cells of the adrenal medulla paraganglia are believed to develop from cells of the neural crest. Paraganglia are richly vascularized. They are regarded as endocrine glands that serve as alternative sites for the production of catecholamines in the fetus, and in early postnatal life, when the adrenal medulla is not yet fully differentiated. Because of their histochemical and ultrastructural features the cells of paraganglia are included in the APUD cell system (page 313). Most of the paraganglia retrogress with age, but some persist into adult life.

Cells similar to those of paraganglia are also present within some sympathetic ganglia. (They are called SIF or small intensely fluorescent cells). Here they are believed to act as interneurons.

Some workers include the para-aortic bodies and carotid bodies described below amongst paraganglia.

Para-aortic bodies

These are two elongated bodies that lie, one on each side of the aorta, near the origin of the inferior mesenteric artery. The two masses may be united to each other by a band passing across the aorta.

These bodies have a structure similar to that of the adrenal medulla. The cells secrete noradrenalin. The aortic bodies retrogress with age.

The Carotid Bodies

These are small oval structures, present one on each side of the neck, at the bifurcation of the common carotid artery (i.e., near the carotid sinus). The main function of the carotid bodies is that they act as chemoreceptors that monitor the oxygen and carbon dioxide levels in blood. They reflexly control the rate and depth of respiration through respiratory centres located in the brainstem. In addition to this function the carotid bodies are also believed to have an endocrine function.

The carotid bodies contain a network of capillaries in the intervals between which there are several types of cells. The carotid bodies have a rich innervation (see below).

The most conspicuous cells of the carotid body are called *glomus cells* (or type I cells). These are large cells that have several similarities to neurons as follows.

(a) They give off dendritic processes.

(b) Their cytoplasm contains membrane bound granules which contain a number of neuropeptides. In the human carotid body the most prominent peptide present is encephalin. Others present include dopamine, serotonin, catecholamines, VIP and substance P.

(c) The cells are in synaptic contact with afferent nerve terminals of the glossopharyngeal nerve. Chemoreceptor impulses pass through these

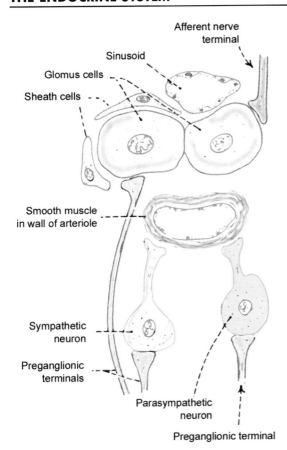

Fig. 20.16. Scheme to show some features of the structure of the carotid body.

fibres to the brain. Some glomus cells also show synaptic connections with the endings of preganglionic sympathetic fibres, and with other glomus cells.

(d) The organisation of endoplasmic reticulum in them shows similarities to that of Nissl substance.

(e) They arc surrounded by sheath cells that resemble neuroglial elements. Because of these similarities to neurons, and because of the possibility that the cells release dopamine (and possibly other substances) they are sometimes described as neuroendocrine cells (and are included in the APUD cell category). The exact significance of the glomus cells, and of their nervous connections, is not understood at present.

They could possibly be sensory receptors sensitive to oxygen and carbon dioxide tension. Dopamine released by them may influence the sensitivity of chemoreceptor nerve endings. They may also serve as interneurons.

Apart from the glomus cells other cells present in the carotid bodies are as follows.

(a) Sheath cells (or type II cells) that surround the glomus cells.

(b) A few sympathetic and parasympathetic postganglionic neurons.

(c) Endothelial cells of blood vessels, and muscle cells in the walls of arterioles.

(d) Some connective tissue cells.

The carotid body is richly innervated as follows.

(1) Afferent nerve terminals from the glossopharyngeal nerve form synapses with glomus cells.

(2) Preganglionic sympathetic and parasympathetic fibres end on the corresponding ganglion cells. Some preganglionic sympathetic fibres end by synapsing with glomus cells.

(3) Postganglionic fibres arising from the sympathetic and parasympathetic nerve cells within the carotid body innervate muscle in the walls of arterioles.

The precise mechanism by which the carotid bodies respond to changes in oxygen and carbon dioxide tension is not understood. It is not certain as to which cells, or nerve terminals are responsible for this function.

THE DIFFUSE NEUROENDOCRINE OR APUD CELL SYSTEM

Apart from the discrete endocrine organs considered in this chapter there are groups of endocrine cells scattered in various parts of the body. These cells share some common characteristics with each other, and also with the cells of some discrete endocrine organs. All these cells take up precursor substances from the circulation and process them (by decarboxylation) to form amines or peptides. They are, therefore, included in what is called the *APUD* (Amine Precursor Uptake and Decarboxylation) *cell system*. These peptides or amines serve as hormones. Many of them also function as neurotransmitters. Hence the APUD cell system is also called the *diffuse neuroendocrine system*. The cells of this system contain spherical or oval membrane bound granules with a dense core. There is an electronlucent halo around the dense core.

Some of the cells included in the APUD or diffuse neuroendocrine systems also give a positive chromaffin reaction (page 311). They were earlier referred to as cells of the *chromaffin system*. However, they appear to be closely related functionally to other cells that are not chromaffin, and the tendency is to consider all these cells under the common category of diffuse neuroendocrine cells.

The diffuse neuroendocrine system is regarded as representing a link between the autonomic nervous system on the one hand, and the organs classically recognized as endocrine on the other, as it shares some features of both. The effects of the amines or peptides produced by the cells of the system are sometimes 'local' (like those of neurotransmitters) and sometimes widespread (like those of better known hormones).

The list of cell types included in the APUD cell system, as well as of their secretions, is large. As stated above even some discrete endocrine glands are now included under this heading. A partial list is given below.

1. Various cells of the adenohypophysis producing the hormones enumerated on page 301.

2. Neurons in the hypothalamus that synthesize the hormones of the neurohypophysis (oxytocin, vasopressin); and the cells that synthesize releasing factors controlling the secretion of hormones by the adenohypophysis.

3. The chief cells of the parathyroid glands producing parathyroid hormone.

4. The C- cells (parafollicular cells) of the thyroid, producing calcitonin.

5. Cells of the adrenal medulla (along with some outlying chromaffin tissues) that secrete adrenalin and noradrenalin. These include the SIF cells of sympathetic ganglia (page 312).

6. Cells of the gastro-entero-pancreatic endocrine system described on page 247. This system includes cells of pancreatic islets producing insulin, glucagon and some other amines. It also includes endocrine cells scattered in the epithelium of the stomach and intestines producing one or more of the following: 5-hydroxytryptamine, glucagon, dopamine, somatostatin, substance P, motilin, gastrin, cholecystokinin, secretin, vasoactive intestinal polypeptide (VIP), and some other peptides (page 246).

7. Glomus cells of the carotid bodies producing dopamine and noradrenalin.

8. Melanocytes of the skin producing promelanin.

9. Some cells in the pineal gland, the placenta, and modified myocytes of the heart called *myoendocrine cells.*

10. Renin producing cells of the kidneys.

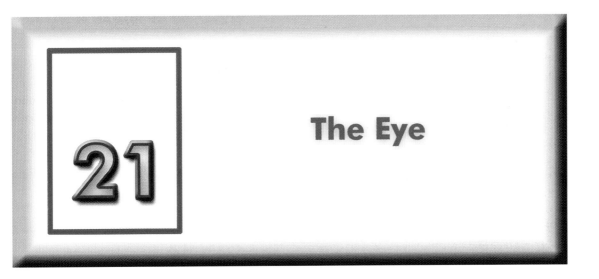

The Eye

21

Preliminary Remarks

The eyes are peripheral organs for vision. Each eyeball is like a camera. It has a *lens* which produces images of objects that we look at. The images fall on a light sensitive membrane called the *retina*. Cells in the retina convert light images into nervous impulses which pass through the optic nerve, and other parts of the visual pathway, to reach visual areas in the cerebral cortex. It is in the cortex that vision is actually perceived.

The main parts of the eyeball are shown (as seen in section) in Fig. 21.1. The outer wall of the eyeball is formed (in its posterior five sixths) by a thick white opaque membrane called the *sclera*. In the anterior one sixth of the eyeball the sclera is replaced by a transparent disc called the *cornea*. The cornea is convex forwards. Deep to the sclera there is a *vascular coat* (or *uvea*), which has the following subdivisions. The part lining the inner surface of most of the sclera is thin and is called the *choroid*. Near the junction of the sclera with the cornea the vascular coat is thick and forms the *ciliary body*. The ciliary body is in the form of a ring. The 'inner' margin of the ring is continuous with the peripheral margin of a pigmented diaphragm which is called the *iris*. The iris lies between the cornea (in front) and the lens (behind). In the centre of the iris there is an aperture called the *pupil*. The retina forms the inner-most layer of the eyeball.

The space between the iris and the cornea is called the *anterior chamber*, while the space between the iris and the front of the lens is called

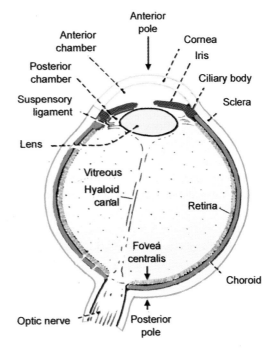

Fig. 21.1. Section across the eyeball to show its main parts.

the *posterior chamber*. These chambers are filled by a fluid called the *aqueous humour*. The part of the eyeball behind the lens is filled by a jelly-like substance called the *vitreous body*. For further details of the general structure of the eyeball see the author's TEXTBOOK OF HUMAN ANATOMY.

forms the *fibrous tunic* of the eyeball. Apart from providing protection to delicate structures within the eye, it resists intraocular pressure and maintains the shape of the eyeball. Its smooth external surface allows eye movements to take place with ease. The sclera also provides attachment to muscles that move the eyeball.

THE SCLERA

The sclera consists of white fibrous tissue (collagen). Some elastic fibres, and connective tissue cells (mainly fibroblasts) are also present. Some of the cells are pigmented.

Externally, the sclera is covered in its anterior part by the ocular conjunctiva, and posteriorly by a fascial sheath (or *episclera*). The deep surface of the sclera is separated from the choroid by the *perichoroidal space*. Delicate connective tissue present in this space constitutes the *suprachoroid lamina* (or *lamina fusca*, page 318).

Anteriorly, the sclera becomes continuous with the cornea at the *corneoscleral junction* (also called *sclerocorneal junction* or *limbus*). A circular channel called the *sinus venosus sclerae* (or *canal of Schlemm*) is located in the sclera just behind the corneoscleral junction (Fig. 21.2). A triangular mass of scleral tissue projects towards the cornea just medial to this sinus. This projection is called the *scleral spur*.

The optic nerve is attached to the back of the eyeball a short distance medial to the posterior pole. Here the sclera is perforated like a sieve, and the area is, therefore, called the *lamina cribrosa*. Bundles of optic nerve fibres pass through the perforations of the lamina cribrosa.

The sclera (along with the cornea) collectively

THE CORNEA

The cornea is made up five layers (Fig. 21.3).

(**1**) The outermost layer is of non-keratinized stratified squamous epithelium (corneal epithelium). The cells in the deepest layer of the

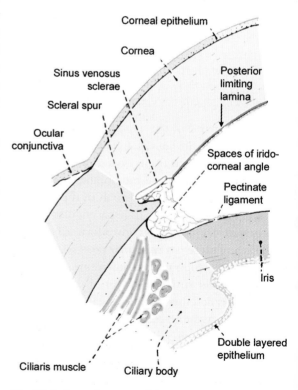

Fig. 21.2. Some features of the eyeball to be seen at the junction of the cornea with the sclera.

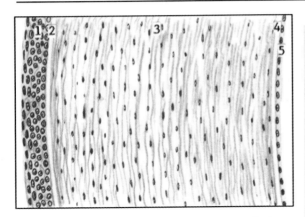

Fig. 21.3. Section through cornea. 1-Stratified squamous epithelium. 2-Anterior limiting lamina. 3-Substantia propria. 4-Posterior limiting lamina. 5-Cuboidal epithelium.

epithelium are columnar; in the middle layers they are polygonal; and in the superficial layers they are flattened. The cells are arranged with great regularity.

> With the EM the cells on the superficial surface of the epithelium show projections either in the form of microvilli or folds of plasma membrane. These folds are believed to play an important role in retaining a film of fluid over the surface of the cornea.

> At the periphery of the cornea the epithelium becomes continuous with that lining the ocular conjunctiva. The corneal epithelium regenerates rapidly after damage.

(2) The corneal epithelium rests on the *anterior limiting lamina* (also called *Bowman's membrane*). With the light microscope this lamina appears to be structureless, but with the EM it is seen to be made up of fine collagen fibrils embedded in matrix.

(3) Most of the thickness of the cornea is formed by the *substantia propria* (or *corneal stroma*). The substantia propria is made up of collagen fibres embedded in a ground substance containing sulphated glycosaminoglycans.

The collagen fibres are of Type II collagen (page 59). They are arranged with great regularity and form lamellae. The fibres within one lamellus are parallel to one another, but the fibres in adjoining lamellae run in different directions forming obtuse angles with each other. The transparency of the cornea is because of the regular arrangement of fibres, and because of the fact that the fibres and the ground substance have the same refractive index.

Fibroblasts are present in the substantia propria. They appear to be flattened in vertical sections through the cornea, but are seen to be star-shaped on surface view. They are also called *keratocytes* or *corneal corpuscles*.

(4) Deep to the substantia propria there is a thin homogeneous layer called the *posterior limiting lamina* (or *Descemet's membrane*). It is a true basement membrane.

At the margin of the cornea the posterior limiting membrane becomes continuous with fibres that form a network in the angle between the cornea and the iris (*irido-corneal angle*). The spaces between the fibres of the network are called the *spaces of the irido-corneal angle*. Some of the fibres of the network pass onto the iris as the *pectinate ligament* (Fig. 21.2).

(5) The posterior surface of the cornea is lined by a single layer of flattened cells that constitute the *endothelium of the anterior chamber*. This layer is in contact with the aqueous humour of the anterior chamber.

> The endothelial cells are adapted for transport of ions. They possess numerous mitochondria. They are united to neighbouring cells by desmosomes and by occluding junctions. The cells pump out excessive fluid from cornea, and thus ensure its transparency.

The cornea has no blood vessels or lymphatics. It receives nutrition from vessels around its periphery. The cornea has a rich nerve supply. The nerve fibres, which are non-myelinated, form

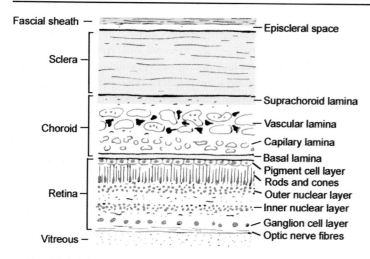

Fig. 21.4. Scheme to show the various layers of the eyeball.
Compare with Fig. 21.5.

a plexus deep to the corneal epithelium, and in the substantia propria. Free nerve endings are present in the epithelium.

THE VASCULAR COAT OR UVEA

We have seen that deep to the sclera there is a vascular coat which consists of the choroid, the ciliary body and the iris. These are considered below.

THE CHOROID

The choroid consists of (a) the **choroid proper**, (b) the **suprachoroid lamina** which separates the choroid proper from the sclera, and (c) the **basal lamina (membrane of Bruch)** which intervenes between the choroid proper and the retina (Figs. 21.4, 21.5).

The Choroid Proper

The choroid proper consists of a network of blood vessels supported by connective tissue in which many pigmented cells are present, giving the choroid a dark colour. This colour darkens the interior of the eyeball. The pigment also prevents reflection of light within the eyeball. Both these factors help in formation of sharp images on the retina.

The choroid proper is made up of an outer **vascular lamina** containing small arteries and veins, and lymphatics; and an inner **capillary lamina** (or **choroidocapillaris**). The connective tissue supporting the vessels of the vascular lamina is the **choroidal stroma**. Apart from collagen fibres it contains melanocytes, lymphocytes and mast cells. The capillary lamina is not pigmented. Nutrients diffusing out of the capillaries pass through the basal lamina to provide nutrition to the outer layers of the retina.

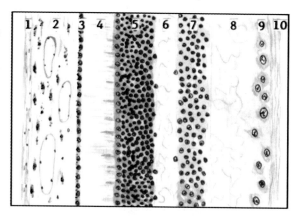

Fig. 21.5. Section through eyeball showing its layers. 3 to 10 belong to the retina. 1-Sclera. 2-Choroid. 3-Pigment cell layer. 4- Rods and cones. 5-Outer nuclear layer. 6-Outer plexiform layer. 7-Inner nuclear layer. 8-Inner plexiform layer. 9-Layer of ganglion cells. 10-Layer of optic nerve fibres.

The Suprachoroid Lamina

The suprachoroid lamina is also called the *lamina fusca*. It is non-vascular. It is made up of delicate connective tissue containing collagen, elastic fibres, and branching cells containing pigment. A plexus of nerve fibres is present. Some neurons may be seen in the plexus.

The Basal Lamina

With the light microscope the basal lamina (or *membrane of Bruch*) appears to be a homogeneous layer. However, with the EM the membrane is seen to have a middle layer of elastic fibres, on either side of which there is a layer of delicate collagen fibres. The membrane is united on the outside to the capillary layer (of the choroid proper); and on the inside to the basement membrane of pigment cells of the retina. Nutrients passing from the capillary layer to the outer layers of the retina have to pass through this membrane. The basal lamina is said to provide a smooth surface on which pigment cells and receptors of the retina can be arranged in precise orientation.

THE CILIARY BODY

The ciliary body represents an anterior continuation of the choroid. It is a ring-like structure continuous with the periphery of the iris. It is connected to the lens by the suspensory ligament. The ciliary body can be divided into a posterior flat part (*pars plana*) called the *ciliary ring*, and an anterior part (*pars plica*) made up of radially arranged *ciliary processes*.

The ciliary body is made up of vascular tissue, connective tissue and muscle. The muscle component constitutes the *ciliaris muscle*. The ciliaris muscle is responsible for producing alterations in the convexity of the lens (through the suspensory ligament) enabling the eye to see objects at varying distances from it. In other words the ciliaris is responsible for accommodation. The inner surface of the ciliary body is lined by a double layered epithelium which represents a forward continuation of the retina.

The ciliary processes are radially arranged ridges formed by folding of tissue. Each fold has a core of connective tissue and blood vessels, and a covering of double layered epithelium. The ciliary folds secrete the aqueous humour. They may also produce some components of the vitreous body.

THE IRIS

The iris is the most anterior part of the vascular coat of the eyeball. It forms a diaphragm placed immediately in front of the lens. At its periphery it is continuous with the ciliary body. In its centre, there is an aperture the *pupil*.

The iris is composed of a stroma of connective tissue containing numerous pigment cells, and in which are embedded blood vessels and smooth muscle. Some smooth muscle fibres are arranged circularly around the pupil and constrict it. They form the *sphincter pupillae*. Other fibres run radially and form the *dilator pupillae*. The posterior surface of the iris is lined by a double layer of epithelium continuous with that over the ciliary body. We have seen that this epithelium represents a forward continuation of the retina. The cells of this epithelium are deeply pigmented.

The pupil regulates the amount of light passing into the eye. In bright light the pupil contracts, and in dim light it dilates so that the optimum amount of light required for proper vision reaches the retina.

THE RETINA

Subdivisions of the Retina

To understand the structure of the retina brief reference to its development is necessary. The retina develops as an outgrowth from the brain (diencephalon). The proximal part of the diverticulum remains narrow and is called the *optic stalk*. It later becomes the optic nerve. The distal part of the diverticulum forms a rounded hollow structure called the *optic vesicle*. This vesicle is invaginated by the developing lens (and other surrounding tissues) so that it gets converted into a two layered *optic cup*. At first, each layer of the cup is made up of a single layer of cells. The outer layer persists as a single layered epithelium which becomes pigmented. It forms the *pigment cell layer* of the retina (Fig.21.8). Over the greater part of the optic cup the cells of the inner layer multiply to form several layers of cells that become the *nervous layer of the retina.* In the anterior part, both layers of the optic cup remain single layered. These two layers line (a) the inner surface of the ciliary body forming the *ciliary part of the retina*; and (b) the posterior surface of the iris forming the *iridial part of the retina*.

Opposite the posterior pole of the eyeball the retina shows a *central region* about 6 mm in diameter. This region is responsible for sharp vision. In the centre of this region an area about 2 mm in diameter has a yellow colour and is called the *macula lutea*. In the centre of the macula lutea there is a small depression that is called the *fovea centralis*. The floor of the fovea centralis is often called the *foveola*. This is the area of clearest vision.

We have seen that the optic nerve is attached to the eyeball a short distance medial to the posterior pole. The nerve fibres arising from the

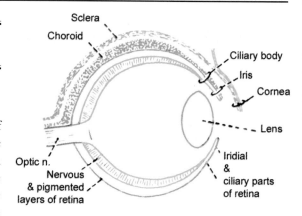

Fig. 21.6. Scheme to show some features of the developing eye.

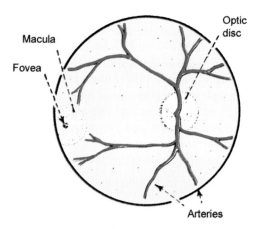

Fig. 21.7 Some features of the retina as seen through an ophthalmoscope. Note the arteries emerging through the optic disc. Veins are omitted for sake of clarity.

retina converge to this region, where they pass through the lamina cribrosa. When viewed from the inside of the eyeball this area of the retina is seen as a circular area called the *optic disc*.

Basic Structure of the Retina

When we examine sections through the retina (stained by haematoxylin and eosin, Fig. 21.5) a number of layers can be distinguished. The significance of the layers becomes apparent, however, only if we study the retina using special

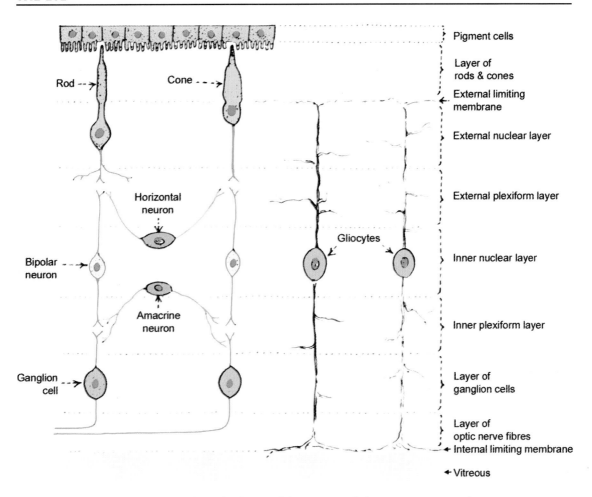

Fig. 21.8. Scheme to show the layers of the retina and the main structures therein.

methods. A highly schematic presentation of the layers of the retina, and of the cells present in them is shown in Fig. 21.8. The retina can be said to have an external surface which is in contact with the choroid, and an internal surface which is in contact with the vitreous. Beginning from the external surface the following layers can be made out.

1. Pigment Cell Layer

This consists of a single layer of cells containing pigment. Processes from pigment cells extend into the next layer (Details on page 323).

2. Layer of Rods and Cones

The rods are processes of rod cells, and cones are processes of cone cells. These cells are described below. The tips of the rods and cones are surrounded by processes of pigment cells.

3. External Nuclear Layer

The external nuclear layer contains the cell bodies and nuclei of rod cells and of cone cells.

These cells are photoreceptors that convert the stimulus of light into nervous impulses. Each rod cell or cone cell can be regarded as a modified neuron. It consists of a cell body, a peripheral (or external) process, and a central (or internal) process. The peripheral process is rod shaped in the case of rod cells, and cone shaped in the case of cone cells. These processes lie in the layer of rods and cones described above. The central process of each rod cell or cone cell is an axon. It extends into the external plexiform layer (see below) where it synapses with dendrites of bipolar neurons (see below). (Note: Rod cells and cone cells are commonly referred to simply as rods and cones). For further details of the structure of rods and cones see page 324.

4. External Plexiform Layer

The external plexiform layer (or **outer synaptic zone**) consists only of nerve fibres that form a plexus. The axons of rods and cones synapse here with dendrites of bipolar neurons (see below). Processes of horizontal cells (see below) also take part in these synapses.

5. Internal Nuclear Layer

The internal nuclear layer contains the cell bodies and nuclei of three types of neurons.

(a) The **bipolar neurons** give off dendrites that enter the external plexiform layer to synapse with the axons of rod and cone cells; and axons that enter the internal plexiform layer (see below) where they synapse with dendrites of ganglion cells (see below).

(b) The **horizontal neurons** give off processes that run parallel to the retinal surface. These processes enter the outer plexiform layer and synapse with rods, cones, and dendrites of bipolar cells.

(c). The **amacrine cells** also lie horizontally in the retina. Their processes enter the inner plexiform layer where they synapse with axons of bipolar cells, and with dendrite of ganglion cells. (Also see retinal gliocytes, below).

6. Internal Plexiform Layer

The **internal plexiform layer** (or **inner synaptic zone**) consists of synapsing nerve

fibres. The axons of bipolar cells synapse with dendrites of ganglion cells; and both these processes synapse with processes of amacrine cells. The internal plexiform layer also contains some horizontally placed **internal plexiform cells**; and also a few ganglion cells.

7. Layer of Ganglion Cells

The layer of ganglion cells contains the cell bodies of ganglion cells. We have seen that dendrites of these cells enter the internal plexiform layer to synapse with processes of bipolar cells and of amacrine cells. Each ganglion cell gives off an axon that forms a fibre of the optic nerve.

8. Layer of Optic Nerve Fibres

The layer of optic nerve fibres is made up of axons of ganglion cells. The fibres converge on the optic disc (page 320) where they pass through foramina of the lamina cribrosa to enter the optic nerve.

Retinal Gliocytes

Apart from bipolar, horizontal and amacrine neurons, the internal nuclear layer (described above) also contains the nuclei of retinal gliocytes or **cells of Muller** (Fig. 21.8). These cells give off numerous protoplasmic processes that extend through almost the whole thickness of the retina. Externally, they extend to the junction of the layer of rods and cones with the external nuclear layer. Here the processes of adjoining gliocytes meet to form a thin **external limiting membrane**. Internally, the gliocytes extend to the internal surface of the retina where they form an **internal limiting membrane**. This membrane separates the retina from the vitreous. The external and internal limiting membranes are sometimes described as additional layers of the retina (increasing their number to ten).

The retinal gliocytes are neuroglial in nature.

they support the neurons of the retina and may ensheath them. They probably have a nutritive function as well. Some astrocytes are also present in relation to retinal neurons.

Appearance of the Retina in Sections

Having considered the structures comprising the various layers of the retina it is now possible to understand the appearance of the retina as seen in sections stained by haematoxylin and eosin (Fig. 21.5). The inner and outer nuclear layers can be made out even at low magnification. The outer nuclear layer is thicker, and the nuclei in it more densely packed than in the inner nuclear layer. We have seen that this (outer nuclear) layer contains the nuclei of rods and cones. The cone nuclei are oval and lie in a single row adjoining the layer of rods and cones. The remaining nuclei are those of rods.

The nuclei in the inner nuclear layer belong (as explained above) to bipolar cells, horizontal cells, amacrine cells, and gliocytes.

The layer of ganglion cells is (at most places) made up of a single row of cells of varying size. The cell outlines are indistinct, but the nuclei can be made out. They are of various sizes. On the whole they are larger and stain more lightly than nuclei in the inner and outer nuclear layers.

The layer of pigment cells resembles a low cuboidal epithelium. All the nuclei in this layer are of similar size, and lie in a row.

The remaining layers (layers of rods and cones, inner and outer plexiform layers, and the layer of optic nerve fibres) are seen as light staining areas in which no detail can be made out. The layer of rods and cones may show vertical striations.

We will now consider the individual cells of the retina in greater detail.

FURTHER CONSIDERATION OF THE RETINA

Pigment Cells

Pigment cells appear to be rectangular in vertical section, their width being greater than their height. In surface view they are hexagonal. The nucleus is basal in position. The pigment in the cytoplasm is melanin. With the EM it can be seen that the surface of the cell shows large microvilli which contain pigment. These microvilli project into the intervals between the processes of rods and cones. Each pigment cell is related to about a dozen rods and cones. The plasma membrane at the base of the cell shows numerous infoldings.

The functions attributed to pigment cells include the following.

(a) The absorption of excessive light and avoidance of back reflection.

(b) They may play a role in regular spacing of rods and cones and may provide mechanical support to them.

(c) They have a phagocytic role. They 'eat up' the ends of rods and cones (which are constantly growing: see below).

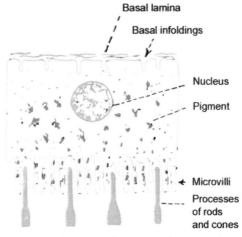

Fig. 21.9. Scheme to show some features of a pigment cell of the retina.

The Rods and Cones

There are about seven million cones in each retina. The rods are far more numerous. They number more than 100 million. The cones respond best to bright light (photopic vision). They are responsible for sharp vision and for the discrimination of colour. Rods can respond to poor light (scotopic vision) and specially to movement across the field of vision.

The density of rods and cones in different parts of the retina is shown schematically in Fig. 21.10. Note the following points.

(a) The density of cones is greatest in the fovea (about 1.5 million/mm²). Their density decreases sharply in proceeding to the margin of the central area, but thereafter the density is uniform up to the ora serrata (about 5000/mm²).

(b) The density of rods is greatest at the margin of the central area (about 1.5 million/mm²). It decreases sharply on proceeding towards the

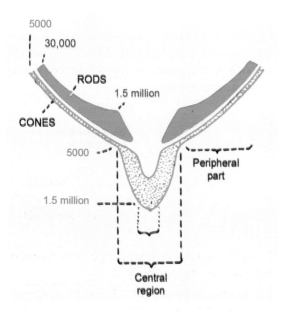

Fig. 21.10. Scheme to show the relative number of rods and cones in different parts of the retina. The figures represent number of receptors per mm².The diagram is not drawn to scale.

margin of the central area. There are no rods in the foveola. The density of rods also decreases in passing towards the ora serrata (where it is about 30,000/mm²).

From what has been said above about the layers of the retina it will be clear that light entering the eye has to pass through several layers of the retina to reach the rods and cones. This 'inverted' arrangement of the retina is necessary as passage of light in the reverse direction would be obstructed by the layer of pigment cells.

The macula lies exactly in the optical axis of the eyeball. When any object is viewed critically its image is formed on the macula. In this context, it is interesting to note that the fibres of the optic nerve do not pass over the macula, but skirt its edges. The macular area is also devoid of blood vessels. Because of these reasons photoreceptors in the macula have better exposure to light than in other parts of the retina. At the fovea centralis even the other layers of the retina are 'swept aside' to allow light to fall directly on the cones.

Each rod is about 50 μm in length and about 2 μm thick. Cones are about 40 μm in length and 3-5 μm thick.

Ultrastructure of Rod and Cone Cells

The ultrastructure of rod cells and of cone cells is similar and is, therefore, considered together. We have seen that each rod or cone cell consists of a cell body containing the nucleus, and of external and internal processes. Further details of the structure of a rod cell are shown in Fig. 21.12. Note the following.

The cell body (lying in the external nuclear layer) gives off two 'fibres', inner and outer. The **outer fibre** passes outwards up to the external limiting membrane and becomes continuous with the rod process, or the cone process. The process itself can be divided into an **inner segment**, and an **outer segment**. The outer segment is the real photo-receptor element. It contains a large

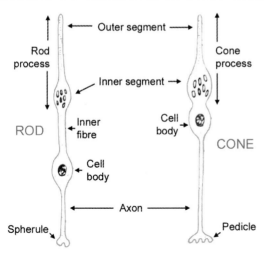

Fig. 21.11. Scheme to show the main parts of rods and cones.

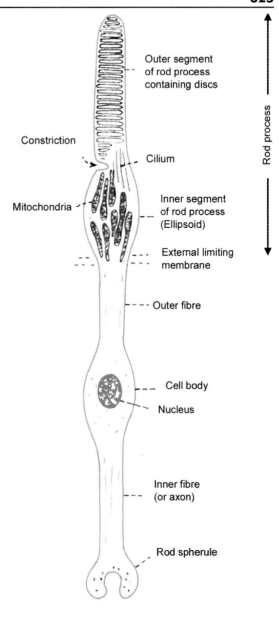

Fig. 21.12. Structure of a rod cell as seen by EM.

number of membranous discs stacked on one another. It is believed that the discs are produced by the cilium (see below) and gradually move towards the tip of the outer segment. Here old discs are phagocytosed by pigment cells.

The outer segments of rods and cones contain photo-sensitive pigments that are concerned with the conversion of light into nerve impulses. The pigments are believed to be bound to the membranes of the sacs of the outer segments. The pigment in the rods is *rhodopsin*, and that in the cones is *iodopsin*. Cones are believed to be of three types: red sensitive, green sensitive, and blue sensitive. Iodopsin has, therefore, to exist in three forms, one for each of these colours. However, the three types of cones cannot be distinguished from one another on the basis of their ultrastructure.

The inner segment of the rod or cone process is wider than the outer segment. It contains a large number of mitochondria which are concentrated in a region which is called the *ellipsoid*.

At the junction of the inner and outer segments of the rod or cone process there is an indentation of the plasma membrane on one side, so that the connection becomes very narrow. This narrow part contains a fibrillar *cilium* in which the microfibrils are orientated as in cilia elsewhere.

This cilium is believed to give rise to the flattened discs of the outer segment.

We have seen that the part of the rod cell between the cell body and the external limiting membrane is the outer fibre. The length of the outer fibre varies from rod to rod, being greatest in those rods that have cell bodies placed 'lower down' in the external nuclear layer. The outer fibre is absent in cones, the inner segment of the cone process being separated from the cone cell body only by a slight constriction.

The **cell bodies** of rod cells and of cone cells show no particular peculiarities of ultrastructure.

The **inner fibres** of rod and cone cells resemble axons. At its termination each rod axon expands into a spherical structure called the **rod spherule**, while cone axons end in expanded terminals called **cone pedicles**. The rod spherules and cone pedicles form complex synaptic junctions with the dendrites of bipolar neurons, and with processes of horizontal cells. Each rod spherule synapses with processes of two bipolar neurons, and with processes of horizontal neurons.

Each cone pedicle has numerous synapses with processes from one or more bipolar cells, and with processes of horizontal cells. In many situations the cone pedicle bears several invaginations which are areas of synaptic contacts. Each such area receives one process from a bipolar dendrite; and two processes, one each from two horizontal neurons. Such groups are referred to as **triads**. Each cone pedicle has 24 such triads. Apart from triads the cone pedicle bears numerous other

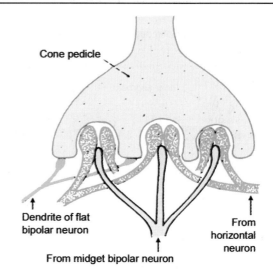

Fig. 21.14. Cone pedicel showing a number of synaptic areas, each area receiving three terminals.

synaptic contacts in areas intervening between the triads. These areas synapse with dendrites of diffusebipolar cells. Some pedicles also establish synaptic contacts with other cone pedicles.

The Bipolar Neurons

Bipolar cells of the retina are of various types. The terminology used for them is confusing as it is based on multiple criteria. The main points to note are as follows.

1. The primary division is into bipolars that synapse with rods (rod-bipolars), and those that synapse with cones (cone-bipolars).

2. As there are three types of cones, responding to the colours red, green and blue we can distinguish three corresponding types of cone bipolars (red cone bipolar, green cone bipolar, blue cone bipolar).

3. When a photoreceptor (rod or cone) is exposed to light it releases neurotransmitter at its synapse with the bipolar cell. Some bipolars respond to neurotransmitter by depolarization (and secretion of neurotransmitter at their synapses with ganglion cells). These are called ON-bipolars as they are 'switched on' by light.

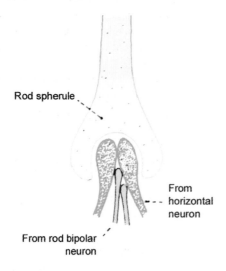

Fig. 21.13. Rod spherule synapsing with terminals of rod bipolar cells and horizontal cells.

Other bipolars respond to release of neurotransmitter by hyperpolarization. In other words they are 'switched off' by light and are called OFF-bipolars.

4. On the basis of structural characteristics, and the synapses established by them, cone bipolars are divided into three types: *midget*, *blue cone* and *diffuse*.

(a) A midget bipolar establishes synapses with a single cone (which may be red or green sensitive). Some midget bipolars synapse with indented areas on cone pedicles forming triads (Fig. 21.14). These are ON-bipolars. Other midget bipolars establish 'flat' synapses with the cone pedicle (and are also referred to as flat-bipolars). These are OFF-bipolars.

(b) A blue cone bipolar connects to one blue cone, and establishes triads. It may be of the ON or OFF variety.

(c) Diffuse cone bipolars establish synapses with several cone pedicels. They are not colour specific.

Axons of rod bipolar neurons synapse with up to four ganglion cells, but those of one midget bipolar neuron synapse with only one (midget) ganglion cell, and with amacrine neurons.

The Ganglion Cells

We have seen that the dendrites of ganglion cells synapse with axons of bipolar cells, and also with processes of amacrine cells. The axons arising from ganglion cells constitute the fibres of the optic nerve.

Ganglion cells are of two main types. Those that synapse with only one bipolar neuron are *mono-synaptic*, while those that synapse with many bipolar neurons are *polysynaptic*. Monosynaptic ganglion cells are also called *midget ganglion cells*. Each of them synapses with one midget bipolar neuron. We have seen that midget bipolars in turn receive impulses from a single cone. This arrangement is usual in the central region of the retina, and allows high resolution of vision to be attained.

Polysynaptic ganglion cells are of various types. Some of them synapse only with rod bipolars (*rod ganglion cells*). Others have very wide dendritic ramifications that may synapse with several hundred bipolar neurons (*diffuse ganglion cells*). This arrangement allows for summation of stimuli received through very large numbers of photoreceptors facilitating vision in poor light. On physiological grounds ganglion cells are also classified as 'ON' or 'OFF' cells.

The Horizontal Neurons

We have seen that horizontal neurons establish numerous connections between photoreceptors. Some of them are excitatory, while others are inhibitory. In this way these neurons play a role in integrating the activity of photorecepors located in adjacent parts of the retina. As they participate in synapses between photoreceptors and bipolar neurons horizontal neurons may regulate synaptic transmission between these cells.

Horizontal neurons are of two types, *rod horizontals* and *cone horizontals*, depending on whether they synapse predominantly with rods or cones. Each horizontal cell gives off one long process, and a number of short processes (7 in case of rod horizontal cells, and 10 in case of cone horizontal cells). The short processes are specific for the type of cell: those of rod horizontals synapse with a number of rod spherules, and

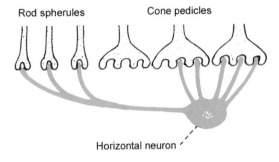

Fig. 21.15. Scheme to show the connections of a cone horizontal neuron.

those of cone horizontals synapse with cone pedicles. The long processes synapse with both rods and cones (which are situated some distance away from the cell body of the horizontal neuron). The long and short processes of horizontal cells cannot be distinguished as dendrites or axons, and each process probably conducts in both directions.

The Amacrine Neurons

The term amacrine is applied to neurons that have no true axon. Like the processes of horizontal cells those of amacrine neurons also conduct impulses in both directions. Each cell gives off one or two thick processes which divide further into a number of branches. Different types of amacrine neurons are recognized depending upon the pattern of branching. We have seen that the processes of amacrine neurons enter the internal plexiform layer where they may synapse with axons of several bipolar cells, and with the dendrites of several ganglion cells. They also synapse with other amacrine cells. At many places an amacrine process synapsing with a ganglion cell is accompanied by a bipolar cell axon. The two are referred to as a *dyad*.

The amacrine cells are believed to play a very important role in the interaction between adjacent areas of the retina resulting in production of sharp

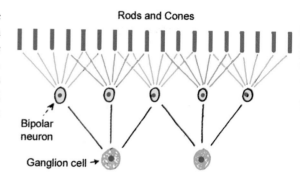

Fig. 21.17. Scheme to show how impulses arising in several photoreceptors concentrate on one ganglion cell.

images. They are also involved in the analysis of motion in the field of vision.

Internal plexiform cells (present in the internal plexiform layer) represent a third variety of horizontally oriented neurons in the retina.

Apart from integration of impulses from rods and cones horizontal, amacrine and internal plexiform cells act as 'gates' that can modulate passage of inputs from rods and cones to ganglion cells. In this connection it is to be noted that processes of amacrine neurons are interposed between processes of bipolar cells and ganglion cells, while processes of horizontal cells are interposed between photoreceptors and bipolar cells.

Some Further Remarks About Connections of Retinal Neurons

1. While there are well over a hundred million photoreceptors in each retina there are only about one million ganglion cells, each giving origin to one fibre of the optic nerve. (The bipolar cells are intermediate in number between photoreceptors and ganglion cells). In passing from the photoreceptors to the ganglion cells there has, therefore, to be considerable convergence of impulses. Each ganglion cell would be influenced by impulses originating in several photoreceptors. On functional considerations it would be expected that such convergence would be most marked near

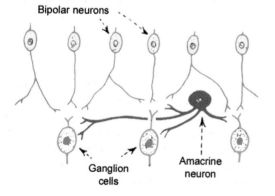

Fig. 21.16. Simplified scheme to show the connections of an amacrine neuron.

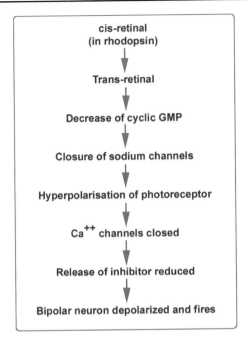

cis-retinal
(in rhodopsin)

↓

Trans-retinal

↓

Decrease of cyclic GMP

↓

Closure of sodium channels

↓

Hyperpolarisation of photoreceptor

↓

Ca^{++} channels closed

↓

Release of inhibitor reduced

↓

Bipolar neuron depolarized and fires

Fig. 21.18. Flow diagram to show sequence of events leading to firing of a bipolar neuron of the ON-type in response to light.

the periphery of the retina; and that it would involve the rods much more than the cones. It has been estimated that in the peripheral parts of the retina one ganglion cell may be connected to as many as 300 rods or to ten cones. Convergence leads to summation of impulses arising in many photoreceptors and allows vision even in very dim light. It would also be expected that convergence would be minimal in the macula, and absent in the foveola, to allow maximal resolution.

2. The second highly important fact about intra-retinal connections is the presence of numerous arrangements for interaction of adjacent regions of the retina as follows.

(a) Firstly, cone pedicles establish numerous contacts with other cone pedicles and with adjacent rod spherules.

(b) Except in the fovea, most photoreceptors are connected to more than one bipolar cell. In turn each bipolar cell is usually connected to more than one ganglion cell.

(c) The vertically arranged elements of the retina (photoreceptors, bipolar cells, ganglion cells) are intimately interconnected to adjacent elements through horizontal neurons and amacrine neurons.

Mechanism of Firing of Bipolar Neurons

1. When no light falls on the retina photoreceptors are depolarized. Exposure to light causes hyper-polarization.

2. When a photoreceptor is depolarized it releases inhibitor at its junction with a bipolar neuron. This prevents the bipolar neuron from firing. Release of inhibitor is controlled by voltage gated calcium channels.

3. Hyperpolarization of photoreceptor, caused by exposure to light, leads to closure of Ca^{++} gates and release of inhibitor is stopped. This causes the bipolar neuron to fire. As explained earlier, this description applies to ON-bipolars.

4. Rhodopsin, present in photoreceptors, is a complex of a protein **opsin** and **cis-retinal** which is sensitive to light. When exposed to light cis-retinal is transformed to trans-retinal. This leads to decrease in concentration of cyclic GMP which in turn leads to closure of sodium channels. Closure of sodium channels results in hyperpolarization (of photo-receptor) (Fig. 21.18).

Blood Retina Barrier

The blood vessels which ramify in the retina do not supply the rods and cones. These are supplied by diffusion from choroidal vessels. The endothelial cells of capillaries in the retina are united by tight junctions to prevent diffusion of substances into the rods and cones. This is referred to as the blood-retina barrier.

THE LENS

The surface of the lens is covered by a highly elastic lens capsule. Deep to the capsule the lens is covered on its anterior surface by a lens epithelium. The cells of the epithelium are cuboidal. However, towards the periphery of the lens the cells become progressively longer. Ultimately they are converted into long fibres that form the substance of the lens. The lens contains about 2000 such fibres.

The substance of the lens is made up of a firm inner part called the *nucleus*, and a pliable outer part the *cortex*. Both parts are made up of a number of layers or laminae. Each lamina consists of long lens fibres that are derived from the anterior epithelium. The lens fibres are made up of special transparent proteins called *crystallins*. The fibres are hexagonal in cross section and have a regular geometric arrangement. They are attached to each other by their edges. For this purpose the edges bear knobs that fit into sockets on adjoining fibres.

When the lens is examined from the front, or from behind, three faint lines are seen radiating from the centre to the periphery. In the fetus these lines form a 'Y' which is upright on the front of the lens, and inverted at the back. The lines become more complex in the adult These lines are called *sutural lines*. They are made up of amorphous material. The ends of lens fibres are attached at these lines. Each lens fibre starts on one surface at such a line, and follows a curved course to reach the opposite surface where it ends by joining another such line.

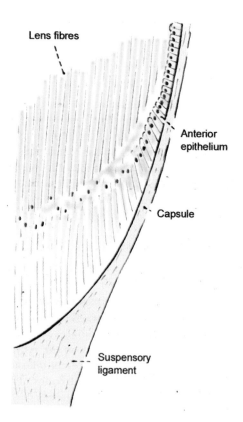

Fig. 21.19. Section through part of the lens near its margin.

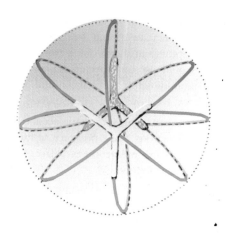

Fig. 21.20. Schematic diagram to show the arrangement of fibres within the lens. Note the Y-shaped lines on the front and back of the lens.

ACCESSORY VISUAL ORGANS

The accessory visual organs include the extraocular muscles, and related fascia; the eyebrows; the eyelids; the conjunctiva and the lacrimal gland. The structure of extraocular muscles corresponds to that of skeletal muscle elsewhere in the body; and the structure of eyebrows is similar to that of hair in other parts of the body. The remaining structures are considered below.

The Eyelids

The basic structure of an eyelid is shown in Fig. 21.21. The various structures in it are as follows.

(1) Anteriorly, there is a layer of true skin with which a few small hair and sweat glands are associated. The skin is thin.

(2) Deep to the skin there is a layer of delicate connective tissue which normally does not contain fat.

(3) Considerable thickness of the lid is formed by fasciculi of the palpebral part of the orbicularis oculi muscle (skeletal muscle).

(4) The 'skeleton' of each eyelid is formed by a mass of fibrous tissue called the *tarsus*, or *tarsal plate*.

(5) On the deep surface of the tarsal plate there are a series of vertical grooves in which *tarsal glands* (or *Meibomian glands*) are lodged. Occasionally, these glands may be embedded within the tarsal plate. Each gland has a duct that opens at the free margin of the lid. The tarsal glands are modified sebaceous glands. They produce an oily secretion a thin film of which spreads over the lacrimal fluid (in the

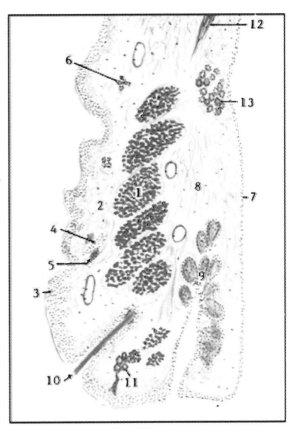

Fig. 21.21. Eyelid. 1-Core of skeletal muscle. 2-Dense connective tissue. 3-Skin. 4-Hair follicle. 5-Sebaceous gland. 6-Sweat gland. 7-Palpebral conjunctiva. 8-Tarsal plate. 9-Tarsal glands. 10-Eyelash. 11-Ciliary gland. 12-Levator palpebrae superioris. 13-Acessory lacrimal glands.

conjunctival sac) and delays its evaporation.

(6) Modified sweat glands, called *ciliary glands* (or *glands of Moll*), are present in the lid near its free edge. Sebaceous glands present in relation to eyelashes constitute the *glands of Zeis*. Accessory lacrimal glands are often present just above the tarsal plate (*glands of Wolfring*).

(7) The inner surface of the eyelid is lined by the palpebral conjunctiva which is described below.

The Conjunctiva

The conjunctiva is a thin transparent membrane which covers the inner surface of each eyelid (*palpebral conjunctiva*) and the anterior part of the sclera (*ocular conjunctiva*). At the free margin of the eyelid the palpebral conjunctiva becomes continuous with skin; and at the margin of the cornea the ocular conjunctiva becomes continuous with the anterior epithelium of the cornea. When the eyelids are closed the conjunctiva forms a closed *conjunctival sac*. The line along which palpebral conjunctiva is reflected onto the eyeball is called the *conjunctival fornix*: superior, or inferior. The ducts of the lacrimal gland open into the lateral part of the superior conjunctival fornix. Lacrimal fluid keeps the conjunctiva moist. Accessory lacrimal glands are present near the superior conjunctival fornix (*glands of Krause*).

Conjunctiva consists of an epithelial lining that rests on connective tissue. Over the eyelids this connective tissue is highly vascular and contains much lymphoid tissue. It is much less vascular over the sclera.

The epithelium lining the palpebral conjunctiva is typically two layered. There is a superficial layer of columnar cells, and a deeper layer of flattened cells. At the fornix, and over the sclera, the epithelium is three layered there being an additional layer of polygonal cells between the two layers mentioned above. The three layered epithelium changes to stratified squamous at the sclerocorneal junction.

The Lacrimal Gland

The structure of the lacrimal gland is similar to that of a serous salivary gland (Fig. 21.22). It is a compound tubuloalveolar gland and consists of a number of lobes that drain through about twenty ducts.

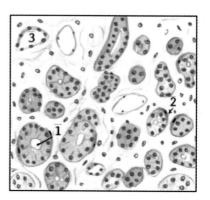

Fig. 21.22. Lacrimal gland. 1-Lumen of acinus. 2-Myoepithelial cell. 3-Duct.

Sections of the lacrimal gland can be distinguished from those of serous salivary glands because of the following features. (**a**) The acini are larger, and have wider lumina..

(**b**) All cells appear to be of the same type. They are low columnar in shape and stain pink with haematoxylin and eosin. (**c**) The profiles of the acini are often irregular or elongated.

(**d**) The walls of adjacent acini within a lobule may be pressed together, there being very little connective tissue between them. However, the acini of different lobules are widely separated by connective tissue. Myoepithelial cells are present as in salivary glands.

Small ducts of the lacrimal gland are lined by cuboidal or columnar epithelium. Larger ducts have a two layered columnar epithelium or a pseudostratified columnar epithelium.

EM studies on the human lacrimal gland reveal that the secretory cells may be of several types, including both mucous and serous cells.

The gland is innervated mainly by parasympathetic fibres which end in relation to secretory cells as well as myoepithelial cells. Sympathetic nerves are also present, but their role is uncertain.

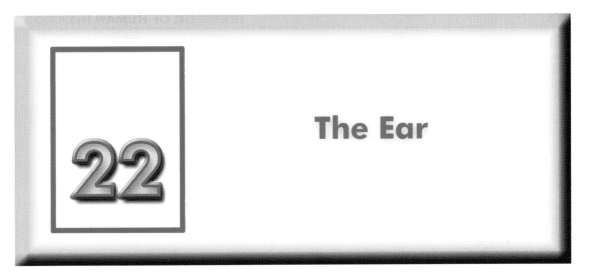

The Ear

Preliminary Remarks

Anatomically speaking, the ear is made up of three main parts called the **external ear**, the **middle ear**, and the **internal ear**. The external and middle ears are concerned exclusively with hearing. The internal ear has a **cochlear part** concerned with hearing; and a **vestibular part** which provides information to the brain regarding the position and movements of the head.

The main parts of the ear are shown in Fig.22.1. The part of the ear that is seen on the surface of the body (i.e., the part that the lay person calls the ear) is anatomically speaking, the **auricle** or **pinna**. Leading inwards from the auricle there is a tube called the **external acoustic meatus**. The auricle and the external acoustic meatus together form the **external ear**. The inner end of the external acoustic meatus is closed by a thin membranous diaphragm called the **tympanic membrane**. This membrane separates the external acoustic meatus from the middle ear.

The **middle ear** is a small space placed deep within the petrous part of the temporal bone. It is also called the **tympanum**. Medially, the middle ear is closely related to parts of the internal ear. The cavity of the middle ear is continuous with that of the nasopharynx through a passage called the **auditory tube**. Within the cavity of the middle ear there are three small bones or **ossicles**: the **malleus**, the **incus**, and the **stapes**. They form a chain that is attached on one side to the tympanic membrane, and at the other end to a part of the internal ear.

The **internal ear** is in the form of a complex system of cavities lying within the petrous temporal bone. It has a central part called the **vestibule**. Continuous with the front of the vestibule there is a spiral shaped cavity called the

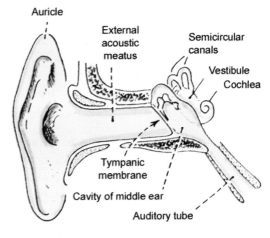

Fig. 22.1. Diagram to show the main parts of the ear.

cochlea. Posteriorly, the vestibule is continuous with three *semicircular canals*.

Sound waves travelling through air reach the ears. In many lower animals in whom the auricle is large and mobile, it may help in directing the sound waves into the external acoustic meatus. The auricle is of doubtful functional significance in man. Sound waves striking the tympanic membrane produce vibrations in it. These vibrations are transmitted through the chain of ossicles present in the middle ear to reach the internal ear. Specialized end organs in the cochlea act as transducers which convert the mechanical vibrations into nervous impulses. These impulses travel through the cochlear nerve to the brain. Actual perception of sound takes place in the brain.

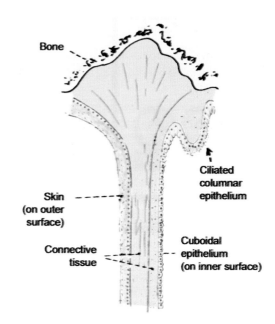

Fig. 22.2. Structure of tympanic membrane.

THE EXTERNAL AND MIDDLE EAR

The Auricle

The auricle consists of a thin plate of elastic cartilage (page 92) covered on both sides by true skin (Fig. A49). The skin is closely adherent to the cartilage. Hair follicles, sebaceous glands, and sweat glands are present in the skin.

The External Acoustic Meatus

The wall of the external acoustic meatus is made up partly of elastic cartilage (in its outer part) and partly of bone (in its inner part). The meatus is lined by skin. The skin lining the bony part is thin and is firmly adherent to the underlying bone. In the cartilaginous part the skin is thick and contains hair, sebaceous glands, and ceruminous glands. The ceruminous glands

secrete the wax of the ear. They are modified sweat glands lined by a columnar, cuboidal or squamous epithelium.

The Tympanic Membrane

The tympanic membrane has three layers. The middle layer is made up of fibrous tissue, which is lined on the outside by skin (continuous with that of the external acoustic meatus), and on the inside by mucous membrane of the tympanic cavity.

The fibrous layer contains collagen fibres and some elastic fibres. The fibres are arranged in two layers. In the outer layer they are placed radially, while in the inner layer they run circularly.

The mucous membrane is lined by an epithelium which may be cuboidal or squamous. It is said that the mucosa over the upper part of the tympanic membrane may have patches of ciliated columnar epithelium, but this is not borne out by EM studies.

The Tympanic Cavity

The walls of the tympanic cavity are formed by bone which is lined by mucous membrane. The mucous membrane also covers the ossicles. The lining epithelium varies from region to region. Typically it is cuboidal or squamous. At places it may be ciliated columnar. The ossicles of the middle ear consist of compact bone, but do not have marrow cavities.

The Auditory Tube

The wall of the auditory tube is partly bony (lateral part) and partly cartilaginous (medial part, nearer the nasopharynx). The bone or cartilage is covered by mucous membrane which is lined by ciliated columnar epithelium. Near the pharyngeal end of the tube the epithelium becomes pseudostratified columnar. Goblet cells and tubulo-alveolar mucous glands are also present. A substantial collection of lymphoid tissue, present at the pharyngeal end, forms the *tubal tonsil* (page 190).

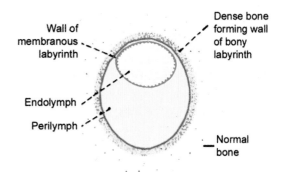

Fig. 22.3. Basic structure of internal ear as seen in a section through a semicircular canal.

semicircular canal (Fig.22.3). The space bounded by bone is *bony labyrinth*. Its wall is made up of bone that is more dense than the surrounding bone. Its inner surface is lined by periosteum. Lying within the bony labyrinth there is a system of ducts which constitute the *membranous labyrinth*. The space within the membranous labyrinth is filled by a fluid called the *endolymph*. The space between the membranous labyrinth and the bony labyrinth is filled by another fluid called the *perilymph*.

The bony labyrinth consists of a central part called the *vestibule* (Fig. 22.4). The vestibule is

THE INTERNAL EAR

Preliminary Remarks

Some elementary facts about the internal ear have been recorded on page 333. We have seen that the internal ear is in the form of a complex system of cavities within the petrous temporal bone. Because of the complex shape of these intercommunicating cavities the internal ear is also called the *labyrinth*.

The basic structure of the labyrinth is best understood by looking at a transverse section through a relatively simple part of it e.g., a

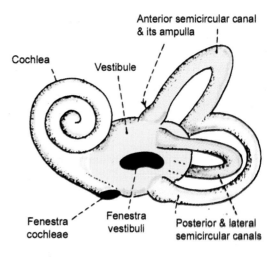

Fig. 22.4. Bony labyrinth as seen from the lateral side.

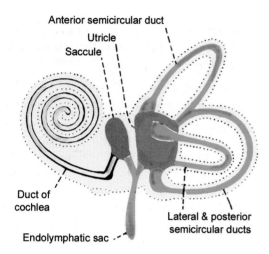

Fig. 22.5. Parts of the membranous labyrinth.

continuous anteriorly with the **cochlea**; and posteriorly with three **semicircular canals**.

The cochlear part of the bony labyrinth is divisible into two parts. One part, the **scala vestibuli** opens into the vestibule; while the second part called the **scala tympani** opens into the middle ear through an aperture called the **fenestra cochleae.**

The parts of the membranous labyrinth are shown in Fig. 22.5. Within each semicircular canal the membranous labyrinth is represented by a **semicircular duct**. The part of the membranous labyrinth present in the cochlea is called the **duct of the cochlea**. The part of the membranous labyrinth that lies within the vestibule is in the form of two distinct membranous sacs called the **saccule** and the **utricle**. Some further details are shown in Fig. 22.5.

The wall of the membranous labyrinth is trilaminar. The outer layer is fibrous and is covered with **perilymphatic cells.** The middle layer is vascular. The inner layer is epithelial, the lining cells being squamous or cuboidal. Some of the cells (called **dark cells**) have an ultrastructure indicative of active ionic transport. They probably control the ionic composition of endolymph.

The Bony Cochlea

The cochlea has a striking resemblance to a snail shell. It is basically a tube that is coiled on itself for two and three-fourth turns. The 'turns' rest on a solid core of bone called the **modiolus**.

[Because of the spiral nature of the cochlea the mutual relationships of the structures within it differ in different parts of the cochlea. A structure that is 'inferior' in the upper part of the canal becomes 'superior' in the lower part. For descriptive convenience the structures lying next to the modiolus are described as 'inner' and those away from it as 'outer'. These terms as used here are not equivalents of 'medial' and 'lateral' as normally used. The words 'superior' and 'inferior' indicate relationships as they exist in

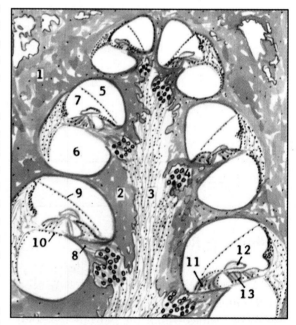

Fig. 22.6A. Cochlea (low power view). 1-Petrous temporal bone. 2-Modiolus. 3-Canal for passage of cochlear nerve fibres. 4-Spiral ganglion. 5-Scala vestibuli. 6-Scala tymapni. 7-Duct of cochlea. 8-Spiral lamina. 9-Vestibular membrane. 10-Basilar membrane. 11-Spiral limbus. 12-Membrana tectoria. 13-Organ of Corti.

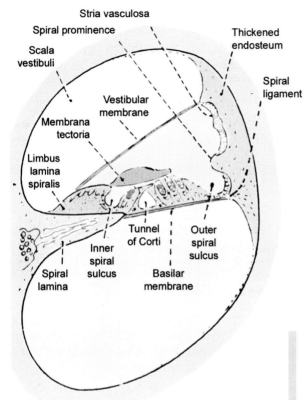

Fig. 22.6B. Section across one turn of the cochlea to
show some of its features.

the lowest (or basal) turn of the cochlea].

In sections through the middle of the cochlea
the cochlear canal is cut up six times as shown
in Fig. 22.6A. Some of the features seen in any of
these sections are shown in Fig. 22.6B. We find
that the cochlear canal is partially divided into
two parts by a bony lamina that projects outwards
from the modiolus. This bony projection is called
the *spiral lamina*. Passing from the tip of the
spiral lamina to the opposite wall of the canal
there is the *basilar membrane*.

The spiral lamina and the basilar membrane
together divide the cochlear canal into two parts
(upper and lower in the figure). The lower part
is the *scala tympani*. When traced proximally,
the scala tympani reaches the medial wall of the

middle ear at the fenestra cochleae, which
is closed by the *secondary tympanic
membrane*.

The part of the cochlear canal above the
basilar membrane is further divided into
two parts by an obliquely placed
vestibular membrane (of Reissner). The
part above the vestibular membrane is the
scala vestibuli. When traced proximally
it becomes continuous with the vestibule.
At the apex of the cochlea the scala vestibuli
becomes continuous with the scala
tympani. The triangular space between the
basilar and vestibular membranes is called
the *duct of the cochlea*. This duct
represents the membranous labyrinth of
the cochlea.

The vestibular membrane consists of a basal
lamina lined on either side by squamous cells.
Some of the cells show an ultrastructure indicative
of a fluid transport function. The cells of the
membrane form a barrier to the flow of ions
between endolymph and perilymph so that these
two fluids have different concentrations of
electrolytes.

The basilar membrane is divisible into two parts.
The part supporting the organ of Corti is the *zona
arcuata*. The part lateral to the zona arcuata is
the *zona pectinata*. The zona arcuata is made
up of a single layer of delicate filaments of
collagen. The zona pectinata is made up of three
layers of fibres.

SPECIALIZED END ORGANS IN
THE MEMBRANOUS LABYRINTH

The internal ear is a highly specialized end
organ that performs the dual functions of hearing
and of providing information about the position
and movements of the head. The impulses in
question are converted into nerve impulses by a
number of structures that act as transducers.

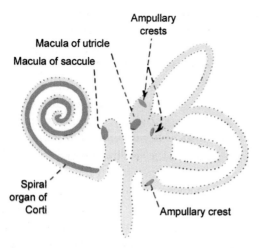

Fig. 22.7. End organs in the membranous labyrinth.

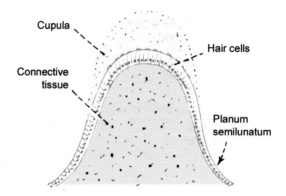

Fig. 22.8. Structure of an ampullary crest.

specialized mechano-receptors, and *supporting* (or *sustentacular*) *cells*.

These are as follows.

The end organ for hearing is the *spiral organ (of Corti)*. It lies in the duct of the cochlea, just above the basilar membrane. Information about changes in position of the head is provided by end organs called *maculae* (singular = *macula*) present in the utricle and saccule. Information about angular movements of the head is provided by end organs called the *ampullary crests* (or *cristae ampullae*). One such crest is present in each semicircular duct. One end of each semicircular duct is dilated to form an *ampulla*, and the end organ lies within this dilatation. These end organs are described below.

Ampullary Crests

One ampullary crest is present in the ampullated end of each of the three semicircular ducts. Each crest is an elongated ridge projecting into the ampulla, and reaching almost up to the opposite wall of the ampulla. The long axis of the crest lies at right angles to that of the semicircular duct. The crest is lined by a columnar epithelium in which two kinds of cells are present. These are *hair cells* which are

The Hair Cells

The hair cells occupy only the upper half of the epithelium. The luminal surface of each hair cell bears 'hairs'. When examined by EM the 'hair' are seen to be of two types as follows.

(a) There is one large kinocilium which is probably non-motile.

(b) There are a number of stereocilia (large microvilli).

These 'hair' extend into a gelatinous (protein polysaccharide) material which covers the crest and is called the *cupula*. The hair processes of the hair cells are arranged in a definite pattern the orientation being specific for each semicircular duct. This orientation is of functional importance.

Each hair cell is innervated by terminals of afferent fibres of the vestibular nerve. Efferent fibres that can alter the threshold of the receptors are also present.

Hair cells can be divided into two types depending on their shape and on the pattern of nerve endings around them. Type I hair cells are flask shaped. They have a rounded base and a short neck. The nucleus lies in the expanded basal part. The basal part is surrounded by a goblet shaped nerve terminal (or *calix*). Type II hair cells are columnar. Both types of hair cells receive nerve terminals which are afferent (non-granular) as well as efferent (granular).

Both in the ampullae of semicircular ducts, and in the maculae of the utricle and saccule, each hair cell is polarized with regard to the position of the kinocilium relative to the stereocilia. Each hair cell (in an ampulla) can be said to have a side that is towards the utricle, and a side that faces in the opposite direction. In the lateral semicircular duct, the kinocilia lie on the side of the cells which are towards the utricle; while in the anterior and posterior semicircular ducts the kinocilia lie on the opposite side. When stereocilia are bent towards the kinocilium the cell is hyperpolarized. It is depolarized when bending is away from the kinocilium. Depolarization depends on the opening up of Ca^{++} channels.

The Supporting Cells

The supporting (or sustentacular) cells are elongated and may be shaped like hour glasses (narrow in the middle and wide at each end). They support the hair cells and provide them with nutrition. They may also modify the composition of endolymph.

Functioning of Ampullary Crests

The ampullary crests are stimulated by movements of the head (specially by acceleration). When the head moves, a current is produced in the endolymph of the semicircular ducts (by inertia). This movement causes deflection of the cupula to one side distorting the hair cells. It appears likely that distortion of the crest in one direction causes stimulation of nerve impulses, while distortion in the opposite direction produces inhibition. In any given movement the cristae of some semicircular ducts are stimulated while those of others are inhibited. Perception of the exact direction of movement of the head depends on the precise pattern formed by responses from the various cristae.

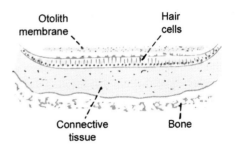

Fig. 22.9. Structure of a macula.

The Maculae

We have seen that the utricle and saccule of each ear have specialized structures called maculae. These are not raised (like the cristae), but are flat areas of specialized epithelium. The epithelium has a structure very similar to that in ampullary crests, the main difference being that calcareous particles (called **otoliths** or **statoconia**) are present in the gelatinous covering. The gelatinous covering is, therefore, called the **otolith membrane** or **membrana statoconiorum**.

The macula of the utricle and that of the saccule are placed at right angles to each other. They also differ in the orientation of hair cells. Each hair cell is polarized in reference to a raised ridge (called the **striola**) that runs along the long axis of the macula dividing it into two halves. In the utricle the kinocilium of each hair cell lies on the side (of the cell) nearest to the striola, but in the saccule the kinocilium is on the side away from the striola.

The maculae give information about the position of the head and are organs of **static balance**. In contrast the ampullary crests are organs of **kinetic balance**. The macula of the saccule may be concerned with the reception of low frequencies of sound. Impulses arising from the ampullary crests and the maculae influence the position of the eyes. They also have an influence on body posture (through the vestibular nuclei).

Planum Semilunatum

On each side of each ampullary crest the epithelium of the semicircular duct shows an area of thickened epithelium that is called the planum semilunatum. The importance of this area is that (amongst other cells) it contains certain dark cells that have an ultrastructure similar to cells (elsewhere in the body) that are specialized for ionic transport. The cells bear microvilli and have deep infoldings of their basal plasma membrane. The areas between the folds are occupied by elongated mitochondria. (Compare with structure of cells of the distal convoluted tubules of the kidney). The dark cells are believed to control the ionic content of the endolymph. Similar cells are also present elsewhere in the membranous labyrinth. The planum semilunatum may secrete endolymph.

The Cochlear Duct

We have seen that the cochlear duct is a triangular canal lying between the basilar membrane and the vestibular membrane. We may now note some further details (Figs. 22.6B, 22.10).

1. The endosteum on the outer wall of the cochlear canal is thickened. This thickened endosteum forms the outer wall of the duct of the cochlea. The basilar and vestibular membranes are attached to this endosteum. The thickened endosteum shows a projection in the region of attachment of the basilar membrane: this projection is called the *spiral ligament*. A little above the spiral ligament the thickened endosteum shows a much larger rounded projection into the cochlear duct: this is the *spiral prominence*. The spiral prominence forms the upper border of a concavity called the *outer spiral sulcus*.

Between the spiral prominence and the attachment of the vestibular membrane the thickened endosteum is covered by a specialized epithelium that is called the *stria vascularis*. The region is so called because there are capillaries within the *within* the thickness of the epithelium. (This is the only such epithelium in the whole body). The epithelium of the stria vascularis is made up of three layers of cells: marginal, intermediate and basal. The cells of the marginal layer are called *dark cells*. They are in contact with the endolymph filling the duct of the cochlea. These cells have a structure and function similar to that of the dark cells already described in the planum semilunatum. These dark cells may be responsible for the formation of endolymph. The basal parts of the dark cells give off processes that come into intimate contact with the intraepithelial capillaries. The capillaries are also in contact with processes arising from cells in the intermediate and basal layers of the stria vascularis.

2. We have seen that the spiral lamina is a bony projection into the cochlear canal. Near the attachment of the spiral lamina to the modiolus there is a spiral cavity in which the *spiral ganglion* is lodged. This ganglion is made up of bipolar cells. Central processes arising from these cells form the fibres of the cochlear nerve. Peripheral processes of the ganglion cells pass through canals in the spiral lamina to reach the spiral organ of Corti (described below).

3. The periosteum on the upper surface of the spiral lamina is greatly thickened to form a mass called the *limbus lamina spiralis* (or *spiral limbus*).

The limbus is roughly triangular in shape. It has a flat 'lower' surface attached to the spiral lamina; a convex 'upper' surface to which the vestibular membrane is attached; and a deeply concave 'outer' surface. The concavity is called the *internal spiral sulcus*. This sulcus is bounded above by a sharp *vestibular lip* and below by a *tympanic lip* which is fused to the spiral lamina.

The Spiral Organ of Corti

The spiral organ of Corti is so called because (like other structures in the cochlea) it extends in a spiral manner through the turns of the cochlea. In sections it is seen to be placed on the basilar membrane and to be made up of epithelial cells that are arranged in a complicated manner. The cells are divisible into the true receptor cells or *hair cells*, and supporting elements which are given different names depending on their location. The cells of the spiral organ are covered from above by a gelatinous mass called the *membrana tectoria*.

From Fig. 22.10 it will be clear that the cells of the spiral organ enclose a triangular cavity called the *tunnel of Corti* (or *cuniculum internum*). The base of the tunnel lies over the basilar membrane. It has a sloping inner wall that is formed by *internal rod cells*; and a sloping outer wall that is formed by *external rod cells*. To the internal side of the inner rod cells there is a single row of *inner hair cells*. The inner hair cell is supported by tall cells lining the tympanic lip of the internal spiral sulcus. On the outer side of each external rod cell there are three or four *outer hair cells*. The outer hair cells do not lie directly on the basilar membrane, but are supported by the *phalangeal cells* (*of Dieters*) which rest on

the basilar membrane. To the outer side of the outer hair cells and the phalangeal cells, there are tall supporting cells (*cells of Hensen*). Still more externally the outer spiral sulcus is lined by cubical cells (*cells of Claudius*).

A narrow space the *cuniculum externum* intervenes between the outermost hair cells and the cells of Hensen. A third space, the *cuniculum medium* (or *space of Nuel*) lies between the outer rod cell and the outer hair cells. The spaces are filled with perilymph (or *cortilymph*).

We will now examine some of the structures mentioned above in greater detail.

Rod Cells

Each rod cell (or *pillar cell*) has a broad *base* (or *foot plate*, or *crus*) that rests on the basilar membrane; an elongated middle part (*rod* or *scapus*); and an expanded upper end called the *head* or *caput*.

The bases of the rod cells are greatly expanded and contain their nuclei. The bases of the inner and outer rod cells meet each other forming the base of the tunnel of Corti. The heads of these cells also meet at the apex of the tunnel. Here a convex prominence on the head of the outer rod cell fits into a concavity on the head of the inner

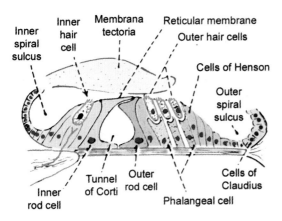

Fig. 22.10. Diagram to show the cells in the organ of Corti. .

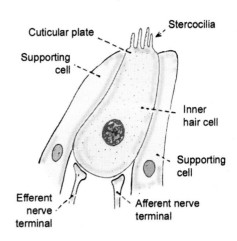

Fig. 22.11. Diagram to show an inner hair cell of the organ of Corti.

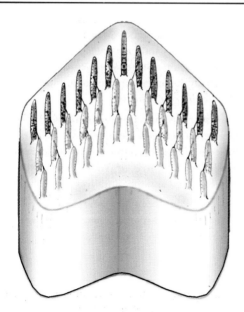

Fig. 22.12. Surface view of a hair cell showing stereocilia arranged in three rows that form a 'V'

rod cell. The uppermost parts of the heads are expanded into horizontal plates called the **phalangeal processes**. These processes join similar processes of neighbouring cells to form a continuous membrane called the **reticular lamina** (see below).

The Hair Cells

The hair cells are so called because their free 'upper' or apical ends bear a number of 'hair'. The hair are really stereocilia (page 25). Each cell is columnar or piriform. The hair cells are distinctly shorter than the rod cells. Their apices are at the level of the reticular lamina. Their lower ends (or bases) do not reach the basilar membrane. They rest on phalangeal cells. The plasma membrane at the base of each hair cell forms numerous synaptic contacts with the terminations of the peripheral processes of neurons in the spiral ganglion. Some efferent terminals are also present (page 344).

The apical surface of each hair cell is thickened to form a **cuticular plate** the edges of which are attached to neighbouring cells.

With the EM the 'hair' of hair cells are seen to be similar to microvilli. Each hair has a covering of plasma membrane within which there is a core of microfilaments. Each hair is cylindrical over most of its length, but it is much narrowed at its base. The hair can, therefore, bend easily at this site.

The hair on each hair cell are arranged in a definite manner. When viewed from 'above' they are seen to be arranged in the form of the letter 'V' or 'U' (Fig. 22.12). Each limb of the 'V' has three rows of hairs. The hairs in the three rows are of unequal height being tallest in the 'outer' row, intermediate in the middle row, and shortest in the 'inner' row. The 'V' formed by the hairs of various hair cells are all in alignment, the apex of the 'V' pointing towards the 'outer' wall of the cochlear canal. At the point corresponding to the apex of the 'V' there is a centriole lying just under the apical cell membrane, but a true kinocilium is not present (unlike hair cells of ampullary crests, page 338).

The above description applies to both inner and outer hair cells. We may now note some differences between the two.

The inner hair cells are piriform (flask shaped) and relatively short; while the outer hair cells are cylindrical and longer. The lower end of each outer hair cell fits into a depression on the upper end of a phalangeal cell, but the inner hair cells do not have such a relationship. The 'hair' of the outer hair cells are somewhat longer and more slender than those on inner hair cells. They are arranged as a shallow 'U' rather than a 'V'. Occasionally, the outer hair cells may have more than three rows of hair, and the rows may assume the shape of a 'W' (instead of a 'V'). We have seen that in all hair cells the apex of the 'V' (formed by the rows of hair) points towards the 'outer' wall of the cochlear canal (i.e., away from the modiolus). The direction of the 'V' is sometimes described in relation to the tunnel of Corti. In the inner hair cells the 'V' points towards the tunnel, while in the case of the outer cells it points away from the tunnel.

The direction of the 'V' is of functional importance. Like hair cells of the maculae and cristae, those of the cochlea are polarized. Bending of stereocilia towards the apex of the 'V' causes depolarization, while the reverse causes hyperpolarization. Ionic gradients associated with depolarization and hyperpolarization are maintained because apices of hair cells and surrounding cells are tightly sealed by occluding junctions.

The Outer Phalangeal Cells and Reticular Lamina

These are the cells that support the outer hair cells. They lie lateral to the outer rod cells. Their bases rest on the basilar membrane. Their apical parts have a complicated configuration. The greater part of the apex forms a cup-like depression into which the base of an outer hair cell fits. Arising from one side (of the apical part) of the cell there is a thin rod-like **phalangeal process**. This process passes 'upwards', in the interval between hair cells, to reach the level of the apices of hair cells. Here the phalangeal process expands to form a transverse plate called the **phalanx**. The edges of the phalanges of adjoining phalangeal cells unite with each other to form a membrane called the **reticular lamina**. (The reticular lamina also receives contributions from the heads of hair cells). The apices of hair cells protrude through apertures in this lamina.

The cell edges forming the reticular lamina contain bundles of microtubules embedded in dense cytoplasm. Adjacent cell margins are united by desmosomes, occluding junctions and gap junctions. The reticular lamina forms a barrier impermeable to ions except through the cell membranes. It also forms a rigid support between the apical parts of hair cells thus ensuring that the hair cells rub against the membrana tectoria when the basilar membrane vibrates.

The Membrana Tectoria

The membrana tectoria lies over the internal spiral sulcus and over the hair cells of the spiral

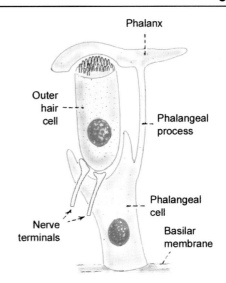

Fig. 22.13. Diagram to show an outer hair cell and a phalangeal cell.

organ. It consists of delicate fibres embedded in a gelatinous matrix. This material is probably secreted by cells lining the vestibular lip of the limbus lamina spiralis (page 340). A narrow gap separates the membrana tectoria from the reticular lamina. The stereocilia of external hair cells are in contact with the membrana tectoria.

SOME ELEMENTARY FACTS ABOUT THE MECHANISM OF HEARING

Sound waves travelling through air pass into the external acoustic meatus and produce vibrations in the tympanic membrane. These vibrations are transmitted through the chain of ossicles to perilymph in the vestibule. In this process the force of vibration undergoes considerable amplification because (a) the chain of ossicles acts as a lever; and (b) the area of the tympanic membrane is much greater than that of the foot plate of the stapes (increasing the force per unit area).

Movement of the stapes (towards the vestibule) sets up a pressure wave in the perilymph. This wave passes from the vestibule into the scala vestibuli, and travels through it to the apex of the cochlea. At this point (called the *helicotrema*) the scala vestibuli is continuous with the scala tympani. The pressure wave passes into the scala tympani and again traverses the whole length of the cochlea to end by causing an outward bulging of the secondary tympanic membrane. In this way vibrations are set up in the perilymph, and through it in the basilar membrane. Movements of the basilar membrane produces forces that result in friction between the 'hairs' of hair cells against the membrana tectoria. This friction leads to bending of the 'hairs'. This bending generates nerve impulses that travel through the cochlear nerve to the brain.

The presence of efferent terminals on the hair cells probably controls the afferent impulses reaching the brain. It can also lead to sharpening of impulses emanating from particular segments of the spiral organ by suppressing impulses from adjoining areas.

It has to be remembered that the transverse length of the basilar membrane is not equal in different parts of the cochlear canal. The membrane is shortest in the basal turn of the cochlea, and longest in the apical turn (quite contrary to what one might expect). Different segments of the membrane vibrate most strongly in response to different frequencies of sound thus providing a mechanism for differentiation of sound frequencies. Low frequency sounds are detected by hair cells in the organ of Corti lying near the apex of the cochlea, while high frequency sounds are detected by hair cells placed near the base of the cochlea.

The intensity of sound depends on the amplitude of vibration. For further details of the mechanism of hearing consult a textbook on physiology.

Index

G

Gall bladder, 253
Ganglia, 163
    autonomic, 164
    sensory, 163
Gene, structural, 32
Genitalia, external. female, 297
Giantism, 116
Gland
    adrenal, 309
    apocrine, 53
    buccal, 225
    cardiac, 237
    ceruminous, 206
    ciliary, 206, 331
    compound, 51
    compound tubular, 51
    compound tubulo-alveolar, 51
    ductless, 51
    eccrine, 53
    endocrine, 51, 299
    epicrine, 53
    exocrine, 51
    gastric, 235
    labial, 225
    lacrimal, 332
    mammary, 297
    Meibomian, 331
    merocrine, 53
    mucous, 52
    multicellular, 51
    of Moll, 331
    of Wolfring, 331
    of Zeis, 331
    palatine, 225
    parathyroid, 308
    parotid, 225
    pineal, 304
    pyloric, 237
    racemose, 51
    saccular, 51
    salivary, 225
    sebaceous, 202
    serous, 52

Gland (Continued)
    simple, 51
    simple alveolar, 51
    simple tubular, 51
    sublingual, 225
    submandibular, 225
    suprarenal, 309
    sweat, 204
    tarsal, 331
    thecal, 289
    thyroid, 306
    unicellular, 51
Glomerulus, 259
    synaptic, 142
Glucagon, 254
Glycocalyx, 5
Glycosaminoglycans, 57, 58
Goblet cell, 46, 52, 240
Golgi complex, 16
Golgi tendon organ, 158
Granulocyte, 72, 85
Grey matter, 145

H

Haemoglobin, 71
Haemopoiesis, 82
Hair follicle, 201
Hassall, corpuscles of, 188
Haversian system, 98, 101, 110
Heart, 176
Hemidesmosome, 9, 11
Henle, loop of, 259, 266
Heterochromatin, 25
Hilus, neurovascular, 122
Histaminocyte, 64
Histiocyte, 63
Histochemistry, 2
Hormone
See under individual endocrine glands
Hyaloplasm, 14
Hydroxyapatite, 101

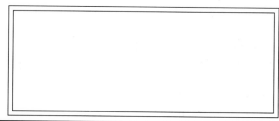